Atlas of
Phonomicrosurgery
and Other Endolaryngeal Procedures
for Benign and Malignant Disease

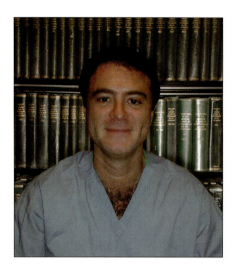

Steven M. Zeitels, MD, FACS, is an Associate Professor in the Department of Otology and Laryngology at Harvard Medical School; Director of the Division of Laryngology in the Department of Otolaryngology of Massachusetts Eye and Ear Infirmary; Clinical Associate in Surgery in the Thoracic Surgery Division of Massachusetts General Hospital; Staff Surgeon at Boston Veterans Administration Medical Center; and Consulting Staff at Boston Children's Hospital Medical Center. In addition, Dr. Zeitels serves as Laryngologist to the Voice Departments of the Berklee College of Music, Boston University School of Fine Arts, New England Conservatory and Boston Conservatory, as well as to the Boston Lyric Opera, visiting vocalists with the Boston Symphony Orchestra, and the American Repertory Theatre of Harvard University.

Dr. Zeitels has been a prolific surgical innovator designing a number of new procedures as well as two laryngoscopes that have been patented. This inclination arose from a long-term development of ambidextrous skills in the art and craft of cutting, sewing, carving, and constructing leather into a variety of creative forms. His major research interests include laryngeal microsurgery, especially as it relates to minimally invasive surgical oncology; phonosurgery and voice disorders; medical and surgical management of performing artists; design and development of endoscopic instruments; and the history of laryngology and head and neck surgery. Dr. Zeitels has contributed more than 100 articles, book chapters, and videotapes in these areas and presents frequently at regional, national, and international conferences. He has been the visiting professor at 13 departments, universities, and hospitals including, Memorial Sloan Kettering, University of Cincinnati, University of Utah, University of Navarra in Pamplona, Spain, and Tel Aviv University in Israel.

Dr. Zeitels has received a number of honors and awards for his achievements including the Casselberry Award from the American Laryngological Association and a Boston University Trustee Scholarship. Among his many national and international guest lectureships, he has served as the Lewis H. Wright Memorial Distinguished Lecturer for the American Society of Anesthesiology; Sylvan Stool History of Medicine Lecturer for the University of Pittsburgh School of Medicine, Arnold Grossman Lecturer in Laryngology for Montreal General Hospital and McGill University, and guest lecturer for the first annual meeting of the Brazilian Society of Laryngology and Voice.

Dr. Zeitels is a committed academic surgeon working locally, nationally, and internationally to advance laryngology and head and neck surgery. Under his direction, a Division of Laryngology, which had not been in existence since the retirement of Harris P. Mosher in the early 20th century, was reestablished at the Massachusetts Eye and Ear Infirmary and Harvard. He currently serves as the Treasurer of the American Broncho-Esophagological Association.

Atlas of Phonomicrosurgery

and Other Endolaryngeal Procedures for Benign and Malignant Disease

Steven M. Zeitels, MD, FACS

Associate Professor
Department of Otology and Laryngology
Harvard Medical School

Director, Division of Laryngology and Associate Medical Director, Voice Laboratory
Massachusetts Eye and Ear Infirmary
Boston, Massachusetts

SINGULAR

THOMSON LEARNING

Australia   Canada   Mexico   Singapore   Spain   United Kingdom   United States

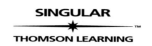

SINGULAR

THOMSON LEARNING

Atlas of Phonomicrosurgery and Other Endolaryngeal Procedures for Benign and Malignant Disease
by Steven M. Zeitels, MD, FACS

Business Unit Director:
William Brotmiller

Acquisitions Editor:
Marie Linville

Editorial Assistant:
Kristin Banach

Executive Marketing Manager:
Dawn Gerrain

Channel Manager:
Tara Carter

Production Manager:
Barbara Bullock

Production Editor:
Sandy Doyle

Library of Congress
Cataloging-in-Publication Data
Zeitels, Steven M., 1957–
Atlas of Phonomicrosurgery and other endolaryngeal procedures for benign and malignant disease/Steven M. Zeitels.
  · p. ; cm.
Includes bibliographic references and index.
ISBN 0-7693-0131-2 (alk. paper)
1. Larynx—surgery—Atlases. 2. Microsurgery—Atlases.
[DNLM: 1. Larynx—surgery—Atlases.
2. Laryngeal Diseases—surgery—Atlases.
3. Laryngeal Neoplasms—surgery—Atlases. 4. Microsurgery—Atlases. 5. Vocal Cords—surgery—Atlases.
WV 17 Z48a 2001]
RF516.Z45 2001
671.5'33—dc21   00-0300050

NOTICE TO THE READER

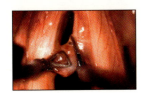

Contents

Premalignant and Malignant Vocal Fold Lesions

Supraglottal Surgery

Conclusion

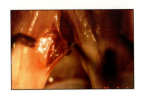

Foreword

Over the past decade, I have been greatly impressed with the consistent and superb activities of Dr. Zeitels in the field of laryngology. He has contributed greatly toward improving instruments for endolaryngeal surgeries; advancing surgical techniques for varying vocal fold diseases; phonosurgeries for singers and performing artists; endoscopic treatments for glottic, supraglottic, and hypopharyngeal carcinomas; and improvements in the arytenoid adduction procedure.

The most important point in modern phonosurgery is to employ procedures that are non-invasive or the least invasive to the layered structure of the vibrating portion of the vocal fold. Preservation of the superficial layer of the lamina propria around the vocal fold edge is the key for a favorable postsurgical vocal function. Dr. Zeitels has employed and developed surgical procedures based on this concept, including the subepithelial infusion, epithelial cordotomy, and epithelial microflap technique.

A unique aspect of this particular book is the fact that clear color photographs demonstrating surgical procedures for many cases of different laryngeal pathologies are beautifully presented. Needless to say, visual demonstrations are particularly useful for understanding the key principles of surgical procedures. I believe that students, residents, and practicing surgeons who are learning microsurgical procedures will benefit greatly from this atlas. Specialized phonosurgeons may get some ideas to improve their technique and surgical skill.

This atlas, which is published in the beginning of the 21st century, explores and advances the basic concepts and techniques of phonosurgery that were established during the latter third of the 20th century. What are the challenges and advances in phonosurgery in the 21st century? I expect Dr. Zeitels will be one of the leading laryngologists in the new century who provides answers to these questions.

Minoru Hirano, MD, PhD.
President and Professor Emeritus of Kurume University
Kurume, Japan

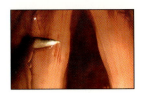

Foreword

Steven Zeitels' *Atlas of Phonomicrosurgery* is unique. No one else in the history of laryngology has had the patience and equipment needed to shoot the 40,000 photographs that were necessary to compile a surgical atlas of this quality. The result is an extraordinary contribution to laryngology.

Dr. Zeitels' Atlas begins with a succinct overview of the history of laryngeal surgery, focused through the eyes of the author, who is regarded widely as laryngology's finest and most scholarly historian. His clinically relevant historical review evolves into an understanding of current treatment paradigms, including philosophy, technique, and surgical instrumentation. However, the vast majority of the book is devoted to elegant photographic documentation of laryngeal pathology and techniques of endoscopic surgery.

Dr. Zeitels presents not only images of numerous variations in appearance of benign and malignant pathology, but also photographs of surgical procedures, with instruments in situ. The surgical techniques are state-of-the-art, and the image quality is outstanding. These pictures provide invaluable insights for surgeons trying to understand or teach the latest surgical methodology. For example, the section on management of varices and ectasias illustrates clearly the technique for resecting individual blood vessels from the vocal fold. Such photographs provide information superior to that contained in the drawings usually used to illustrate these procedures. The same is true for the photographs depicting resections of cancer, subepithelial cysts, and a variety of other common and unusual lesions. The pictures are cropped perfectly and consistently, and they are arranged in an order that is convenient for the clinician and logical to a practicing phonosurgeon.

This Atlas represents a herculean, 10-year, scholarly accomplishment that makes an unprecedented clinical and historical contribution to otolaryngology. It should be in the library of every surgeon who operates upon the vocal folds.

Robert T. Sataloff, MD, DMA
Professor, Otolaryngology, Thomas Jefferson University
Chairman, Otoloaryngology, Head and Neck Surgery,
The Graduate Hospital
Chairman, Board of Directors, The Voice Foundation

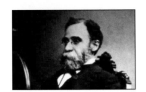

Preface

This atlas of endolaryngeal surgery represents the culmination of a decade of investigations designed to enhance endoscopic management of laryngeal pathology in adults. Surprisingly, there has been scant photodocumentation of the details of microlaryngeal procedures. This occurred because most surgeons have photographed the operations by means of a separate telescope through the lumen of the laryngoscope, which precludes simultaneous tissue instrumentation. All of the microlaryngeal photography herein was obtained from a sidearm of the microscope to simulate the surgeon's proximal view during the procedure. This was facilitated by prototype laryngoscopes that were developed to improve exposure.

Although transoral treatment paradigms will continue to evolve, this text should serve as an enduring compilation of magnified images of laryngeal pathology. Photographs at various magnifications are frequently displayed to portray different perspectives and because surgeons are accustomed to working at different powers. Because the text is intended to serve as a pictorial reference of clinical pathology, there is duplication of the types of lesions to demonstrate subtle clinical variations. Many of the cases are displayed to exhibit the interface between the deep surface of lesion and the underlying normal vocal fold tissue, which facilitates understanding of how pathology arises within the layered microstructure.

The first chapter provides readers with an overview of pertinent historical advances in the development of laryngology and endolaryngeal surgery. Laryngology was one of the earliest examples of surgical and medical specialization. Surgical manipulation of the larynx has fueled the development of the discipline since its origin and this continues today. In turn, transoral/endoscopic management of the upper aerodigestive tract provided a foundation for minimally invasive surgery because the pharynx and larynx were natural passages. A primary focus of 19th century laryngology was mirror-guided management of laryngeal airway obstruction, primarily from infectious diseases of the upper aerodigestive tract. This continued into the early 20th century when Kirstein, Killian, and Jackson popularized direct endolaryngeal surgery. In the 20th century, mass production of cigarettes led to increasing importance of laryngeal neoplasia. The primary emphasis in laryngology appropriately has been on airway safety, swallowing function, and the treatment of cancer. At this point, a majority of the important problems in these areas have been solved by previous generations of laryngologists so that **phonosurgery** has evolved to the forefront as a primary 21st century challenge.

There has been an inextricable linkage between laryngology and human voice production since Manuel García's[1] presentation, *Observations on the Human Voice,* in 1855. Although procedures to enhance the voice have been described since the inception of the specialty, presently, there is renewed interest and funding to support multidisciplinary investigations in phonatory disorders.

Chapter 2 discusses principles and theories of phonomicrosurgical management, especially as it relates to performing artists. The surgical restoration of impaired vocal fold vibration will probably always be the foundation of voice surgery. Except for epithelial lesions such as cancer and papilloma, most pathology of the vocal folds occurs in association with traumatic voice use. Reticent individuals rarely develop vocal fold lesions. We currently live in a communication-based society in which the human voice is a fundamental component of a majority of jobs. This has led to increasing numbers of professional voice users and, in turn, more pathology.

Current methodology in voice surgery arose from the convergence of physiological principles of laryngeal sound production with procedural innovations that enhance oscillation of the vocal folds. The microsurgical approach is based on identifying (visualization and palpation) the layer(s) affected by the pathology to maximally preserve the vocal folds' layered microstructure (epithelium and laminae propria). In benign pathology, the surgical goal is to excise lesions without disturbing normal tissue, and in malignant tumors, the goal is to minimize oncologically sound cancer margins to optimize postresection function.

Phonosurgery represents a group of procedures to improve or maintain the human voice. The term was created by Hans von Leden over 35 years ago and has attracted tremendous interest during the last decade. This has been catalyzed by advances in surgical technology both in lasers and hand instrumentation. Chapter 3 details many of the salient issues regarding instrumentation with current state-of–the-art suggestions. There is an extensive section on theories of laryngoscope design and positioning because the scope provides the gateway to the pathology and since optimal endoscopic exposure is often the rate-limiting factor for precise surgical intervention. Except for miniaturization, until recently, laryngeal hand instrumentation had undergone little change throughout most of this century. However, new models in other minimally invasive surgical paradigms are now catalyzing development of microlaryngoscopic instruments. These technological improvements will likely lead to a variety of procedural innovations in the first decade of the 21st century.

The philosophy underlying the management of benign lesions is discussed in Chapters 4–10. Nodules, polyps, varices, and ectasias (Chapters 4–6) are often encountered separately or in combination and represent a spectrum of traumatic vascular and soft-tissue injury. Although nodules and polyps can often be excised successfully by means of amputation, whenever possible, a subepithelial resection approach has become the author's standard method. Although symptomatic varices and ectasias are classically treated by cauterization, new techniques are demonstrated using cold-instrument dissection. The subepithelial resection method is further illustrated for the management of subepithelial vocal fold cysts in Chapter 7. New approaches for the treatment of granulomas including the use of botulinum toxin for arytenoid lesions are described in Chapter 8. A variety of patients with Reinke's edema are illustrated in Chapter 9. Resection and cytoreduction techniques are discussed for respiratory papillomatosis (Chapter 10), the most common benign epithelial disorder. This chapter serves as an introduction to the technique for removing epithelial atypia.

Vocal fold injury including scar, sulcus, web, and synechia are detailed in Chapter 11. The treatment of laryngeal airway obstruction as a result of posterior glottic impairment is discussed in Chapter 12. Unusual vocal fold lesions are depicted in Chapter 13 and a spectrum of complex cases with multiple lesions are illustrated in Chapter 14.

An extensive discussion of vocal fold atypia and cancer is presented in Chapters 15 and 16. The graded phonomicrosurgical resection approach is delineated along with an explanation of the associated oncological and functional outcomes. Microlaryngoscopic supraglottal surgery has rarely been displayed photographically. Therefore, both benign and malignant supraglottic lesions are reviewed in Chapters 17 and 18.

The main focus of this text is phonomicrosurgery since it is the most common reason to perform endolaryngeal surgery and since it is one of the most dynamically evolving subspecialties with a rich heritage and an exciting future. Because of the vigorous motor function of the larynx, a majority of vocal fold pathology is the result of vocal overuse and abuse. As in all forms of trauma, surgery should prevail as the mainstay of treatment. Therefore, unlike treating problems such as cancer, foreseeable scientific and medical breakthroughs are unlikely to result in a decline in endolaryngeal surgery. Furthermore, indications for surgical intervention will probably expand as the field of molecular laryngology develops and as methods to reconstitute the layered microstructure evolve. Ultimately, this will result in vocal rejuvenation procedures.

Steven M. Zeitels, MD, FACS

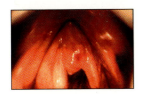

Acknowledgments

The author would like to express his gratitude to Ramon Franco for his indefatigable effort and skill in the preparation of the photographs. These surgical images would not have been possible without the dedication and assistance of Mary Williams, Elizabeth Stahl, and Carey Shiney in the operating room. My collaboration with Robert E. Hillman (discussing issues of voice science) catalyzed the design of a number of the procedures demonstrated in this text. His associates in our voice laboratory, Glenn Bunting, Patricia Doyle, Janice Eng, and Mary Klemack provided outstanding voice rehabilitation for the patients while Virginia Griffin provided specialized nursing care. The Harvard laryngology fellows, Ilan Hochman, Rosemary Desloge, John Jarboe, and Ramon Franco induced provocative discussion that provided the stimulus for many of the new developments. Rox Anderson and William Farinelli have provided us with unique insights into new uses of a variety of lasers in laryngology. This work emanated from the invaluable mentorship bestowed by M. Stuart Strong, Charles W. Vaughan, Gerald B. Healy, and Geza Jako in the art, craft, and science of rigid endoscopy of the upper aero-digestive tract. Finally, my parents Natalie and Harry Zeitels (1919–2000) provided unyielding support.

This work is dedicated to Gerald B. Healy, the consummate academic surgeon, whose wisdom has influenced generations of laryngologists. He has catalyzed my thoughts, ideas, and aspirations, since my days in medical school and residency, and he continues to serve as a critical source of inspiration.

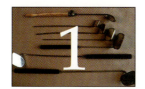

1

History

THE ORIGIN OF ENDOSCOPIC SURGERY OF THE LARYNX

The origin and growth of laryngology is inextricably linked to the development of endoscopic surgery of the larynx. Phillip Bozzini (1773–1809; Figure 1–1)[2] was the first individual to suggest that visually controlled endoscopic surgery was possible and is therefore considered to be the father of minimally invasive surgery. In 1807, at the age of 34, he described the *Lichtleiter* (light conductor) (Figure 1–2), which was composed of a universal handle that incorporated a candle and a reflector as an extracorporeal light source. He attached a variety of cannulae to the handle to facilitate the examination of accessible orifices (ie, throat, urethra, rectum). This concept was a revolutionary advance in medical and surgical science but his work continues to be largely unrecognized. The laryngeal cannula consisted of an additional mirror that allowed visualization of the lower pharynx and larynx. Unfortunately, Bozzini's method was not embraced by

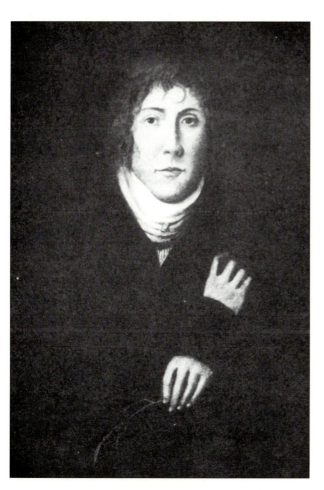

Fig 1–1. Phillip Bozzini: self portrait (1773–1809).

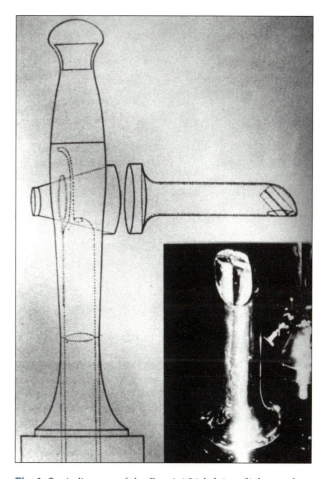

Fig 1–2. A diagram of the Bozzini Lichtleiter (light conductor) with the associated laryngeal speculum. The inset photograph in the bottom right is the actual speculum. (Courtesy of the American College of Surgeons.)

the medical community and he died in 1809 before the validity of his approach was established.

There were a number of other reports of mirror laryngoscopy in the first half of the 19th century;[3–9] however, none was widely acknowledged or accepted. Most notable were the descriptions by Babington,[5] Liston,[7] and Avery.[9] Babington first used the term glottoscope (1829; Figure 1–3) for his instrument, which consisted of a variety of mirrors as well as a retracting spatula to distract the tongue base. By retracting the tongue base out of the visual field, Babington's glottoscope became the first device to employ internal distention of supraglottal tissues[10,11] to enhance visualization of the glottis. Liston's[7] brief description in 1837 of mirror laryngoscopy for the assessment of laryngeal edema was important because he introduced the concept of heating the mirror to avoid condensation on the reflecting surface. In 1844 Avery[9] designed a laryngeal cannula similar to Bozzini's; however, he employed an artificial light source separate from the device in the form of a headlight (Figure 1–4). This remarkable device employed a perforated concave mirror to reflect the illumination into the oropharynx to facilitate visualization of the larynx.

The isolated reports of mirror laryngoscopy arose from the need to observe the airway. Infectious diseases were a formidable problem that could cause membranous laryngeal airway obstruction.[12,13] Horace Green (1802–1866; Figure 1–5) dedicated his career to this problem and spent time with Trousseau and Belloc[12] in Europe. He received his medical training in Vermont but ultimately practiced in New York City, where he became the first specialist for throat and respiratory diseases in the United States. Green described transoral application of caustics to the larynx to treat infectious inflammatory disorders of the laryngeal membranes.[14–17] However, he was maligned by his contemporaries, who did not believe that his transoral interventions were possible.[18–20] Later, Green resolved this by placing a whalebone probang transorally through the glottis of a patient who had a tracheotomy until the probang could be observed through the tracheotomy site.

In 1852, Green made his most seminal contribution to laryngology by describing the first direct laryngoscopy and

visually controlled excision of a laryngeal neoplasm. He was managing a child with obstructive sleep apnea. He excised her tonsils, which did not resolve the problem. Subsequently, he inserted a bent tongue spatula (similar to a Macintosh

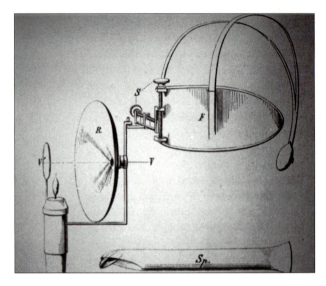

Fig 1–4. John Avery's (1807–1855) laryngoscope (1844). (From MacKenzie, M.: *The Use of the Laryngoscope in Diseases of the Throat with an Appendix on Rhinoscopy*. London, UK: J and A Churchill; 1865.)

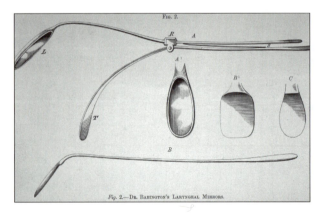

Fig 1–3. Benjamin Guy Babington's (1794–1866) glottoscope (1829). (From MacKenzie, M.: *The Use of the Laryngoscope in Diseases of the Throat with an Appendix on Rhinoscopy*. London, UK: J and A Churchill; 1865.)

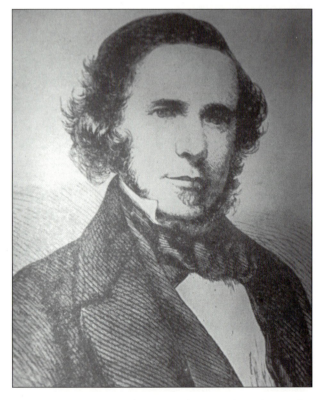

Fig 1–5. Horace Green (1802–1866): The Father of American Laryngology.

laryngoscope; Figure 1–6) and was able to observe a ball-valving fibroepithelial polyp obstructing the glottal aperture. Using sunlight for illumination, he was able to successfully observe and resect the lesion because of the favorable cephalad position of the child's larynx. He reported the case in detail in his landmark textbook, *On the Surgical Treatment of Polypi of the Larynx and Oedema of the Glottis*.[21] The book contained a drawing of what the artist could view from the procedure (Figure 1–7).

Both Bozzini and Green were courageous figures in medical history, as their work was not accepted by their contemporaries, who could not replicate their techniques. Both were branded as charlatans by the general medical establishment. Although Bozzini died shortly after his manuscript was published, Green lived through the initial period of the origin of laryngology and he was vindicated. Louis Elsberg, the first President of the American Laryngological Association, dedicated that organization's first meeting in 1879[18] to Green and referred to him as the "Father of American Laryngology" because of his brilliant skill and courageous contributions.

Manuel García (1805–1906; Figures 1–8 and 1–9), the renowned vocal pedagogist, reported auto-laryngoscopy to the Royal Society of London in 1855.[1] This investigation was catalyzed by his desire to better understand singing phonation. In his paper entitled, "Observations on the Human Voice," Garcia made important contributions to the understanding of laryngeal sound production, especially with regard to rhythmic pulsation of the expiratory airstream. Clerf[20] believed that García's emphasis on observations and deductions regarding laryngeal physiology led to the subsequent widespread adoption of mirror laryngoscopy by physicians, which had not occurred as a result of prior 19th century descriptions of the technique.

There is little debate that laryngology was born from the investigations of the acclaimed classical voice teacher. In addition to inspiring the genesis of this new field in medicine, García maintained active engagement with laryngologists as the field developed from its infancy. This is evidenced in Mackenzie's text, *The Hygiene of the Vocal Organs*.[22] The tremendous esteem that laryngologists held for García was vividly illustrated in Mackinlay's[23] description of the celebration for the maestro's 100th birthday in 1906 (Figure 1–10). Laryngologists commissioned John Singer Sargent to paint García (see Figure 1–9) for his centennial birthday. It appears that García was too frail to remain stable for the entire process. Sargent is reported to have used a photograph (see Figure 1–8) as a model for the majority of the painting, while the head and hands were derived from the live sitting.

In 1857, Turck (Figure 1–11) explored, but then abandoned the clinical application of mirror laryngoscopy. He could not obtain a reliable image because, like García, he was depending on the sun; unfortunately it was often overcast in Pesth in the autumn. Shortly thereafter, his colleague Czermak (Figure 1–12) borrowed the same mirrors and commenced further investigations, which were highly successful. Czermak reintroduced the artificial light source and the perforated concave mirror (Figure 1–13). A feud developed between Czermak[24] and Turck[25] over priority for the medical

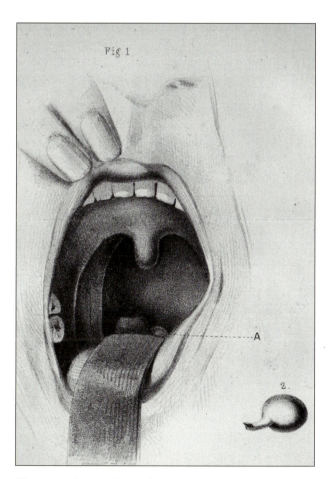

Fig 1–6. A laryngeal polyp excised at direct vision by Green. (From Green: *On the Surgical Treatment of Polypi of the Larynx, and Oedema of the Glottis.*)

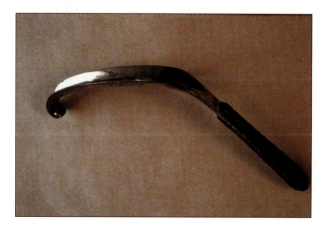

Fig 1–7. Nineteenth century tongue spatula similar to that used by Green. Note the curve on the end for placement within the vallecular glossoepiglottica. It bears great resemblance to a standard anesthesia-type spatula laryngoscope but without self-contained illumination. (Courtesy of the Massachusetts Eye and Ear Infirmary.)

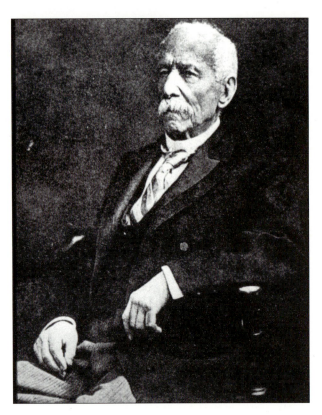

Fig 1–8. A photograph of García as an elderly gentleman. Since García was too old to sit for the entirety of the Sargent portrait, this is likely to be the photograph that Sargent used to complete the famous portrait.

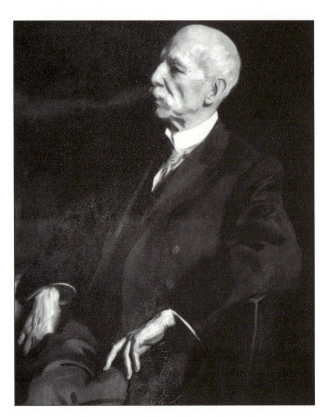

Fig 1–9. Manuel García (1805–1906). This portrait was done by John Singer Sargent at the celebration of the maestro's centennial birthday. (Courtesy of the Rhode Island School of Design.)

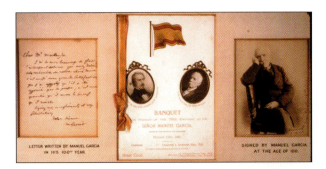

Fig 1–10. Memorial from the Centennial birthday celebration of Manuel García. (Courtesy of Jack Gluckman: University of Cincinnati Department of Otolaryngology.)

application of mirror laryngoscopy. The most important aspect of the dispute between Turck and Czermak was that the bitter quarrel fueled attention in the Western world toward the fledgling field of laryngology. Both pioneers immediately concentrated on educating physicians in the technique of laryngoscopy by convening clinics throughout Europe. This dissemination of knowledge led to a watershed of new instruments (Figures 1–14 to 1–16) and contributions.

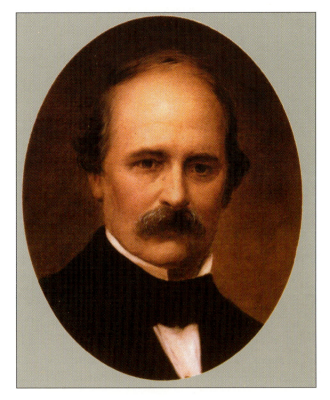

Fig 1–11. Ludwig Turck (1810–1868).

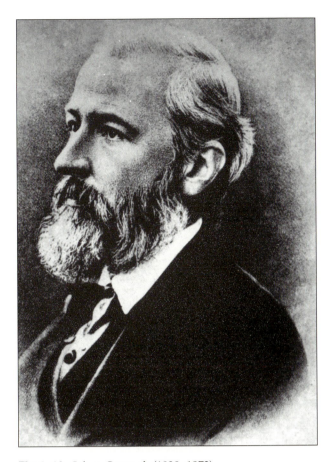

Fig 1–12. Johan Czermak (1828–1873).

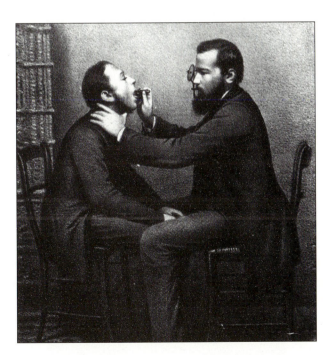

Fig 1–13. Woodcut drawing of Czermak performing mirror laryngoscopy. Note that the mirror is stabilized through an attachment that fits between the teeth. Also note that he is applying external laryngeal counterpressure with his left thumb.

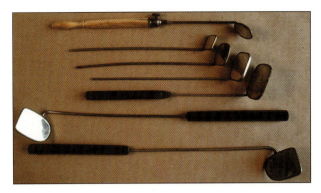

Fig 1–14. Assorted 19th century laryngeal mirrors. (Courtesy of the Massachusetts Eye and Ear Infirmary.)

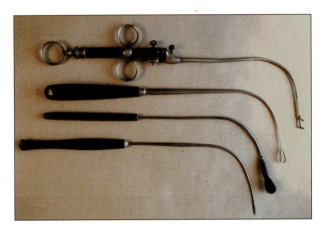

Fig 1–15. Assorted 19th century hand instrumentation. Superiorly a polyptome by Stoerk. Also seen are a curette, a silver nitrate brush, and a lancet knife. (Courtesy of the Massachusetts Eye and Ear Infirmary.)

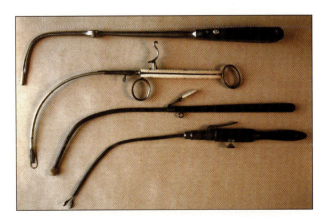

Fig 1–16. Other assorted 19th century laryngoscopic hand instrumentation. Superiorly, a cocaine pledget holder designed by Elsberg is seen. Below that is a polyp guillotine. The lower two instruments were designed by MacKenzie. The bottom instrument was utilized to resect polyps and the probe above it was utilized to apply electric current in the treatment of vocal fold paralysis. (Courtesy of the Massachusetts Eye and Ear Infirmary.)

In 1859 Stoerk[26] reported the first laryngoscopically controlled manipulation, which involved the topical application of silver nitrate to the larynx. In 1860 Lewin[27] was the first to report laryngoscopically guided management of laryngeal tumors. In his series of 50 neoplasms, he excised 3 and applied caustics to 4. Mackenzie (Figure 1–17)[28] introduced mirror laryngoscopy to Great Britain after attending Czermak's clinic. He acquired acclaim as a surgical innovator and a prolific author.[29,30] In 1886 Fraenkel (Figure 1–18)[31] published the first report of a transoral resection of a laryngeal cancer.

In the United States, laryngoscopy and laryngology were initially slow to develop due to the concurrent outbreak of the Civil War. Near the end of the conflict, Louis Elsberg (1837–1885; Figure 1–19), who attended the Jefferson Medical College in 1860, published the first formal American manuscript in laryngology and endolaryngeal treatment in 1864.[32] Soon thereafter, he received the Gold Medal from the American Medical Association for his paper entitled, "Laryngoscopal Surgery Illustrated in the Treatment of Morbid Growths Within the Larynx" (Figure 1–20).[33]

Similar to virtually all laryngologists of the day, Elsberg was a physician and not a trained surgeon. At the conclusion of his Civil War service as a surgeon in the Union Navy and Army, Jacob Da Silva Solis-Cohen (1838–1927; Figure 1–21) was influenced to become a laryngologist by his boyhood friend and medical-school classmate, Elsberg. To the best that this author can document, Solis-Cohen was the first formally

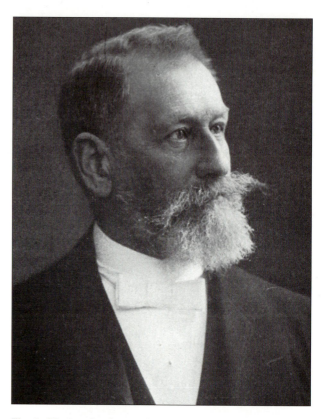

Fig 1–18. Bernhard Fraenkel (1836–1911). (Courtesy of the *Annals of Otology, Rhinology and Laryngology*.)

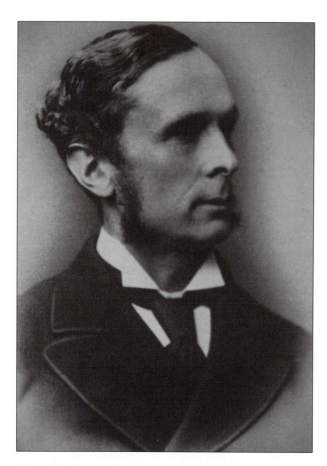

Fig 1–17. Sir Morell MacKenzie (1837–1892).

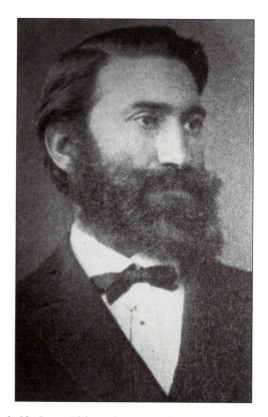

Fig 1–19. Louis Elsberg (1837–1885), first president of the American Laryngological Association.

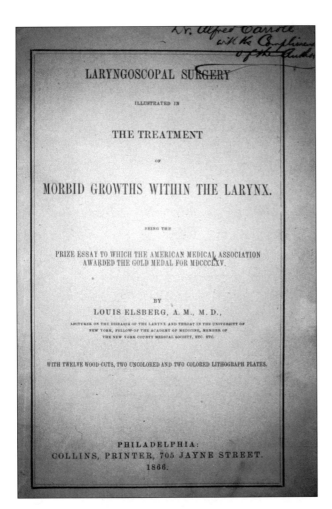

Fig 1–20. Elsberg's award-winning manuscript describing endolaryngeal surgery.

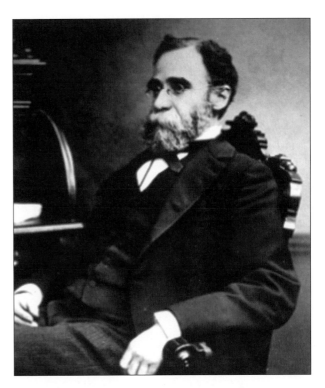

Fig 1–21. Jacob Da Solis-Cohen (1838–1927), second president of the American Laryngological Association. (Courtesy of the College of Physicians: Philadelphia.)

trained surgeon to become a laryngologist. Since surgical procedures in the larynx have primarily fueled the development of laryngology, Solis Cohen's professional development became a critical turning point in the history of laryngology, laryngeal surgery, and ultimately phonosurgery.

Solis-Cohen introduced his rigorous surgical training and war-time experience to the fledgling medical specialty of laryngology, and most likely, he was the first specialist head and neck surgeon in history.[34] Unlike preeminent general surgeons, such as Billroth, who often performed extensive surgery in the head and neck, Solis-Cohen operated solely in this area, which was a primary factor for his many formidable accomplishments. He was probably the first individual to cure a laryngeal cancer, which was done by means of a laryngofissure and hemilaryngectomy in 1867.[34,35] At the age of 29, he performed the procedure, having never previously witnessed it, and in the company of a hostile gallery that included Samuel Green and Joseph Pancoast. Green was Solis-Cohen's surgical mentor and was opposed to his surgical specialization in the head and neck. Solis-Cohen was also one of the first individuals to separate the trachea from the neopharynx during the tissue reconstruction subsequent to total laryngectomy. This minimized the perioperative deaths from that procedure and established total laryngectomy as

a viable cancer operation. In turn, Solis-Cohen's new reconstruction facilitated the first description of pharyngoesophageal speech.[36]

Solis-Cohen realized and taught that precise management of the upper aerodigestive tract disorders required endoscopic and open surgical skills. This philosophy was vividly displayed in his magnum opus published in 1872, *Diseases of the Throat: A Guide to the Diagnosis and Treatment,*[37] which was the benchmark for textbooks of its kind for decades. Jackson's *Peroral Endoscopy and Laryngeal Surgery*[38] appears to be modeled after Solis-Cohen's text.

Elsberg and Solis-Cohen helped found the American Laryngological Association (ALA; Figure 1–22) in 1878 (they served as the first and second presidents), which became the model for similar organizations throughout the world. Solis-Cohen had a unique perspective, having trained initially as a surgeon before specializing in upper aerodigestive tract disease, which is the current-day model for otolaryngological training.[34] He lived and contributed actively well into the 20th century and served as the Nestor of American laryngology and laryngeal surgery through its formative period and through the establishment of direct laryngoscopy.

Education in laryngology and laryngeal surgery has been of paramount importance since the origin of the specialty. The clinics taught by Czermak and Turck became the initial model for disseminating knowledge. The forefathers of American laryngology were acutely aware of the importance of education to raise standards of skill. Elsberg's first two presidential addresses were entitled, "Laryngology in America"[18] and "Laryngological Instruction."[39] Solis-Cohen established the first US course in laryngology at the

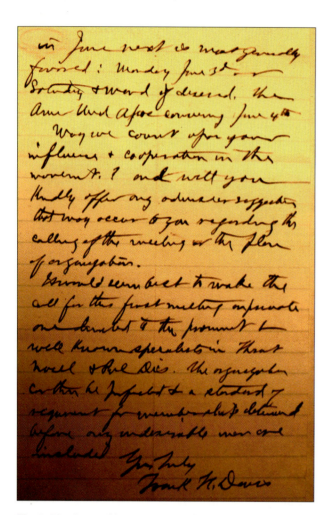

Fig 1–22. Original letter conceiving the origin of the American Laryngological Association. (Courtesy of the Francis Countway Medical Library: Harvard Medical School.)

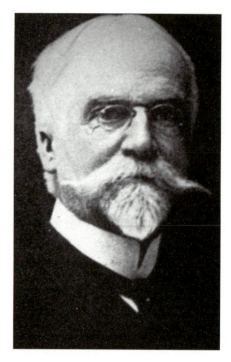

Fig 1–23. Frederick Knight (1841–1909), third president of the American Laryngological Association.

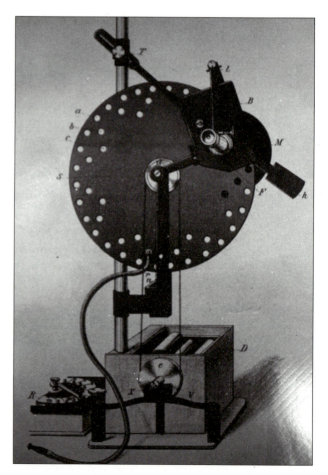

Fig 1–24. Oertel's laryngostroboscope. (From *Archiv für Laryngologie und Rhinologie.*)

Philadelphia School of Anatomy, while Henry Oliver established the first course in a US medical school (Harvard). Frederick Knight (1841–1909; Figure 1–23) carried the responsibility for developing laryngological education and research at Harvard and he reported on this topic in his address as the third president of the ALA. This rich heritage of education in laryngology continues into the present, which was elegantly discussed by Robert Sataloff at the 1999 meeting of the ALA.[40]

The laryngeal stroboscope, which was fundamental for understanding and teaching the physiology underlying laryngeal sound production, was introduced initially by Oertel[41] in 1878. In this brief communication, Oertel outlined the concept; however the device functioned poorly due to the lack of a consistent adjustable power source to regulate the rotating perforated disks (Figure 1–24). His landmark manuscript, published in 1895,[42] described the use of electricity for this purpose, which facilitated the feasibility of the laryngeal stroboscope. Furthermore, Oertel ingeniously fitted the stroboscope with a magnifying telescope. The heuristic value of Oertel's contribution is evidenced today, as the stroboscope is an invaluable instrument in the armamentarium of the laryngeal surgeon.

THE ORIGIN AND DEVELOPMENT OF DIRECT LARYNGOSCOPIC SURGERY: THE 20TH CENTURY

By the end of the 19th century, Kirstein (Figures 1–25 and 1–26)[43,44] reintroduced direct laryngoscopy (autoscopy) and appears to have been unaware of Green's work. Kirstein, who was in private practice, was visionary in his appreciation of the value of his technique, yet he was fully aware of the potential academic resistance both to a different approach for visualizing the larynx and to a new technology. He therefore called his procedure "autoscopy" and avoided calling it laryngoscopy. He wisely concluded in the preface of his text, "Of course, many a laryngologist is convinced that the laryngological technique needs no additions; others may think differently. Only the future can decide this question."[44]

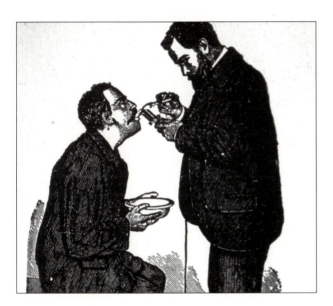

Fig 1–25. Alfred Kirstein performing autoscopy (direct laryngoscopy). Note the "Kirstein position" of the head and neck.

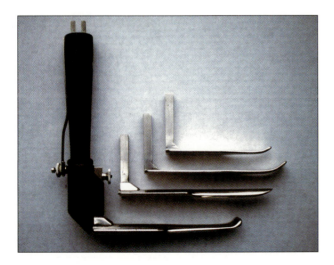

Fig 1–26. Kirstein's autoscope. (Personal collection S.M. Zeitels; gift from M.S. Strong.)

Kirstein's success in precipitating a paradigm shift in endolaryngeal surgery was due to his careful and patient approach to change and to the fact that there was great academic interest in the field of laryngology. This allowed for enough open-minded inspection to embrace the advantages of direct endolaryngeal surgery, which has served us well in the 20th century. In 1895, Kirstein even predicted the enhanced value of autoscopy if it were to be married to the improved imaging techniques that could be provided by magnification and stroboscopy.

Killian (1860–1921; Figure 1–27), who was an academic surgeon, was initially incredulous of Kirstein's claims regarding direct laryngoscopy. After viewing Kirstein's demonstration, Killian became absorbed with the new technique. Not to be outdone, Killian perfected rigid bronchoscopy by 1897, thereby demonstrating direct examination of the airway distal to the larynx. Killian was destined to make other major contributions to direct laryngoscopy in the early 1900s.

All of the substantive improvements in endoscopic surgery of the larynx during the 20th century have enhanced precision. Increased precision is inevitably linked to better exposure of the operative field and in turn enhanced visualization. The important innovations for enhancing laryngeal

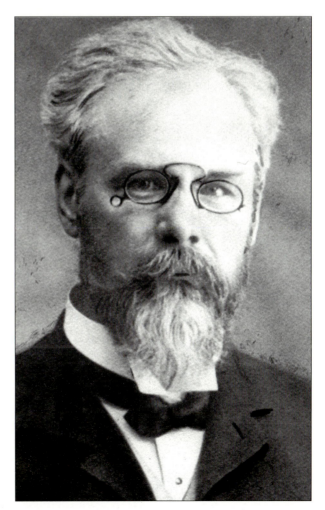

Fig 1–27. Gustav Killian (1860–1961). (Courtesy of the Massachusetts Eye and Ear Infirmary.)

exposure had been introduced by 1925. Jackson (Figure 1–28) employed Kirstein's head and neck position for direct laryngoscopy in the supine position (Figure 1–29).[45,46] Killian[47]

introduced the inverted V laryngoscope blade (Figure 1–30) to conform to the anterior glottal commissure and designed the laryngeal suspension (Figures 1–31 through 1–33)[48–50] that facilitated bimanual surgery. Internal distension was reintroduced (initially by Babington) in the antero-posterior dimension by Haslinger[51] with his bivalve laryngoscope (Figures 1–34 and 1–35) and in the medio-lateral dimension by Jackson[52] with his laryngostat. Although previously used by Czermak, external counter-pressure was formally described

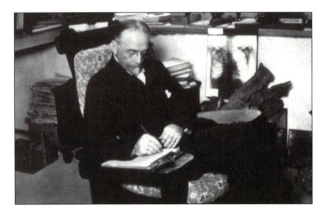

Fig 1–28. Chevalier Jackson (1865–1958). (Courtesy of the Massachusetts Eye and Ear Infirmary.)

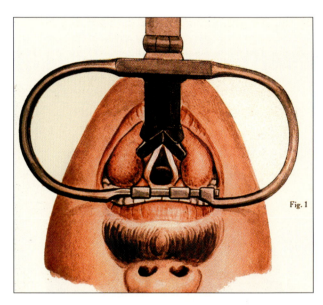

Fig 1–30. Drawing of Killian suspension laryngoscope in place. Note the inverted V spatula. (From Die Schwebelaryngoscopic und ihre praktische.)

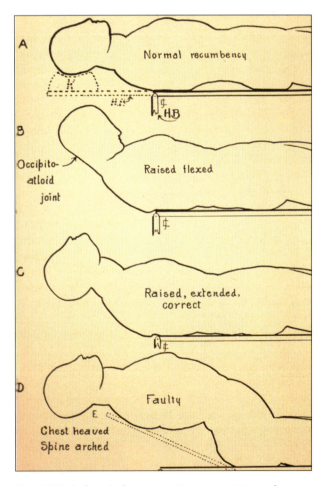

Fig 1–29. Jackson's diagrammatic representation of proper head and neck position for effective supine direct endolaryngeal surgery. (From Jackson and Jackson: *Bronchoscopy, Esophagoscopy, and Gastroscopy.*)

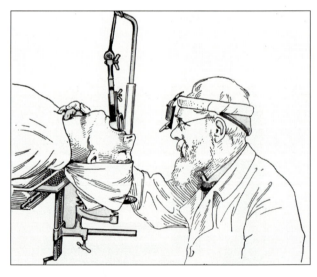

Fig 1–31. Diagrammatic representation of Killian performing suspension microlaryngoscopy. Again, note the incorrect head and neck position and the use of external laryngeal counterpressure. (From Die Schwebelaryngoscopic und ihre praktische.)

by Brünings (Figures 1–33, 1–36, and 1–37).[47,53] All laryngologists utilize one or more of these concepts; recently; however, Zeitels and Vaughan[10] combined them while using *elevated vector suspension*.

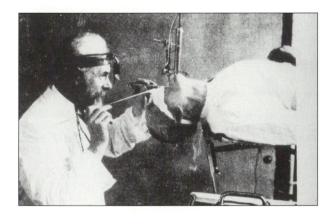

Fig 1–32. Gustav Killian (1860–1921) performing suspension laryngoscopy. Note that he is operating bimanually and that the source of illumination is a headlight. Also note the incorrect head and neck position.

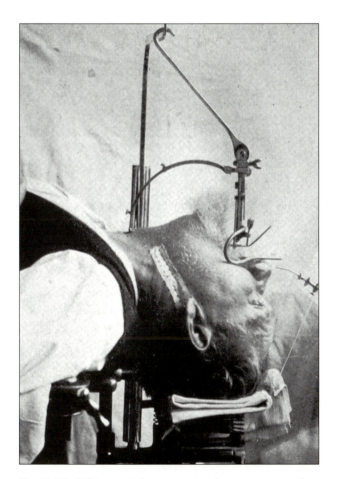

Fig 1–33. Killian spatula suspension laryngoscopy with a retrofitted Brünings external counterpressure device. (Courtesy of the Laryngoscope Journal.)

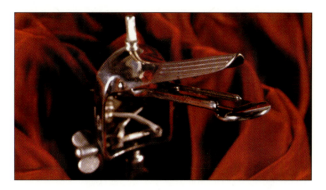

Fig 1–34. Haslinger's distending bivalve laryngoscope. (From the collection of C.S. Karmody.)

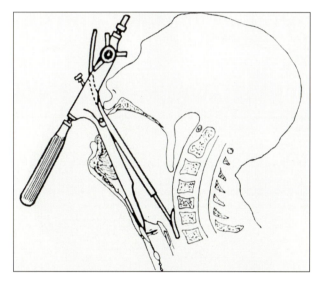

Fig 1–35. Diagrammatic representation of the Haslinger laryngoscope in place revealing anteroposterior internal distention. The handle could be placed at either end of the laryngoscope so that the instrument could be used for sitting or supine direct laryngoscopy. (From the collection of C.S. Karmody.)

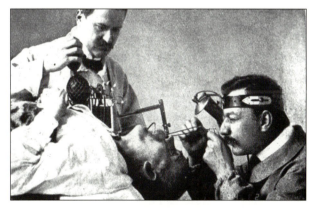

Fig 1–36. Brünings also performed bimanual surgery by utilizing the external counter pressure device as a stabilizing mechanism for his spatula laryngoscope. Again, a headlight was employed for illumination.

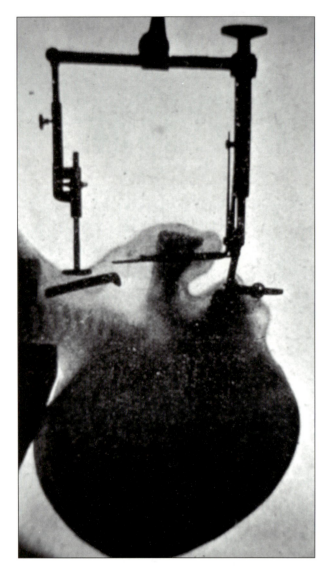

Fig 1–37. A radiograph of a cadaver with a laryngeal dilator placed within the glottal aperture. This facilitated visualization of the functional advantages of Brünings' external counter-pressure device.

Most surgeons throughout the world employ torsion-fulcrum laryngoscope holders to maintain the laryngoscope in position for endolaryngeal surgery. They mistakenly refer to this as suspension laryngoscopy. This misconception appears to have evolved from a manuscript in the early 1950s that referred to a gear-powered torsion-fulcrum holder as a suspension device.[54] Remarkably, there were no references indexed in this report. Prior authors[55–58] and scientific reports discussing these types of devices referred to them using terms such as "fulcrum-lift," "self-retaining," and "stabilizer."

The development of torsion laryngoscope holders arose from functional necessity, but their popularity today largely persists due to habit and custom rather than anatomical science and engineering principles. The forerunners of current laryngoscope holders were designed by Killian's disciples since they had difficulties utilizing the suspension gallows on awake patients with marginal nonendotracheal anesthesia.

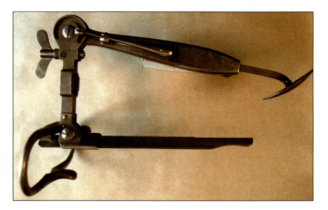

Fig 1–38. Seiffert's spatula laryngoscope. This device is the forerunner for current laryngoscope holders that rest on the chest wall for a stand while fulcruming off the maxilla.

Brünings laryngoscope system (Figures 1–36 and 1–37) pushed off the larynx, whereas Seiffert's instrument (Figure 1–38) utilized the chest wall as a means of support. Remarkably, chest-support torsion-holder systems were used exclusively for spatula laryngoscopes until the late 1940s, at which point they were retrofitted for use with tubular laryngoscopes.[54–58]

The introduction of general endotracheal anesthesia to direct laryngoscopic surgery by 1960[59] should have catalyzed a rebirth in the use of true elevated vector suspension. Detailed discussions of the forces required for optimal exposure of the larynx advocate the use of a suspension-type device from which the patient is hanging.[10,46,60–67] This information was well known to Strong and Vaughan when they fathered the Boston University Suspension Gallows (Pilling Company, Fort Washington, Pa).[63] Unfortunately, this suspension gallows has not gained wide acceptance and has remained primarily in use among the 2 generations of surgeons trained by Strong and Vaughan.

The justification for a return to a suspension gallows is that the most precise endolaryngeal procedure will be accomplished with the widest endoscopic surgical field, which requires the largest laryngoscope that can be placed between the lips and the larynx. Placement of the largest-lumen laryngoscope requires hanging the patient by the soft tissues adjacent to the lower jaw with accompanying general endotracheal anesthesia and muscular paralysis. It cannot be achieved by using the maxilla as a fulcrum and the laryngoscope as a lever.

Around 1960, the surgical microscope was introduced to endoscopic laryngeal surgery by Scalco et al,[68] Jako (Figure 1–39),[69] and Kleinsasser (Figure 1–40).[70] Jako[71] also designed the first set of microlaryngeal hand instruments. Kleinsasser designed hand instrumentation as well and became preeminent in educating surgeons throughout the world in micro-laryngoscopic technique.[70,72] At the same time, Priest[59] introduced the concept of general endotracheal anesthesia to laryngoscopy. These innovations led to a new era of precision because of the stable magnified surgical field. In the early 1970s, Polanyi[73] worked with Jako,[74] Strong,[75] and Vaughan,[76] and coupled the carbon dioxide (CO_2) laser (Figure 1–41) to the surgical microscope. The laser provided precise hemostatic cutting as well as a delivery system that consisted of a

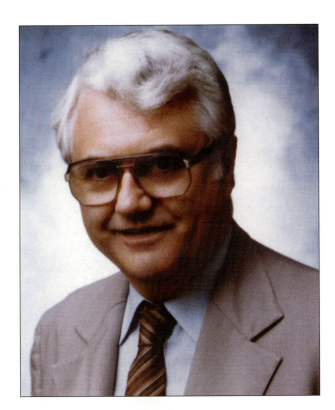

Fig 1–39. Geza Jako (1930–).

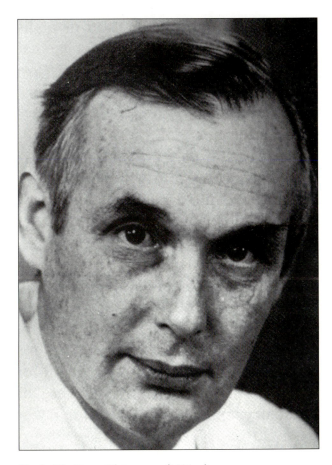

Fig 1–40. Oscar Kleinsasser (1931–).

joystick and a foot-pedal. This in turn allowed for precise bimanual surgery under high magnification, which was problematic for those who had difficulty controlling their nondominant hand in a magnified field.[77]

The aforementioned history reflects the inseparable linkage and interdependence of performing vocal arts, laryngeal physiology, and laryngeal surgery. Hans von Leden's (Figure 1–42)[78–87] career and voluminous scientific

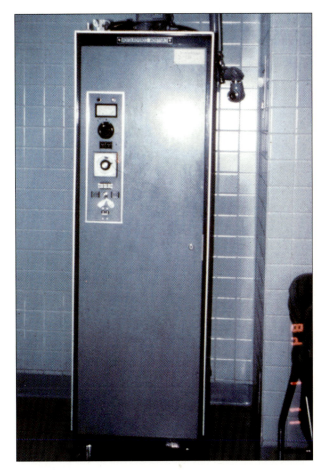

Fig 1–41. Original American Optical carbon dioxide laser used at Boston University.

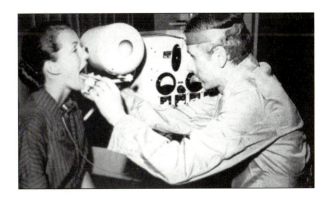

Fig 1–42. Hans von Leden performing laryngeal stroboscopy over 30 years ago.

contributions embody this philosophy and serve as the foundation for modern Phonosurgery, a term he developed in 1963. His seminal contributions have retained their heuristic value through the last 4 decades and he continues to contribute into the present. A number of his collaborating colleagues including Hirano (Figure 1–43) and Isshiki (Figure 1–44) have subsequently established a number of the current phonosurgical treatment paradigms based on their anatomical and physiological approach to laryngeal sound production.

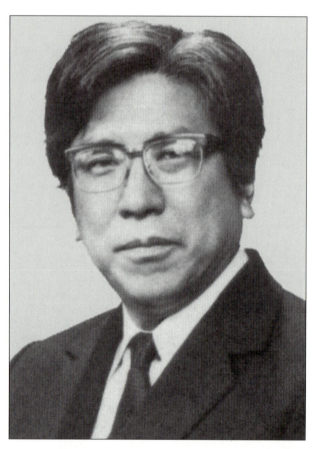

Fig 1–43. Minoru Hirano.

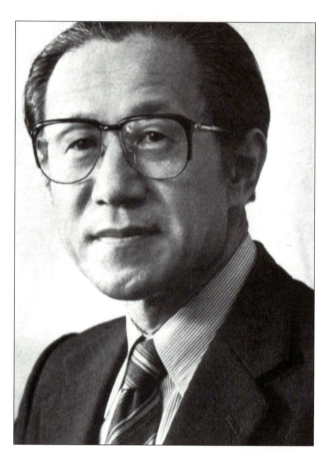

Fig 1–44. Nobuhiko Isshiki.

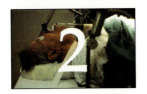

Phonomicrosurgical Management Philosophy Including Performing Artists

OVERVIEW

In the last decade, many substantive advances in endoscopic laryngeal surgery have been based on design innovations in soft-tissue handling, resulting from improved understanding of physiological principles of laryngeal sound production[88,89] and the use of stroboscopy to analyze vocal fold oscillation. This approach, termed **phonomicrosurgery** by the author in 1994,[65] is based on maximally preserving the vocal fold's layered microstructure, the epithelium and laminae propria.

Bishop[90] described the body-cover theory of vocal fold vibration in 1836 by deductive reasoning based on anatomical dissections. Apart from the work of Fournie in1866,[91] this concept was relatively dormant for 140 years until Hirano[88,89] performed his ground-breaking scanning electron microscope analysis of the vocal fold anatomy. These seminal investigations provided the anatomical foundation for the physiological observations that facilitated the design of the majority of current phonosurgical procedures. Precision is paramount in the execution of effective endolaryngeal surgery, especially phonomicrosurgery. The ensuing photographic anthology should serve as a guide for tissue handling and procedural approach.

The majority of endoscopic surgery in the glottis is done to treat benign processes. The most frequent presenting symptoms for glottal disease is hoarseness. Benign lesions typically occur in vocal overdoers and seldomly occur in individuals who are reticent and shy. Many of these individuals will require preoperative and postoperative vocal therapy to unload habits that predisposed them to the original lesion and/or to remove compensatory strategies that developed as a result of the lesion(s). Because the timing and decision about surgery is frequently linked to the response to vocal therapy, the surgeon must know the speech-language pathologist well in order to accurately assess the adequacy of therapy.

The patient must always be warned that it is possible for the voice to be worse subsequent to the surgery[92] and the laryngologist must have an accurate assessment of his or her surgical skills. Furthermore, it is very common for patients to have more pathology than can be appreciated even by stroboscopy.[92,93] Examination in the operating room provides significantly greater magnification, as well as the potential for use of telescopes to examine surfaces that are tangential and/or obscured in the clinic examination. Therefore, consent must be obtained to remove potential pathology that may not be appreciated during the office examination, including both folds. All patients should be prepared for the possibility of vocal deterioration after a phonomicrosurgical procedure. Phonomicrosurgery should be avoided if possible in female patients during the premenstrual period or during menses.

The preoperative workup for phonomicrosurgical procedures should include flexible and rigid laryngeal stroboscopy as well as acoustic and aerodynamic assessment.[94] Telescopic stroboscopy provides superior optics for analyzing the anatomy of the vocal folds, the details of the lesion, and the characteristics of the mucosal wave oscillation. Flexible stroboscopy is superior for analyzing generalized laryngeal configuration and arytenoid motion during sound production, which is necessary for assessing the magnitude of muscle tension that occurs during phonation. This information can usually assist the surgeon intraoperatively and often helps prognosticate the postoperative result.

The aforementioned visual information, along with acoustic and aerodynamic data, provide the surgeon with objective information about laryngeal sound production, which is valuable for discussion with the patient about what to expect from his or her voice. It also provides information to the speech-language pathologist, who may be instituting vocal therapy.

The acoustic and aerodynamic information should be obtained for normal and loud voice tasks. The aerodynamic (pressure, flow, and resistance) efficiency is an excellent indicator of a patient's phonatory effort and stamina. This factor is often overlooked in the preoperative history and postoperative discussions.

Ideally, the complete assessment should be repeated approximately 1 month postoperatively to analyze the result and again at the completion of voice therapy as is appropriate. Finally, the postoperative assessment documents the result since many individuals are prone to develop new lesions.

PATIENT POSITION

Czermak[24,95] introduced the sniffing position while perfecting mirror laryngoscopy (see Figure 1–13). Kirstein adopted the same position for sitting direct laryngoscopy (see Figure 1–25). It was composed of flexion of the cervical spine in relation to the thoracic spine and extension of the head at the atloid-occipital joint. Jackson demonstrated that this position could be achieved in a supine patient (see Figure 1–29) with an assistant supporting the patient's head and neck (Jackson position; Figure 2–1). When surgeons attempt to simulate the Jackson position without an assistant by placing a pillow under the vertex, extension at the atloid-occipital joint can actually be impaired, thus inhibiting proper positioning.

Anesthesiologists employed the Jackson position for endotracheal intubation.[96–100] Recently, this precept was challenged in a study[67] that examined the efficacy of 3 head and neck positions for exposing the glottis with different sized tubular laryngoscopes: (1) extension of the head and neck, (2) (sniffing) extension of the head and flexion of the neck, and (3) flexion of the head and neck.

Although the head-forward flexion-flexion position had been described by Killian[101] for difficult indirect laryngoscopy (Figures 2–2 and 2–3), and Johnston[102] (Figure 2–4) for the difficult sitting direct-laryngoscopy, the sniffing position has been accepted as the ideal configuration for examination of the larynx. As had been noted by Johnston[102] 85 years earlier in his Triological thesis, the recent study[67] demonstrated that flexion of the head and neck[66,67] most reliably achieved the most complete exposure of the anterior glottis, especially with the largest laryngoscope. Hochman et al[66,67] recently demonstrated that pure flexion (Figures 2–5 and 2–6) is the position of choice[67] for the difficult exposure during direct laryngoscopic endotracheal intubation.

The study also confirmed that the interarytenoid region could be adequately exposed in pure extension position with a small laryngoscope in most patients, which is the typical requirement for intubation. Finally, the investigation explained why there was great success at the turn of the century

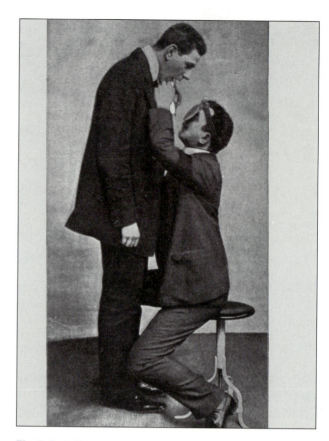

Fig 2–2. Killian position for indirect laryngoscopy. Note the flexion position of the head and neck and the uncomfortable position of the examiner. (From Bruck A. In: Forbes W, trans-ed. *Diseases of the Nose, Mouth, Pharynx,* and *Larynx.* New York, NY: Rebman; 1910:375–376.)

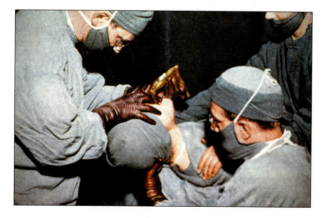

Fig 2–1. Jackson's supine positioning for laryngoscopy with the assistant supporting the head and neck. The head is extended at the atloid-occipital joint and the neck is flexed with relationship to the chest. (From Jackson C, Jackson CV, eds. *Diseases of the Nose, Throat, and Ear.* Philadelphia, Pa: Saunders; 1945:455.)

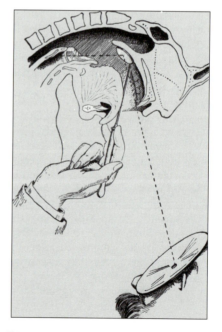

Fig 2–3. Diagrammatic representation of Figure 2–2. (From Bruck A. In: Forbes W, trans-ed. *Diseases of the Nose, Mouth, Pharynx,* and *Larynx.* New York, NY: Rebman; 1910:375–376.)

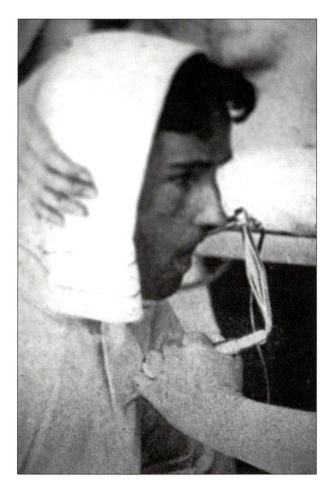

Fig 2–4. The patient is in a flexion position. This is an excellent position for a difficult intubation. The vertex and occiput of the patient's head can rest on the surgeon's chest and abdomen. This is not a good position for performing endolaryngeal surgery. (From Johnston RH. *Laryngoscope.* 1913;23: 607–617 with permission.)

with catheter placement by means of narrow-lumen tubular laryngoscopes for anesthetic endotracheal insufflation.[96,98] Larger endotracheal tubes with distal cuffs would be introduced later. The pure flexion position was technically unfeasible for microlaryngoscopic surgery because the proximal lumen of the laryngoscope is directed toward the ceiling (see Figure 2–5). Therefore, the Jackson position was confirmed experimentally to be the ideal position for microlaryngoscopic surgery.[66,67]

Glottal and Supraglottal Surgery

Suspension microlaryngoscopy is generally performed with general endotracheal anesthesia and paralysis. External counterpressure and internal distension are employed routinely. The smallest endotracheal tube to adequately ventilate the patient is inserted (laser-safe as necessary). When a patient is difficult to intubate, the head and neck are placed in flexion (see Figures 2–4 to 2–6).[66,67] The endotracheal tube provides a stable point from which the largest lumen laryngoscope is intercalated between the endotracheal tube and

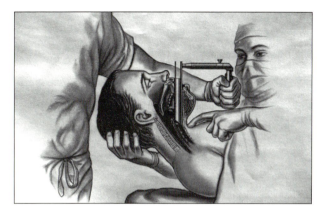

Fig 2–5. Diagrammatic representation of Figure 2–4 with an assistant providing head and neck support as well as external laryngeal counterpressure. (From Hochman II, Zeitels SM. *Operative Tech Otolaryngol Head Neck Surg.* 1998;9:192–195 with permission.)

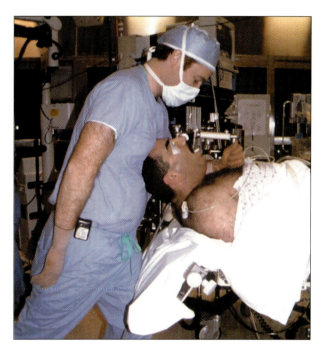

Fig 2–6. A wider image of Figure 2–4. The surgeon supports the weight of the head and neck with the legs rather than with the back. (From Hochman II, Zeitels SM, Heaton JT. *Ann Otol Rhinol Laryngol.* 1998;108:715–724 with permission.)

the infrapetiole region of the supraglottis (for glottal surgery) to internally distend the surgical field (Figure 2–7). For supraglottal surgery, the upper blade of a bivalved laryngoscope is placed against the tongue base or the epiglottis (see Chapter 17).

Jet ventilation is typically used when an endotracheal tube precludes adequate exposure of the pathology or when an intubation can result in further edema of a narrow airway. Our preference has been to use the Hunsaker catheter (Xomed; Figure 2–8), which positions the jet below the vocal folds and maintains the tip in the lumen of the trachea to

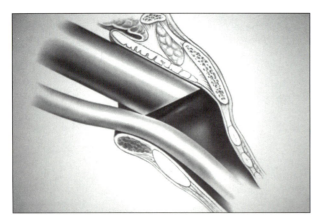

Fig 2–7. Distention of the laryngeal introitus is achieved by intercalating the distal portion of the laryngoscope between the petiole of the epiglottis and the endotracheal tube. (From Hochman II, Zeitels SM. *Operat Tech Otolaryngol Head Neck Surg.* 1998;9:192–195 with permission.)

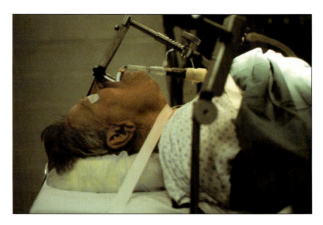

Fig 2–9. Jackson position with the Boston University Suspension Gallows. External counterpressure is applied with 1-inch silk tape.

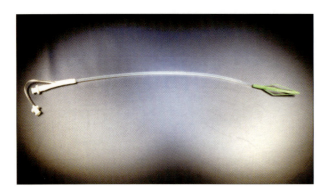

Fig 2–8. Hunsaker jet ventilation catheter.

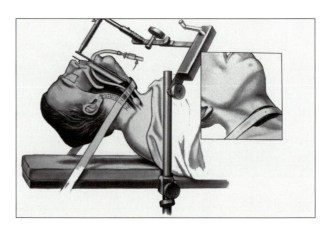

Fig 2–10. Diagrammatic representation of Figure 2–9. (From Hochman II, Zeitels SM. *Operat Tech Otolaryngol Head Neck Surg.* 1998;9:192–195 with permission.)

avoid barotrauma. Disadvantages of jet ventilation include the lack of practicality with many lesions, motion of the surgical field, and the inability to create adequate internal distension of the laryngeal introitus.

The patient is placed in the classic Jackson position with the neck flexed and the head extended at the atloid-occipital joint. The position is maintained with a modified Killian gallows (Pilling Co.) in true elevated-vector suspension (Figures 2–9 and 2–10). External laryngeal counterpressure is first applied manually to determine its value for improving exposure. It is then applied with a laryngeal cushion (Endocraft LLC, Providence, RI) and silk tape, which is stretched from the lower laryngeal framework to the operating table.[10,66,103] The magnitude of the pressure and vector of the force are adjusted to optimize the exposure of the lesion and the anterior glottis. If the CO_2 laser is to be used, both the patient and the endotracheal tube are protected in the appropriate fashion.

An operating microscope fitted with a 400-millimeter front lens is used to examine the glottal surgical field at various magnifications. A majority of lesions that are smaller than 6 mm in size should be resected at the greatest magnification for which the surgeon has the ability to precisely manipulate the tissue. This is typically limited by the surgeon's manual dexterity in the nondominant hand. The numbers on the knob of the surgical microscope that controls magnification do not usually reflect the magnification because of the 400-millimeter lens. The greatest magnification is typically 10×–13×. When working under high magnification, the surgeon should enhance his or her manual dexterity by resting the forearms on a platform or utilize a chair with armrests (Figure 2–11).

In addition to the magnified visual examination, the pathology is palpated with a blunt probe to help assess the texture of the lesion(s) and the depth of deep tissue involvement. In a majority of cases, a specially designed needle (Endocraft LLC; Figures 2–12 and 2–13) is used to perform a subepithelial infusion (Figures 2–14 and 2–15) of saline and 1/10,000 epinephrine[65,104,105] into the superficial lamina propria (SLP). A deleterious systemic response to the infusion

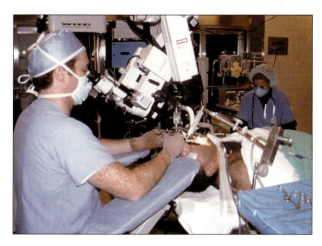

Fig 2–11. The surgeon's arms are stabilized by means of supports that extend from the automated chair. The table, as well as the microscope, should be positioned so that the surgeon's head and neck are in a straight, comfortable position.

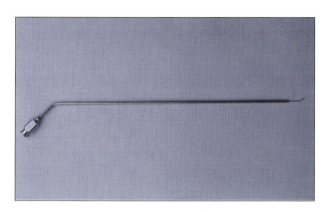

Fig 2–12. Zeitels vocal-fold infusion needle. (Courtesy of Endograft LLC.)

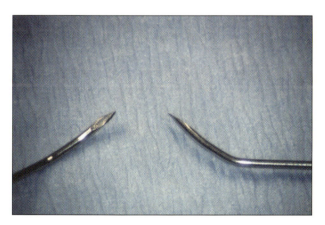

Fig 2–13. The tip of the Zeitels' needle has a specially designed short bevel. (Courtesy of Endograft LLC.)

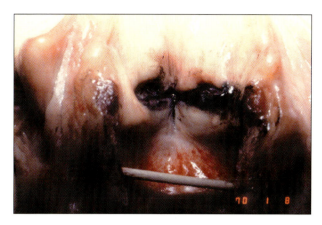

Fig 2–14. Subepithelial infusion of the right superficial lamina propria with India ink in a cadaver. There is some staining on the contralateral side.

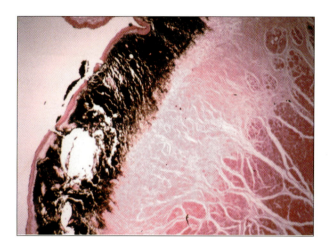

Fig 2–15. The India ink is seen directly at the vocal fold epithelium and superficial to the vocal ligament.

has not been observed in more than 1000 cases. If the epithelial lesion has not invaded and/or obliterated the SLP, the infusion solution will hydrodissect under the lesion and lift it away from the vocal ligament (Figures 2–16 and 2–17). Based on intraoperative observations, our experience has revealed that preoperative stroboscopy is helpful but not always reliable for determining the depth of invasion of epithelial lesions such as keratosis.[106] Preexcisional knowledge about the depth of penetration of the lesion (especially cancer) is critical for selecting instrumentation (cold versus laser) as well as for adjusting the deep margin precisely. Both of these factors are crucial to the patient's postoperative vocal outcome.

During superficial glottal procedures, hemostasis is achieved by topical application of epinephrine-soaked cotton. For deeper glottal lesions and supraglottal lesions, the laser is employed with a defocused spot or electro-coagulation is used. When the surgery is completed, any residual blood or secretions that are in the laryngeal introitus or hypopharynx

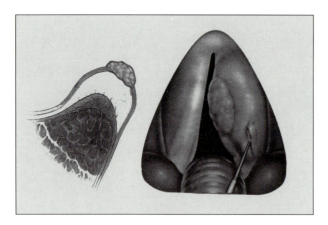

Fig 2–16. Diagrammatic representation of a subepithelial infusion where there is no invasion of the epithelial lesion into the vocal ligament. (From Hartig G, Zeitels SM. *Operat Tech Otolaryngol Head Neck Surg.* 1998;9:214–223 with permission.)

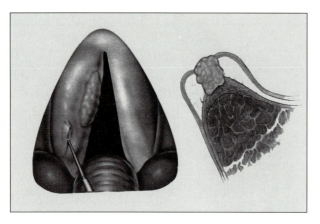

Fig 2–17. Diagrammatic representation of a subepithelial infusion where there is invasion of the epithelial lesion into the vocal ligament. (From Hartig G, Zeitels SM. *Operat Tech Otolaryngol Head Neck Surg.* 1998;9:214–223 with permission.)

are suctioned and the larynx is sprayed with plain lidocaine to avoid laryngospasm during emergence from anesthesia and extubation. Postoperatively, the patient is placed on humidified room air. Endolaryngeal surgery is done as an outpatient procedure unless there is an airway problem or medical-support requirements.

PERIOPERATIVE MANAGEMENT

Perioperative (pre and post) treatment of laryngopharyngeal reflux (LPR)[107,108] is often necessary to optimize the surgical result. This typically consists of diet and behavior modification and frequent use of proton pump inhibitors. Laryngopharyngeal reflux often accompanies laryngeal pathology because the inflammatory mucositis predisposes these tissues to injury from phonatory trauma and/or carcinogens. Most patients sustain laryngopharyngeal mucositis without heartburn because the mucosa above the upper

esophageal sphincter are more sensitive and susceptible to acidic refluxate and gastric enzymes than the epithelium of the esophagus. Essentially, heartburn reflects esophagitis, which is not present in the majority of patients with LPR. Antibiotics, steroids, and/or analgesics are prescribed selectively based on surgeon preference, and the extent of the surgery.

After vocal fold surgery, complete voice rest is advised for a minimum of 10 days after the surgery and modified voice use for 2 weeks. This is adjusted based in part on the extent of the surgery. Atrophy or significant rest-induced hypo/hyperfunction has not been observed. It is not unusual for patients to have temporary tongue numbness and/or dysgeusia in the region of the laryngoscope placement. After 10 days, if postoperative strobovideolaryngoscopy revealed no significant or unexpected findings, the patient is allowed gradual resumption of voice use under the guidance of a speech pathologist. For phonosurgical procedures, the patient has preoperative and postoperative appointments for objective voice assessment and vocal hygiene discussion. Formal voice therapy is administered as necessary.

BENIGN LESIONS OF THE GLOTTIS

Lesions along the rima glottidis impair entrained oscillation by creating stiffness in the diseased vocal fold and by preventing smooth vocal-edge closure. These factors result in an aerodynamically inefficient glottal valve. Phonomicrosurgical procedures are designed to improve aerodynamic efficiency and vocal quality by creating a smooth vocal fold edge that is not excavated with overlying epithelium that is flexible.

Optimal phonomicrosurgical management of benign glottal lesions requires maximal preservation of normal laminae propria and epithelium. Therefore, it is valuable to assess the micro-layers of involvement of any lesion. This should involve both high-magnification visual inspection as well as gentle retraction and palpation. Given the choice of sacrificing or disturbing normal SLP or normal epithelium, it is wiser to preserve normal SLP.

In our experience, there is little difficulty in the growth and regeneration of normal epithelium as is seen after a cordectomy that is left to heal secondarily. We have further noted that normal SLP does not typically regenerate if it has been removed. The exception is found in patients, who have undergone partial cyto-reduction of the SLP for the management of polypoid corditis (Reinke's edema). The voluminous SLP is predisposed to postresection distension if the predisposing factors (smoking, reflux, and vocal abuse) are not controlled.[109]

Our postoperative stroboscopic findings further reveal that if extensive dissection in normal SLP is performed to raise a wide microflap, stiffness will be noted in the field of dissection. Contrary to common belief, Hochman et al[93] demonstrated the location of epithelial incisions had no effect on postoperative mucosal wave pliability. Impaired mucosal wave propogation was related to dissection within the SLP. Epithelium has minimal visco-elasticity and primarily reflects the visco-elastic properties and the oscillation characteristics of the tissues underlying it.

PHONOMICROSURGERY ON PERFORMING ARTISTS

Endolaryngeal resection of lesions on the vocal fold edge in singers and performing artists has been done since the 19th century, after mirror-guided removal of lesions was introduced. The critical pathway for decision making that faced the patient and surgeon then remains unchanged today. Cooperatively, the patient and surgeon must carefully assess whether the lesion(s) are of greater liability to the vocal instrument and career than the operation to excise the lesion(s).[92,110] This judgment requires detailed communication and mutual responsibility for the chosen management course.

Phonomicrosurgery in performing artists has historically been associated with controversy because of variable results as well as divergent opinions about the pathogenesis of lesions and the potential for nonsurgical reversibility. Furthermore, the tremendous societal visibility of performers leads to significant publicity both in and out of the entertainment industry if suboptimal surgical outcomes occur. Paradoxically, excellent results are often obscured by the artists' desire to conceal the injury and reconstruction for fear it will imply that their singing technique is flawed, which could have a career-damaging affect.[111]

Surgical intervention in performing artists presents the laryngologist with a unique set of circumstances. The patient population is typically outgoing, often quite sophisticated from prior laryngological problems, and frequently outspoken about their previous care. A reticent performer is almost an oxymoron. Singers are vocal athletes and therefore should be managed at a level of precision and sophistication commensurate with their needs. The indication for phonomicrosurgical intervention is rarely caused by inherent systemic danger to the patient. Phonomicrosurgery is typically done because there is a functional performing deficit, which is accompanied by a lesion that can be attributed as a major etiological factor.

There is no exact formula for which patients should undergo surgical intervention and/or how long any patient should undergo voice therapy prior to surgery. The timing of surgery and the extent of preoperative voice therapy should be individualized based on lesion characteristics as well as concomitant inflammation from vocal abuse, reflux, infection, menstrual swelling, and smoking. Furthermore, preference of the patient, voice therapist, and surgeon are interdependent influences in the decision-making process. Finally, performance, recording, and traveling schedules frequently delineate the window of opportunity for comprehensive intervention.

Patient bias about management strategies based on previous experiences with their performing colleagues is an extremely important consideration. The surgeon should generally avoid persuading a performer to undergo surgery. Furthermore, surgeons must discuss the possibility that the voice can be made worse by a procedure. This approach engenders a mutual responsibility for the decision of pursuing the elective procedure. Finally, surgeons should generally relate their personal experience with the particular problem, not quoted literature, especially if the patient inquires. In this patient population, unfavorable results will often become widespread information due to collegial networking amongst performing artists.

Patients should not be unduly fearful of surgery since many of them are performing with injured vocal folds and a procedure often provides an opportunity for significant skill advancement.[92,110] Many performers have been masking the lesion-induced vocal aberration by expending tremendous compensatory effort. In addition to acoustical vocal improvement, patients should understand that effort of phonation may decrease and stamina may improve, which are a reflection of enhanced aerodynamic function.

The management of performing artists requires a collaborative team approach, in and out of the operating room. The speech pathologist and/or singing therapist is an especially critical member of the team. Phonomicrosurgery on performing artists should be done primarily under the highest possible magnification and with a laryngoscope that provides the widest aperture of the glottal surgical field. The technique of epithelial cordotomy and subepithelial resection[93] results in maximal preservation of the vocal folds' layered microstructure. This approach was designed to shorten healing time so that performers could return to full activity as soon as possible. Typically, patients commence singing at 3 weeks and can be professionally performing in 5 to 8 weeks.

In a recent study,[110] a retrospective review was performed on 125 performing artists who underwent phonomicrosurgical resection of 256 lesions to assess the efficacy of this approach. All patients underwent cold-instrument resection of a variety of lesions followed by vocal rehabilitation therapy. Virtually all patients with SLP lesions had improvement in their vocal function based on patient satisfaction and this was confirmed by comparing preoperative and postoperative stroboscopic assessments. Phonomicrosurgical resection of small vocal fold lesions is being done with increasing frequency in performing artists due to a variety of improvements in diagnostic assessment, as well as advances in surgical methodology and rehabilitation.

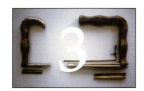

Instrumentation

LARYNGOSCOPES DESIGNED FOR MICROSCOPIC VOCAL FOLD SURGERY

This is an extensive section because laryngoscope design is fundamental to glottic exposure as it provides the pathway for effective and precise vocal fold surgery. The art and craft of direct laryngoscopy, including laryngoscope design, were standard components of laryngological education in the first part of the century but are often neglected today. The current de-emphasis of this teaching occurred as a result of the introduction of general anesthesia with paralysis, which was not typically used for these procedures in the first half of the 20th century. The control over the patient provided by advanced general anesthetic techniques diminished the need for highly skilled rigid endoscopists.

Much of the ensuing discussion is taken from a recent report in the *Annals of Otology Rhinology and Laryngology*.[11] This overview provides the reader with essential information so that he or she can carefully evaluate varied instrumentation. As in all surgery, exposure frequently becomes the variable that limits precision because of suboptimal visualization and tissue maneuverability. The photo-documentation in this book was greatly facilitated by a variety of prototype laryngoscopes. It is often unrecognized that a significant component of the difficulty of phonomicrosurgical procedures for most surgeons is compromised exposure and not tissue handling. Since all otolaryngologists are trained in otologic surgery, they typically have outstanding microscopic manual dexterity, which is the primary premise of phonomicrosurgical dissection within the layered microstructure of the vocal folds.

The microlaryngeal photography in this book was obtained from a sidearm of the microscope to simulate the surgeon's proximal stereoscopic view during each procedure. Although camera-mounted mobile telescopes that are placed within the lumen of a laryngoscope provide outstanding images of tangential tissue surfaces, they are of little value in demonstrating the details of microsurgery because this approach precludes tissue handling. Telescope systems that are mounted within laryngoscope lumens do allow for microsurgical photography. However, these systems were designed primarily to improve the view of the distal lumen of the laryngoscope examining tube, which is not adequate from the surgeon's proximal microscopic vantage. Furthermore, the surgeon is advised to operate from the viewing monitor and forego direct stereoscopic vision and depth perception. Finally, the internal telescope takes up working space within the laryngoscope lumen, which can impair positioning of hand-held instrumentation.

Binocular Laryngoscope Examining Tubes

At the turn of the century, Yankauer[112] appears to be the first to design a binocular laryngoscope tube (Figure 3–1). One is on display in the Wood-Library Museum of the American Society of Anesthesiologists. Approximately 40 years later, Roberts[55,56] described a novel laryngoscope that had detachable binocular tubes (Figure 3–2). These instruments were introduced prior to the era of microlaryngoscopy, which required larger diameter tubes to accommodate to the microscope oculars. Kleinsasser[72] and Jako[69,113] shouldered

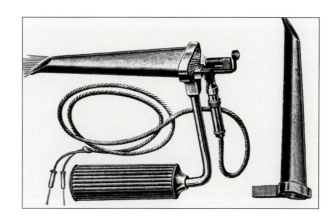

Fig 3–1. Yankauer binocular laryngoscope. (With permission *Laryngoscope Journal*.)

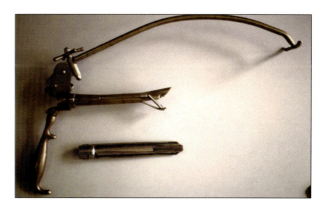

Fig 3–2. Roberts binocular laryngoscope with detachable tubes, distal internal distention phlange, and a self-retaining fulcrum arm. (Collection of Steven M. Zeitels.)

the development of current binocular laryngoscope tubes that are compatible with the surgical microscope. However, there is an ever-present limitation to widening the diameter of the examining tube because increasing its size restricts distal insertion of the laryngoscope.

Internal Distention and Bivalve Laryngoscopes

Internal distention represents the distraction of pharyngeal/supraglottal tissues so that the laryngeal introitus can be visualized more completely. This idea was first applied in 1829 in Babington's glottoscope, which was composed of a laryngeal mirror and an accompanying spatula (see Figure 1–3) to retract the tongue base anteriorly for enhancing endolaryngeal visualization. Antero-posterior internal distention was incorporated into bivalve distending pharyngeal specula (Figure 3–3) designed by Killian and Mosher in the early 20th century. Internal distention does not appear to be formally described for direct laryngoscopy until Haslinger[51,114] introduced the bivalved laryngoscopes (see Figures 1–34 and 1–35). Roberts' ingenious modification of Haslinger's tubular laryngoscope (Figure 3–4) created distal internal distention by means of a hinged flange on the bottom of the laryngoscope tube (see Figure 3–2).

Most subsequent current-day bivalve spatula laryngoscopes[115,116] also employ antero-posterior internal distention. However, the distending force generated at the proximal handle does not successfully transmit to the distal tip of the laryngoscope blade, which is engaging the laryngeal tissues. A great advantage of bivalve laryngoscopes is that hand instrumentation can be brought in easily between the spatula blades and into the scope lumen, which is important when used with lasers that have large delivery systems that are attached to the microscope. More importantly, hand instruments can be angulated between the spatula blades for enhanced tissue retraction in the laryngeal surgical field.

Jackson, Tucker, and Clerf[52] described internal distention with medial to lateral distraction of the vestibular folds to enhance visualization of the musculo-membranous vocal folds during endoscopic glottal surgery. They explained that patients were awake and frequently coughing, and that the laryngostat ensured for an adequate view of the vocal folds. The laryngostat was a teardrop-shaped tubular laryngoscope that conformed to the anterior commissure and maintained the vestibular folds laterally. Priest[59] also discussed the importance of lateral distraction of the vestibular folds in his landmark manuscript, which described direct laryngoscopy with general endotracheal anesthesia.

Illumination

Initial illumination for direct laryngoscopy was sunlight.[21] As a result of the introduction of electricity, Kirstein[43] used a headlight (Figure 3–5) with his initial autoscope spatula. Subsequently, he designed an electrified handle (Figure 3–6) with an proximal incandescent bulb and a prism to direct the light distally.[44] Later, Jackson introduced distal illumination by means of detachable electrified light-carriers (Figure 3–7).[117] Holinger[118] explained that little changed until "Broyles[119] first demonstrated the advantage of fiberoptic light transmission in peroral endoscopes" during his address as the guest of honor of the American Broncho-Esophagological Association in 1962. About the same time, the additional light provided by the surgical microscope, enhanced the self-contained illumination of the direct laryngoscopes. There has not been dramatic change since then.

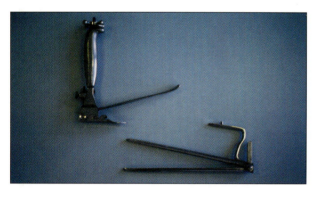

Fig 3–3. Pharynx specula designed by Mosher (*left*) and Killian (*right*). (Courtesy of the Massachusetts Eye and Ear Infirmary.)

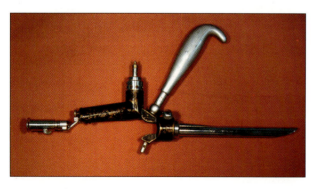

Fig 3–4. Haslinger direct laryngoscope, which incorporates detachable examining tubes. Note the proximal magnifying telescope. (Courtesy of R. García Tapia.)

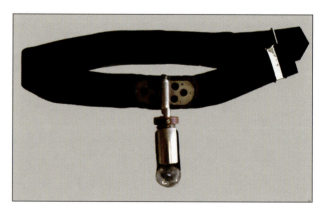

Fig 3–5. Kirstein headlight. (Courtesy of the Massachusetts Eye and Ear Infirmary.)

PARADOXES IN DIRECT LARYNGOSCOPE DESIGN AND TECHNIQUE

Since Kirstein formally introduced the first direct laryngoscope, numerous variations of this instrument have been designed to enhance endolaryngeal surgery and endotracheal intubation. All of these rigid laryngoscopes employ a spatula(s) or a tube to provide visualization of the laryngeal field. The construction and function of more than 50 of these laryngoscopes were analyzed to make the following observations, which reflect design flaws based on current technique requirements. Categorizing the design deficiencies of each instrument is an inefficacious use of time and would likely lead to ill sentiment because most laryngologists and anesthesiologists are content with their instrumentation. Therefore, observations are delineated without ascribing characteristics to specific laryngoscopes. Clinicians will be able to individualize the value of these observations based on their personal preference and experience.

Terminology

Laryngoscope is a generic term for a device, that is used to visualize the larynx. In the 19th century a laryngoscope was a mirror. The anatomy of the larynx is complex enough so that it is reasonable to stratify laryngoscopes by the specific tissues that they are designed to expose. Just as *subglottiscopes*[120] and *supraglottiscopes*[121] have been introduced, it seems prudent to use the term glottiscope if the instrument is fashioned to exclusively to expose the vocal folds. The precedence for the use of term, *glottiscope* (glottoscope), was established by Babington (see Figure 1–3)[5] in 1829, about 30 years before the field of laryngology developed.

Examination Tube/Spatula Design

The Distal Lumen

The distal lumen of most tubular laryngoscopes designed for glottal surgery is circular or oval (Figure 3–8), yet the glottal shape is most similar to a triangle. For this reason,

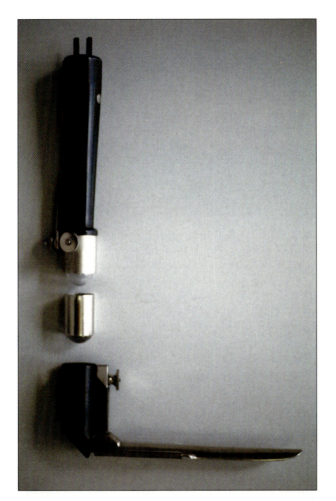

Fig 3–6. Kirstein autoscope. It is composed of proximal illumination in which the handle contains a bulb and a prism. (Collection of S.M. Zeitels.)

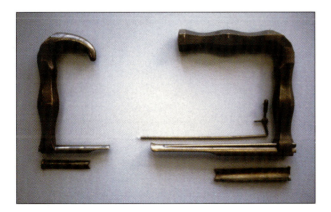

Fig 3–7. Early Jackson laryngoscopes with distal lighting in which the examining tube separates. The handle was ergodynamically designed for manual comfort. The short horizontal component of the C-shaped handle was adequate for the pediatric size but the adult size required lengthening for stability. When assembled, the examining tube is a tube proximally and a spatula distally.

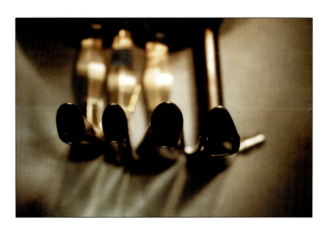

Fig 3–8. The distal lumen of a variety of tubular laryngoscopes designed for glottal surgery. The instrument on the right is a prototype designed by Vaughan and is composed of a rounded triangular configuration.

laryngoscopes are typically situated cephalad to the vestibular folds, precluding internal distention[10] and optimal exposure of the true vocal folds. The inverted "V" concept for spatula laryngoscopes (see Figures 1–30 and 1–34) should be incorporated into tubular laryngoscopes for adequate internal distention of the supraglottal tissues. Jackson et al[52] designed the teardrop-shaped laryngostat to achieve this; however, it was a small-lumen monocular instrument conceived prior to microlaryngoscopy. Broyles and Priest[59] also employed monocular variations of Jackson's laryngostat, that conformed to the anterior commissure while distracting the vestibular folds. Interestingly, a laryngostat was described for use in the first report of rigid laryngoscopy with general endotracheal anesthesia.[59] Later, Vaughan[64] elucidated the importance of this principle for effective exposure in phonomicrosurgery. Using prototype laryngoscopes that adequately expose the anterior commissure, Desloge and Zeitels[122] dispelled some of the myths regarding surgery (for benign and malignant disease) in that region in a series of 115 patients.

Tube Contour

There is no controversy that tubular glottiscopes should taper from a wider proximal lumen to the narrower distal aperture to accommodate the optical properties of the surgical microscope. Many laryngoscopes have a wider proximal aperture than is required for use with the microscope to facilitate angulation of hand instruments. Excessive widening of the proximal lumen can inhibit distal placement of the laryngoscope examining tube[59,67] since the widened proximal lumen cannot be inserted through the oral cavity and within the inner diameter of the mandible (Figure 3–9). This can result in two problems. The distal end of the scope is cephalad to the vestibular folds so that internal distention of these structures is not achieved, and exposure of the vocal folds (especially the superior surface) is not optimal. Additionally, as more of the laryngoscope tube is outside of the oral cavity, the distance between the surgical microscope and the proximal laryngoscope lumen is decreased. This can actually preclude placement of hand instruments despite the 400-mm lens (40 cm working distance). The micro-manipulator of the CO_2 laser is attached to the microscope lens, which also results in the loss of working distance between the microscope and the proximal lumen of the laryngoscope.

Another common design flaw of current tubular laryngoscopes is the perception about what constitutes an "anterior commissure" scope, which is hourglass in configuration (Figure 3–10). These instruments were excellent when they were introduced[123] in the mid-20th century, prior to the use of the surgical microscope or the CO_2 laser. At the time when these laryngoscopes were conceived, they worked quite well because endolaryngeal surgery was done with both the surgeon and the patient (adjusted by the head-holder assistant) being mobile (see Figure 2–1). The hourglass configuration is cumbersome at best during microlaryngoscopy, because neither the patient nor the surgeon are typically moving during the procedure to position for the ideal optical vector.

The hourglass shape was not found in the original tubular laryngoscopes[69,70,72,124] designed for use with the surgical microscopes. Neither the optical pathway of the microscope nor the CO_2 laser[74,75] (introduced later) can bend around the central narrowing. Although Dedo's microscope-compatible laryngoscope (Figure 3–10) was wider than previous "anterior commissure" laryngoscopes, it retained an hourglass configuration limiting full micro-stereoscopic view of the distal lumen. Additionally, to utilize the anterior flare, the microscope must be malpositioned, which can be problematic with the focusing beam of the CO_2 laser (Figures 3–11 through 3–13).[65]

A microscope-compatible laryngoscope is properly contoured when a stereoscopic view through the proximal lumen encompasses the entire distal lumen. In contradistinction, some current laryngoscopes with an hourglass shape have an

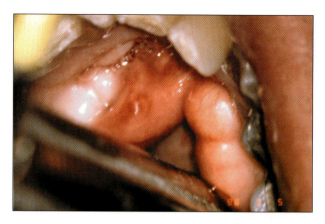

Fig 3–9. The vocal folds could not be exposed in this patient despite the use of a narrow monocular examining tube because of large mandibular torus deformities. After the exostosis was removed, the microlaryngoscopic surgery was performed uneventfully. This case illustrates how a wide examining tube may not be adequately positioned in a narrow mandibular arch.

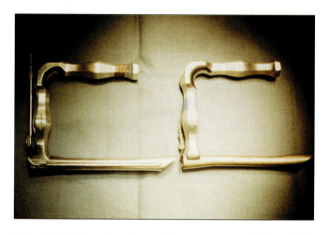

Fig 3–10. Hourglass-shaped laryngoscopes designed by Dedo (*left*) and Holinger (*right*).

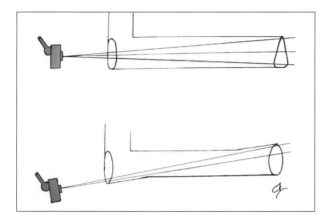

Fig 3–11. Diagrammatic representation of microlaryngoscopic examination through straight-tube and hourglass-tube laryngoscopes. Note that the microscope must be malpositioned to utilize the distal flare for anterior commissure exposure. (From Zeitels SM. *Laryngoscope.* 1995;105:1–51 with permission.)

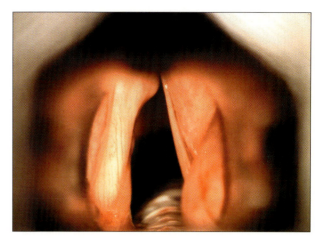

Fig 3–12. (4×) Proximal view through a microscope-compatible hourglass-shaped laryngoscope; Note the sessile polyp anteriorly on the left.

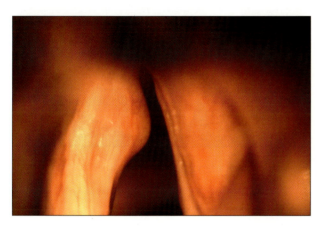

Fig 3–13. (7×) After the microscope has been repositioned as shown in Figure 3–11, the distal flare can be used and the polyp can be seen. Note that the shape of the distal lumen is round and that the right vestibular fold is obscuring the right vocal fold.

internal telescope to bypass the compromised viewing aperture, which reduces the critical intralumenal working area of the laryngoscope. The shaft of accompanying hand instruments were then bent to accommodate the hourglass distal flair, which limits maneuverability of those instruments within the lumen of the laryngoscope. The enigmatic engineering logic of this approach is fraught with interdependent flaws. Furthermore, it has been suggested that the surgeon utilize this laryngoscope by operating from the telescope-generated monitor image since there is difficulty viewing the tip of the bent hand instruments. Conceptually, this disregards magnified 3-dimensional endolaryngeal surgical technique, one of the most critical innovations of the 20th century.

Handle Design

The ideal handle is ergodynamically comfortable for manual gripping and for exertion of force as is necessary. An L-shaped design, as originally described by Kirstein (see Figure 3–6), is adequate for most intubations. Typically, the pharyngeal and supraglottal soft tissues are easily distracted to expose the interarytenoid region and the sniffing position with the head off the table is unnecessary.[67] If the exposure is difficult, a C-shaped handle is ideally suited to apply the appropriate vector force near the distal aspect of the laryngoscope blade. Jackson initially utilized an ergodynamically conformed C-shaped handle with a short horizontal limb (see Figure 3–7). Soon thereafter, a longer horizontal limb was introduced. Killian (see Figure 1–33 and 3–14),[48,125] Lynch (Figures 3–15 and 3–16),[126,127] Thomas,[62] Grundfast et al,[63] and Andrews[128] were keenly aware of this vector-force requirement of the horizontal limb for suspension laryngoscopy. The L-shaped hinged handle probably became popular among anesthesiologists in mobile army hospitals where the laryngoscope was folded into a pocket for versatility. This requirement is less crucial for most conventional hospital settings.

Adjustability and modular design

Despite the fact that the Kirstein's first direct laryngoscope[43] was modular with a universal handle and detachable blades, most current tubular laryngoscopes are single units with fixed handles. There is relatively little variation in laryngoscope blades in any specific model despite the wide variation in anatomy based on age, gender, and pathology of the head and neck. Anatomic variation was recognized by those who designed suspension laryngoscope systems (Killian, Lynch, Seiffert, Roberts), since a plurality of spatula blades were attachable to a universal handle. The lack of a modular universal handle, which is designed to accompany a spectrum of detachable tubes, has limited surgeons' choice, created a more cumbersome operating set up, and increased expense.

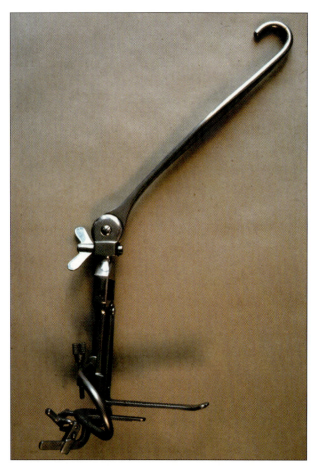

Fig 3–14. Early Killian suspension laryngoscope. (Courtesy of Massachusetts Eye and Ear Infirmary.)

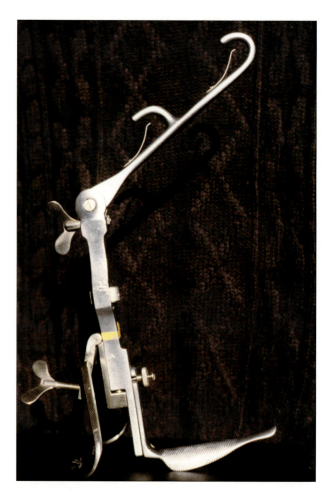

Fig 3–16. Lynch suspension laryngoscope.

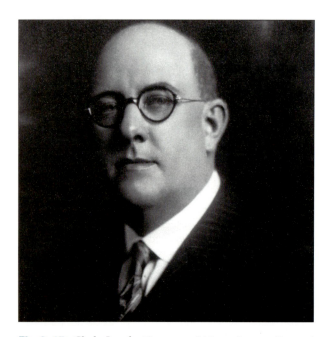

Fig 3–15. Clyde Lynch. (Courtesy of Massachusetts Eye and Ear Infirmary.

THE UNIVERSAL MODULAR (UM) GLOTTISCOPE

The universal modular glottiscope (Figures 3–17 to 3–22) was conceived from a century of direct laryngoscope designs to incorporate the most valuable prior innovations into a uniquely amalgamated instrument. The goal of this glottiscope system is to provide the clinician with a versatile laryngoscope that can optimally expose the vocal folds for diagnosis and instrumental manipulation, regardless of the diversity of human anatomical factors inherent to age, gender, and pathology of the head and neck. As is typically the case when a large number of instruments are available to serve a similar purpose, none has distinguished itself as superior in quality and design for universal acceptance.

The UM glottiscope was computer modeled in the solid modeling program Pro/Engineer (Parametric Technologies Corporation, Waltham, Mass) (Figures 3–20, 3–21, 3–22). Various sections were generated and a smooth surface was interpolated between them. The finite element analysis program Pro/MECHANICA (Parametric Technologies Corporation, Waltham, Mass) was used to determine the structural integrity of the laryngoscope. This program allowed simulation of actual working loads and conditions to be applied to

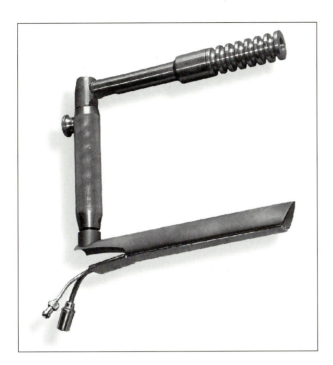

Fig 3–17. Zeitels universal modular UM glottiscope. (Courtesy of Endocraft LLC.)

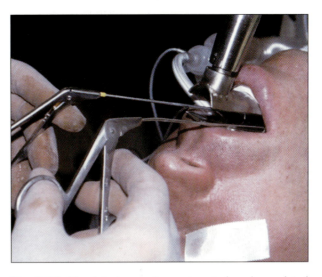

Fig 3–19. Hand instruments are inserted and angulated between the lateral slots. (Courtesy of Endocraft LLC.)

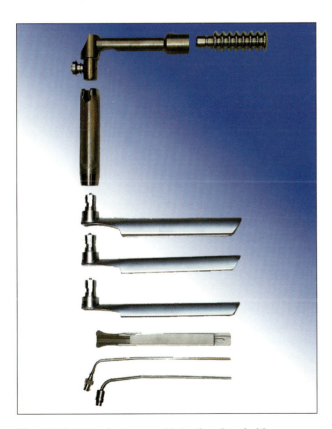

Fig 3–18. UM glottiscope. Note the detachable components: suction cannula, light carrier, base plate, 3 examining tubes, vertical handle, horizontal handle, and handle extension. (Courtesy of Endocraft LLC.)

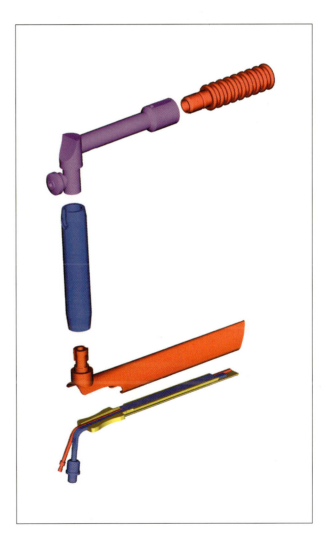

Fig 3–20. Diagrammatic representation of the components of the UM glottiscope. (Courtesy of Endocraft LLC.)

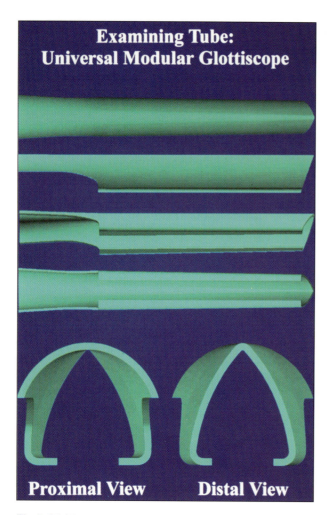

Fig 3–21. Diagrammatic representation of an examining tube from a variety of perspectives. (Courtesy of Endocraft LLC.)

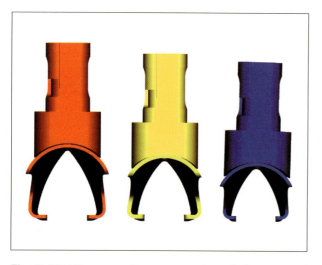

Fig 3–22. Diagrammatic representation of the proximal view through the different-sized examining tubes. (Courtesy of Endocraft LLC.)

the computer model and provided the resulting stresses. The geometry of the laryngoscope was then refined and reanalyzed to provide the maximum strength while maintaining the desired form and fit. Metallurgists were consulted for selecting the ideal composition of the components.

The Distal Lumen of the Laryngoscope Tube

The distal lumen of the UM glottiscope is an isosceles-triangle shape with arcuate sides (Figures 3–21 through 3–25) to create a lancet-arch[129] conformation. Unlike Jackson's laryngostat,[52] which was designed prior to the use of endo-tracheal anesthesia with endolaryngeal vocal fold surgery, the UM glottiscope has a flat planar base. Jackson's laryngostat was appropriately curved at the base to conform to the interarytenoid region. Holinger's anterior commissure scope[123] had a longer distal teardrop-shaped aperture than was found in the laryngostat (formed by increasing the distal flair). This was an important improvement at the time because this shape expanded supraglottal internal distention and, in turn, vocal fold exposure.

However, these experienced laryngologists did not perform laryngoscopy with an endotracheal tube in place. The planar base of the UM glottiscope rests on the endotracheal tube, maintaining the tube between the arytenoids for optimal exposure of the musculo-membranous vocal folds. The arcuate-sided distal-triangular lumen of the UM glottiscope is distinct from most microscope-compatible laryngoscopes, which are circular or oval. This shape is ideal for internal distention of supraglottal tissues because the triangular tube with arcuate sides can be safely intercalated (with reasonable force) between the endotracheal tube and the infrapetiole region of the supraglottis (see Figure 2–7).[10,66] Jet ventilation is not typically used by the author for phonomicrosurgery on the musculo-membranous vocal folds because internal distention is limited without an endotracheal tube and because the surgical field is less stable under high magnification with jetting.

The ideal distal lumen of a glottiscope can be loosely envisioned in the following fashion. In the era prior to general anesthesia, the surgical exposure of the glottal introitus was roughly in the shape of an inverted ice cream cone, which is similar to Holinger's laryngoscope. Today the endotracheal tube is in the location of where the ice cream would be situated so that the UM glottiscope simulates the cone, which has a flat planar base.

Tube Contour

The UM glottiscope tapers from the proximal lumen to the distal one to accommodate the stereoscopic optical properties of the surgical microscope. The narrow arch-shaped contour along the top of the examining tube facilitates insertion through the oral cavity[123,130] and pharynx. Unlike virtually all microscope-compatible tubular laryngoscopes, which further widen the proximal aperture to facilitate angulation of hand instruments, the UM glottiscope has bilateral proximal slots (see Figures 3–17 and 3–19). Creating bilateral slots dramatically increases the degree-of-freedom for positioning hand instrumentation and facilitates the insertion of hand instru-

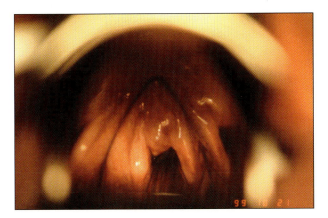

Fig 3–23. (2.5×) Proximal view through the UM glottiscope of a hemorrhagic polyp. Note the complete view of the pathology since there is not an hourglass shape. (Courtesy of Endocraft LLC.)

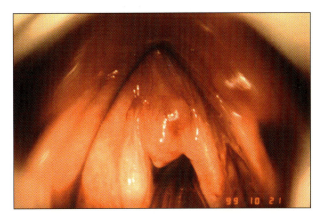

Fig 3–24. (4×) Figure 3–23 at higher magnification; the microscope position has not been altered. (Courtesy of Endocraft LLC.).

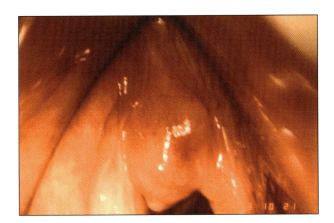

Fig 3–25. (7×) Figure 3–23 at even higher magnification; the microscope position has not been altered. (Courtesy of Endocraft LLC.)

ments into the laryngoscope lumen. Removing the lateral walls of the tube allows UM glottiscope to function uniquely as a bivalved laryngoscope proximally and a tube distally.

As stated earlier, excessive widening of the proximal lumen can inhibit distal positioning of the examining tube adjacent to the superior surface of the vocal folds.[52,59] The widened proximal lumen cannot be inserted through the oral cavity and oropharynx, within the inner diameter of the mandible.[123] When more of the examining tube lies outside the oral cavity, placement of hand instrumentation is impeded because the working distance (exacerbated by the micro-manipulator of a laser) is reduced between the surgical microscope and the laryngoscope. The surgeon may then face the difficulties encountered in the early days of microlaryngoscopy,[68,69,72] when the 400-mm lens was not available.[69,72]

The UM glottiscope is not hourglass in configuration since neither the visual vector from the microscope nor the CO_2 laser can bend around the narrowing. When using the

UM glottiscope, the surgeon only minimally readjusts the microscope to optimize visualization of the glottal surgical field (see Figures 3–23 through 3–25). Also, the aiming beam of the laser remains centered. The hourglass shape was conceived when patients were examined without general anesthesia and the point of constriction was noted to be at the posterior floor of mouth at the junction of the oral cavity and oropharynx.[123] With general endotracheal anesthesia and neuromuscular paralysis, a much larger tube can be placed. Unlike most microscope-compatible laryngoscopes, the superior aspect of the UM glottiscope is lancet-arch shaped to simulate the narrow central tube conformation of Holinger's anterior commissure laryngoscope.

Tube Construction

The flat planar base-plate of the UM glottiscope is detachable (see Figures 3–18 and 3–20) and slides into the upper arch-shaped spatula, which is a primary component of the bilateral slot design. When the base-plate is in place, the distal lumen of the UM glottiscope has the strength of a tubular glottiscope for effective internal distention. Distending bivalve spatulas do not have the structural integrity to maintain the distention forces, which are created proximally and transmitted to the distal end of the spatula blades, at the glottal aperture. The inadequate distal internal-distention of bivalved spatulas is exacerbated if significant external counter pressure is applied to the lower laryngeal framework.[10] Another drawback of bivalved spatulas is that they do not preclude oral and pharyngeal tissues from insinuating between the blades and obscuring visualization of the glottal surgical field.

For ease in difficult intubations as well as for maintenance and cleaning of the instrument, the base-plate of the tube can be separated even while in the patient. The concept of the separation capability of the examining tube was first introduced by Killian (Figure 3–26) and Jackson (see Figure 3–7)[117] at the turn of the century to facilitate the placement of a rigid bronchoscope. The UM glottiscope tube is similarly designed for placement of bronchoscopes, as well as for

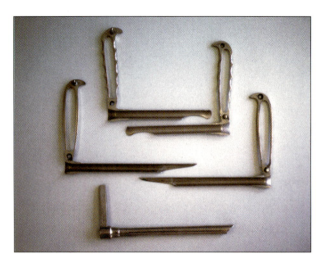

Fig 3–26. Two Killian separating-monocular laryngoscope examining-tubes above and a fixed tube below. (Courtesy of Massachusetts Eye and Ear Infirmary.)

difficult intubations, especially from obstructing carcinomas. Lancet-arch shaped spatula blades with a self-contained distal light-carrier will also be available for routine orotracheal intubations; the handle will contain a power source and will retain the versatile "L" or "C" shape.

Handle Design

Despite the associated expense in raw material and machining, the UM glottiscope handle is hollow and composed primarily of titanium rather than stainless steel because titanium is lighter, which is a desirable property for a laryngoscope. It has long been observed that a lighter laryngoscope improves the surgeon's manual dexterity and instrument-mediated tissue proprioception.[124]

The handle is composed of 3 elements: a vertical limb, a horizontal limb, and an extension piece (see Figures 3–17, 3–18, and 3–20). These elements combine ergodynamic principles of hand stability and comfort because of the potential need for the use of significant force. The vertical limb of the handle has fine knurling, which facilitates stability of the gripping force by increasing the friction coefficient. At the upper aspect of the vertical handle, there is a spring lock mechanism for attachment of the horizontal portion of the UM glottiscope handle or European chest support systems.[72] The spring lock is curved, so that it contours to the inner aspect of the distal phalanges of the fingers.

The horizontal component of the handle fits easily into the vertical limb. It is excavated proximally to accommodate the curve of the index finger. This distributes the force of lifting over a broader area during elevation of the head or neck or distraction of the pharyngeal tissues. For comfort in gripping the laryngoscope, the proximal aspect of the horizontal component has been cut at an angle to support the distal phalanx of the thumb. The shaft of the horizontal component has been designed to be compatible with standard clamp-on fulcrum laryngoscope holders.[54] At the distal end of the

horizontal component, an optional handle-extension can be attached for use with true suspension gallows.[63]

The proximal portion of the extension fits easily into the horizontal handle and is maintained by a novel spring-lock mechanism. The body of the extension handle is composed of a series of circular ridges to act as a support for the arm of the suspension gallows. The plurality of ridges allows for a variety of linear positions to place the suspension arm. This facilitates precise exertion of the appropriate vector of force for different-length laryngoscope tubes.

Adjustability and Modular Design
(see Figures 3–18 and 3–20)

The universal glottiscope was designed as a series of attachable and detachable components for a variety of reasons. First and foremost, this approach allows for precise selection of which components are necessary to purchase and which components are necessary for any individual case, which streamlines surgical efficiency.

Specifically, there are a plurality of tubes that accompany one universal handle. The range of sizes and variations in arch-conformation of the examining tubes facilitate precise accommodation of the glottiscope to the spectrum of human sizes and shapes, irrespective of gender, age, or disease. Therefore, clinicians can select which tube(s) are most likely suitable and valuable to their practice. This is cost effective as well as more orderly in the operating suite. The detachable tubes attach to the vertical handle by means of a unique spring-loaded bayonet-joining system, which facilitates ease of use, as well as strength and stability.

The universality of the components to other conventional equipment allows selective use of portions of this system, which can be joined to other laryngoscopic instrumentation (eg, using the current handle with European bivalved distending laryngoscopes). The modularity also facilitates the use of the UM glottiscope with other European chest-support systems of laryngoscope stabilization. Finally, the modularity minimizes replacement costs if components are lost or broken, or when future innovations are developed.

Illumination and Suction (see Figures 3–18 and 3–20)

Fiberoptic light carriers and suction tubes were designed as easily attachable and detachable devices, which can be placed or removed even when the laryngoscope is positioned in the patient. Standard light transmission cables can be used for attachment to the light carriers. These components have been designed to be situated in the planar base. In turn, instrumentation of the vocal folds is not affected by the position of these components. If desired, the light carrier can be easily removed once the patient is positioned, since the microscope light is usually sufficient for endolaryngeal surgery. Suction tubes are unnecessary if cold instruments are used and can be added if the surgeon converts to a laser procedure.

LARYNGOSCOPES FOR SUPRAGLOTTAL SURGERY

See Chapter 17.

SUSPENSION LARYNGOSCOPY AND TORSION-FULCRUM LARYNGOSCOPE HOLDERS

Suspension laryngoscopy improved the precision of endolaryngeal surgery by allowing for bimanual tissue manipulation, which revolutionized the technique. Killian introduced his suspension laryngoscope (see Figures 1–31 through 1–33) in 1912 and the modified tongue spatula(s) (see Figure 1–30) soon thereafter. However, he placed the patient in pure extension, which was a suboptimal position for exposure of the glottis.

The author has not been able to determine why Jackson never adopted suspension laryngoscopy and accompanying bimanual surgery, or why Killian never adopted the Jackson position to improve exposure. This is surprising considering their academic collaborative relationship. Killian's chapter[125] describing suspension laryngoscopy in Jackson's text, *Peroral Endoscopy and Laryngeal Surgery* is the only section not authored by Jackson.

Killian, Jackson, Kirstein, and Green all retained a similar philosophy; the appropriate application of force during direct laryngoscopy was to the tongue-mandible complex. They did not use the maxilla as a fulcrum for the laryngoscope blade, which would then serve as a lever to expose the anterior glottis. In contradistinction, most surgeons today utilize a torsion laryngoscope holder/stabilizer, which applies the primary force from the chest wall or a stand to the maxilla for obtaining anterior glottal exposure.

Suspension laryngoscopy requires that the patient is hanging from some type of gallows, as described by Killian (see Figures 1–31 to 1–33)[48–50,125] Lynch,[126,127] and Mosher.[112] Torsion-fulcrum stabilizing devices were reported by Killian's disciples, Brünings[53,131] and Seiffert, because they desired to perform bimanual surgery and they found suspension laryngoscopy was too difficult. Brünings cleverly stabilized his spatula laryngoscope by applying external counterpressure to the laryngeal cartilage framework (see Figure 1–36) while Seiffert[132] utilized the chest wall (see Figure 1–38). With a fulcrum laryngoscope stabilizer or holder, the movement of a spatula/tube within the laryngeal introitus to expose the anterior glottis is analogous to an oar where the maxilla is the oarlock.

In the first half of the 20th century, those surgeons who used tubular laryngoscopes, operated with one hand, as described by Jackson. Bimanual surgery with a suspension laryngoscope was done with spatula blades and was practiced by a minority of surgeons, many of whom were directly influenced by Killian and Lynch.[133–135] After World War II, Roberts[55,56] modified Haslinger's tubular laryngoscope (Figure 3–4) and added a chest-support stabilizer (Figure 3–2) to maintain position of the instrument for bimanual endolaryngeal surgery. Later, King[57] and Sommers[58] retrofitted stabilizing devices to Jackson-type C-shaped laryngoscopes.

Subsequent to these reports, Lewy[54] introduced a similar laryngoscope stabilizer with a gear-power advantage, which became quite popular since most otolaryngologists continued to find suspension laryngoscopy difficult to perform without general anesthesia. During the era in which Lewy's laryngoscope holder was introduced (the 1950s), general endotracheal anesthesia was not typically employed in conjunction with direct laryngoscopy. His gear-powered device was easy to use and enabled a large number of surgeons who previously were unsuccessful with suspension techniques to perform bimanual surgery. This was very important for the development of endolaryngeal surgery in the middle part of the century. However, he referred to his laryngoscope holder as a suspension device and that incorrect terminology persists. Webster[136] defines the word suspend as "to hang so as to be free on all sides except at the point of support; as to suspend a ball by a thread."

This misunderstanding of suspension laryngoscopy obscured the tremendous cumulative experience and knowledge of Kirstein, Killian, and Jackson, even to the present. Laryngoscope holders became popular throughout the world in the 1950s and 1960s. The use of these devices should have been supplanted by suspension laryngoscopy in the 1960s when general endotracheal anesthesia with paralysis was popularized with direct laryngoscopy.[59] Improvements in anesthesia brought true suspension laryngoscopy within the purview of most surgeons. Thomas[62] as well as the Boston University group[63] realized this and introduced true suspension systems; however, surgical habits are slow to change. The reader is encouraged to critically review the primary sources regarding laryngoscope holders and suspension gallows to develop an unbiased perspective on the development of this instrumentation.

A return to suspension laryngoscopy would be advantageous to surgeons who use laryngoscope holders/stabilizers. Current phonomicrosurgical techniques are performed optimally by obtaining the widest possible glottal surgical field. This is accomplished by placing the largest diameter, well-designed laryngoscope that can be inserted between the lips and the glottis and can only be achieved if the patient is suspended by the supraglottal/pharyngeal tissues in Jackson position.[64] This approach represents the convergence of Kirstein's, Killian's, and Jackson's techniques and is termed elevated-vector suspension (see Figures 2–9 and 2–10).[65]

MAGNIFIED LARYNGOSCOPY

A magnified view of the larynx was first reported in 1895 by Oertel[42] in his description of the mirror-guided stroboscope (see Figure 1–24). Brünings[137] also utilized a magnified ocular[138] and was the first to employ magnification to enhance direct laryngoscopy. Haslinger also designed a tubular laryngoscope with accompanying telescopic magnification (see Figure 3–4). Kahler's panelectroscope[112] probably had magnification capabilities as well. In the early 1950s, Albrecht used a colposcope for magnified indirect vocal fold examination and for photo-documentation of keratosis. The first published report of the use of the surgical microscope during laryngoscopy was by Scalco, Shipman, and Tabb[68] in 1960; they employed the Lynch spatula suspension laryngoscope for the task. The open spatula design facilitated complete distal stereoscopic viewing. The surgical microscope was a monumental innovation for enhancing the precision of endolaryngeal surgery because it provided high-power magnification with a 3-dimensional stereoscopic field.

Jako[71,139] in the United States and Kleinsasser[70,72] in Europe perfected surgical microlaryngoscopy. While Jako[71] introduced the first set of microlaryngeal hand instruments, Kleinsasser[72] introduced the 400-mm lens. The latter innovation increased the working distance between the microscope lens and the proximal lumen of the laryngoscope, which facilitated the placement of the long-shafted otologic instruments. Both surgeons designed wide-bore examining tubes to accommodate the optical characteristics of the surgical microscope. Strong[140,141] and DeSanto et al[142] systematically discussed microlaryngeal surgery, which broadened its appeal in the United States.

Kleinsasser[72,143] designed his own hand instrumentation and established the foundations for cold-instrument microlaryngoscopic technique, which has recently enjoyed renewed enthusiasm as phonomicrosurgical procedures have increased in popularity.[65,77,88,144–150] Today, most phonomicrosurgical procedures should be performed under high magnification to ensure maximal preservation of the vocal folds' layered microstructure (laminae propria and epithelium).[77,109,151–153]

COLD INSTRUMENTS AND THE CARBON DIOXIDE LASER

Jako[71] designed the first microlaryngoscopic hand instruments about 1962 in collaboration with the Stumar Company. They were otologic instruments with long shafts. Soon thereafter, Kleinsasser introduced more designs. Since then, the most substantial change has been size reduction[154] to facilitate more precise and delicate soft-tissue dissection in the layered microstructure of the vocal fold.

Hand instrumentation for microlaryngoscopic surgery can be classified into 7 types: (1) forceps (Figures 3–27 to 3–29),

(2) scissors (Figure 3–30), (3) dissectors/knives (Figure 3–31), (4) spatulas/mirrors (Figure 3–32), (5) suctions (Figure 3–33), (6) needles (see Figures 2–12, 2–13, and 3–34), and (7) sponge/cotton carriers (Figure 3–35). These instruments may be

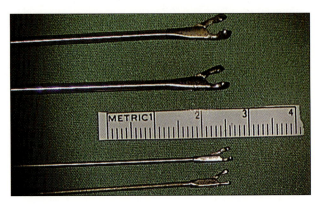

Fig 3–29. Angled cup forceps.

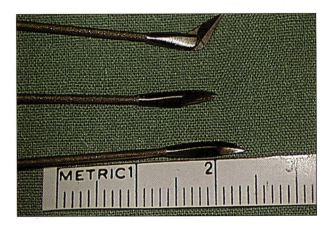

Fig 3–30. Microscissors.

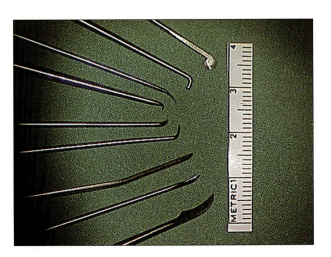

Fig 3–31. Dissectors and knives.

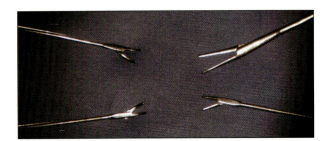

Fig 3–27. Alligator forceps.

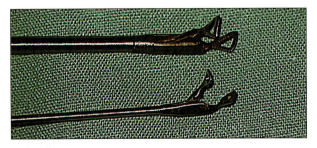

Fig 3–28. Angled triangular forceps.

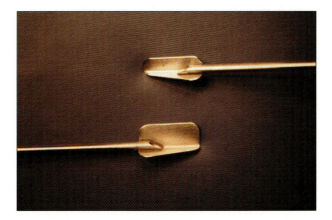

Fig 3–32. Spatulas (cord retractors).

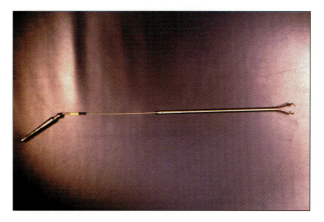

Fig 3–35. Sponge/cotton carrier.

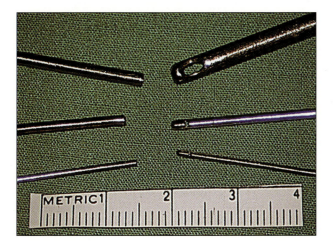

Fig 3–33. Straight-tip and velvet-eye suctions.

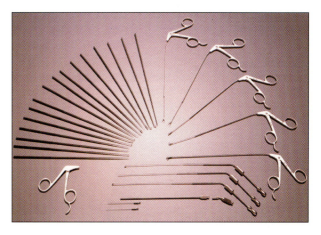

Fig 3–36. Sataloff instrument set. (Medtronic Surgical Products, Jacksonville, Fla.)

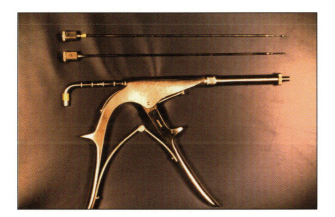

Fig 3–34. Brünings injecting system.

acquired individually or in sets (Figure 3–36). Forceps may be shaped as a cup, triangle, or alligator and the latter can lock to function as a needle holder. Scissors are straight, angled, and curved. Dissectors and knives may attach to separate handles, which allow for 360° rotation. Spatulas may be designed to protect unintentional soft tissue injury or may have a reflecting surface to facilitate laser ablation of tangential surfaces. Suctions can have a perpendicular opening and may have insulation for cauterization. They can also be configured with a distal side port, which is referred to as a whistle-tip or velvet-eye. Needles allow for infusion of thin liquids[65,104,155] or viscous fluids[131] (ie, fat) or may facilitate fine micro-cautery.

During the past decade, there has been controversy regarding the appropriate use of cold instruments and the CO_2 laser. The CO_2 laser provides excellent hemostasis as well as a stable delivery system (joystick and foot-pedal) for those who have difficulty maintaining dexterity in their nondominant hand under high magnification (personal communication: M.S. Strong 1986). In a recent study,[77] it was noted that 77% of 263 glottal procedures were done with cold instruments alone. The thermal trauma of the CO_2 laser was found to be detrimental to the delicate loosely arranged elastic tissue of the superficial lamina propria. The laser was optimally used in more vascular lesions because bleeding would otherwise obscure the operative site and in larger lesions that could not be effectively retracted within the lumen of the laryngoscope.

It should be remembered that Jako introduced both cold instruments and the laser to laryngology and that they were intended to be used synergistically rather than to the exclusion of each other. Both forms of instrumentation are essential in the armamentarium of the endolaryngeal surgeon. In the future, the role of lasers (as an energy source to selectively manipulate different tissue) will probably expand again with further breakthroughs in laser technology.

In the cases that follow, the reader will observe that the author frequently begins glottal surgery with a cold-instrument epithelial incision, which is often referred to as an *epithelial cordotomy*. This initial incision facilitates microscopic exploration of the relationship of the pathology to the superficial lamina propria. During the last decade, this has been a standard approach by the author for the management of pathologies such as cysts, epithelial atypia, and cancer.[65,104,146,151,156] Over the last 4 years, this approach has been extrapolated for the management of nodules, polyps, ectasias, and varices so that a subepithelial resection of these traumatic lesions has become typical.[93,157] Although it takes significantly longer to perform a subepithelial resection because of the grasping limitations of current hand instruments, patients heal very rapidly after this approach because secondary epithelialization is obviated. Amputation is now rarely performed except for the smallest lesions.

FIBEROPTIC AND TELESCOPIC ENDOLARYNGEAL SURGERY WITH LOCAL ANESTHESIA

The author does not ascribe to the philosophy that there are significant advantages to performing most phonosurgical procedures in the clinic setting by means of fiberoptic or telescopic visualization regardless of stroboscopic control. This approach ignores the majority of substantive innovations of the 20th century and is a throwback to 19th century technology. This approach ignores: (1) bimanual precise tissue retraction and cutting, (2) subepithelial dissection and microflap techniques, (3) an immobile stable operating field, (4) adequate magnification, and (5) distraction of supraglottal tissues which can obscure visualization of the operating field. Conversely, this approach encourages: (1) poorly controlled avulsion, (2) secondary healing and epithelialization, and (3) general imprecision. Ironically, the stroboscopic examination at the time of the procedure is of little significance as compared with the examination 4 to 6 weeks after fibrosis and secondary epithelialization have occurred.

The office approach is reasonable for patients who cannot undergo general anesthesia; refuse conventional surgery; cannot be exposed by direct laryngoscopy, which is almost no one if elevated vector suspension is used; require a piecemeal avulsion, such as a cancer biopsy from a large field; or need other procedures that do not require precision. This approach should also be considered if health care resources are not available to administer general anesthesia or to purchase adequate microlaryngoscopic instrumentation.

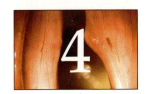

4

Polyps

Vocal fold polyps present in a spectrum of sizes, shapes, and tissue composition. Typically, they are the result of trauma to the superficial lamina propria and most frequently the microvasculature. Polyps are commonly found in the middle portion of the musculo-membranous region because the aerodynamically induced shearing and collision forces on the SLP are greatest in this region. These lesions may be sessile or pedunculated and they may also be vascular, fibrotic, or mixoid. The overlying epithelium is usually normal and can often be preserved partially or totally, as is appropriate.

There is great variation in the magnitude of involvement and replacement of the SLP by these lesions. This critical information is initially assessed by stroboscopy in the clinic, as well as by palpation under anesthesia with high-magnification observation. Frequently, a smaller traumatic fibrovascular lesion will be noted on the opposing surface of the contralateral vocal fold. It can be difficult to determine whether the collision trauma from the polyp induced the smaller lesion or whether there were bilateral lesions in which one grew larger. This differentiation is only of academic interest because, if there is palpable tissue alteration, both lesions should be resected.

When resecting polyps, an epithelial cordotomy adjacent to the lesion provides the definitive information about the nature of the involvement of the normal SLP and is the initial step in the resection of the lesion. This is clearly displayed in the photographs of the cases that follow. Since the epithelium overlying a sessile polyp is typically normal, all or a portion of it is usually preserved to facilitate rapid healing. This approach was recently described by Hochman and Zeitels.[157] Essentially, sessile polyps are being managed similarly to subepithelial cysts. Pedunculated polyps are often amputated by means of retraction and resection by means of microscissors.

Subepithelial infusion of saline and epinephrine enhances the precision of the resection in a large number of these lesions.[104,105] The infusion places tension on the normal mucosa, which facilitates the epithelial cordotomy. The infusion also increases the depth of the SLP and exaggerates the discrepancy of the normal SLP from the denser fibrovascular polyp tissue. These factors enhance maximal preservation of normal SLP during the dissection. The epinephrine in the solution as well as the hydrostatic pressure within the Reinke's compartment improve hemostasis, which is critical when working at high magnification.

As stated earlier, sessile lesions are ideally removed by means of an epithelial microflap and a subepithelial resection of the polyp contents.[157] Pedunculated lesions with a narrow pedicle are optimally resected by retraction and amputation. The surgeon will need to individualize the resection approach based on pathological presentation. Care should be taken to palpate the component of the polyp that is in the SLP so that it is adequately excised. The small (0–3 mm) and medium (3–6 mm) sized lesions can usually be removed with greater precision by cold instruments.[77]

When removing polyps, a small feeding vessel may be encountered. It will usually stop bleeding by gentle application of saline/epinephrine 1/10,000 soaked cotton. Occasionally the CO_2 laser is necessary to microcauterize the vessel. Initial work using a pulsed dye laser (Zeitels, Anderson, Franco, Jarboe, and Farinelli; unpublished data) to coagulate vessels without disturbing the epithelium or SLP is very promising. Larger sessile lesions (>6 mm), which are often difficult to retract within the lumen of the glottiscope, are often best managed with the microspot CO_2 laser.[77] The bleeding that occurs after incising these lesions with cold instruments can obscure the magnified operative field. This results in poor visualization and lack of precision.

Case 4A

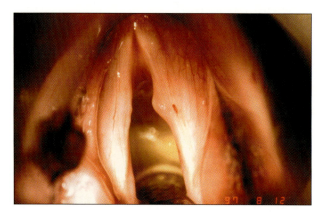

Fig 4–1. (4×) There is a spheroid mass emanating from the medial surface of the right musculo-membranous vocal fold. An ectasia is visible at the supero-lateral surface of the lesion. On the contralateral vocal fold, there is a prominent varix in a similar location with nodular swelling.

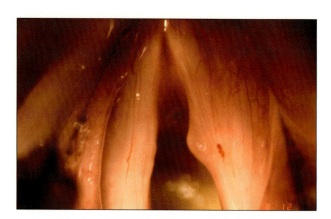

Fig 4–2. (7×) Figure 4–1 at higher magnification.

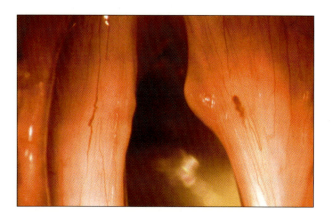

Fig 4–3. (10×) Figure 4–2 at even higher magnification.

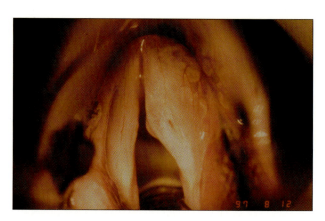

Fig 4–4. (4×) The subepithelial infusion of saline and adrenaline has been performed.

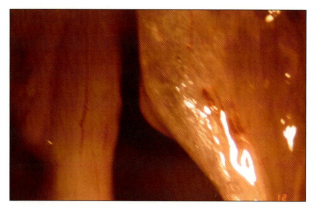

Fig 4–5. (10×) Figure 4–4 at higher magnification. Small bubbles are seen at the translucent epithelium as a result of the mild turbulence created by the subepithelial infusion.

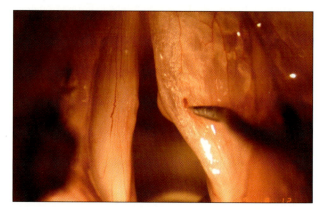

Fig 4–6. (7×) An epithelial cordotomy is performed through the site of the ectasia, so that it can be resected.

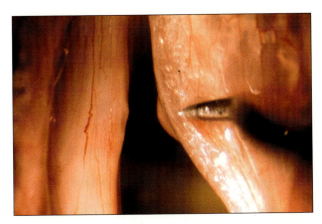

Fig 4–7. (10×) The sharp pick is utilized both to excise the ectasia as well as to create a precise epithelial cordotomy.

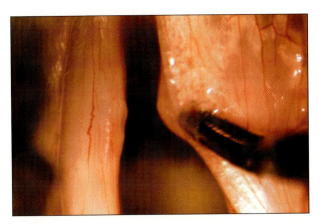

Fig 4–8. (10×) The resultant mass was a fibrovascular polyp. An alligator forceps is used both to explore the cordotomy as well as to begin to mobilize the mass and remove it.

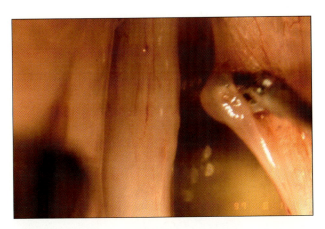

Fig 4–9. (10×) A microcup forceps is placed through the cordotomy for removal of the subepithelial fibrovascular mass. The forceps is well seen through the translucent epithelium.

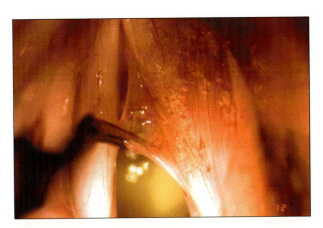

Fig 4–10. (7×) A microalligator forceps is utilized to retract the microflap.

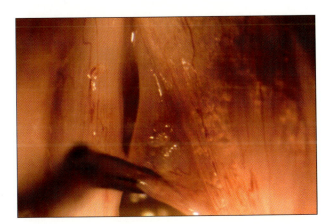

Fig 4–11. (10×) Figure 4–10 at higher magnification, the mass has been completely excised.

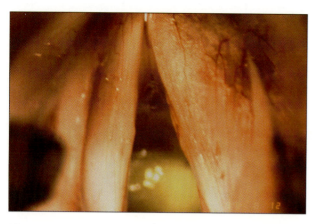

Fig 4–12. (7×) The microflap is repositioned with excellent coaptation of the epithelial edges revealing a smooth and straight vocal fold without loss of epithelium or normal SLP. The contralateral nodular swelling did reveal some fibrovascular changes, which were excised.

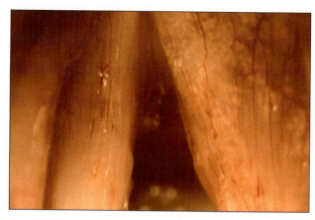

Fig 4–13. (10×) Figure 4–12 at higher magnification.

Case 4B

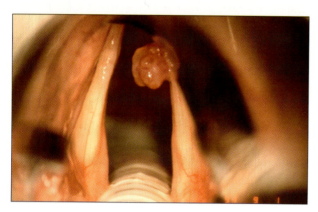

Fig 4–14. (4×) There is a pedunculated hemorrhagic polyp emanating from the right vocal fold. It is poorly exposed through the glottiscope without external laryngeal counterpressure.

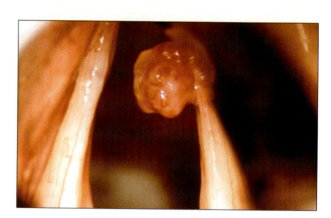

Fig 4–15. (7×) Figure 4–14 at higher magnification.

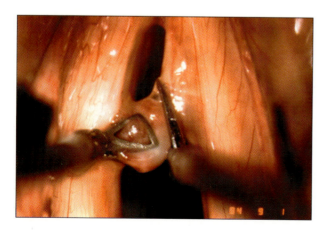

Fig 4–16. (7×) After external laryngeal counterpressure, there is dramatically improved exposure. Since the lesion is now in the mid-region of the distal aperture of the glottiscope, angulation of the hand instruments is facilitated. The narrow pedicle can be both visualized with retraction, as well as palpated with the upturned microscissors. It is therefore amputated rather than performing an epithelial cordotomy. There was a small feeding vessel, which was controlled with a cottonoid soaked in saline and adrenaline.

Case 4C

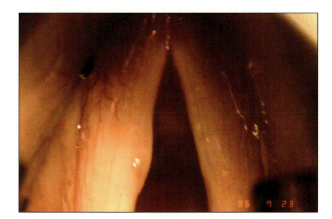

Fig 4–17. (7×) A spheroid mass emanating from the left vocal fold. A light reflex can be seen overlying it. This was a mixoid polyp (pseudocyst).

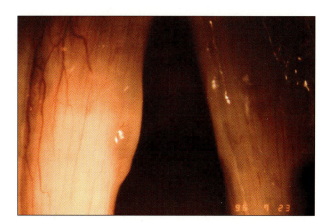

Fig 4–18. (10×) Figure 4–17 at higher magnification. This image as well as palpation suggested a gelatinous polyp rather than a subepithelial cyst.

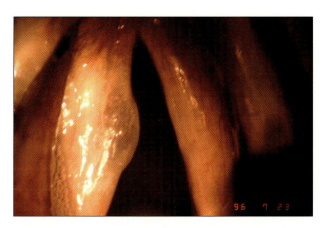

Fig 4–19. (7×) A subepithelial infusion was performed.

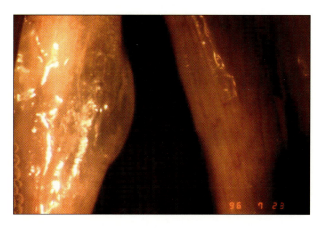

Fig 4–20. (10×) Figure 4–19 at higher magnification.

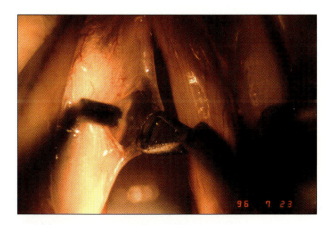

Fig 4–21. (7×) The epithelial cordotomy confirmed that the lesion was a gelatinous polyp, which was resected without difficulty. This image depicts retraction of the microflap as well as the residual normal SLP. The translucent epithelial microflap is well seen.

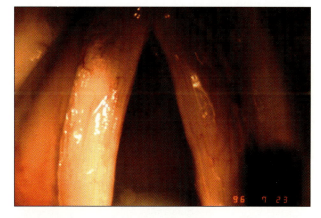

Fig 4–22. (7×) The epithelial microflap is repositioned and there is excellent coaptation of the edges revealing an almost normal appearing vocal fold at the conclusion of the procedure.

Case 4D

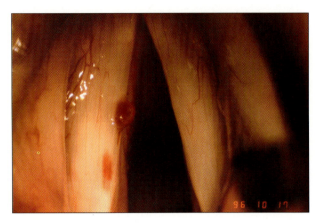

Fig 4–23. (7×) A hemorrhagic ectatic polyp of the left vocal fold in a classical vocalist. More superiorly, there is a contusion of the left vocal fold, which occurred during the intubation.

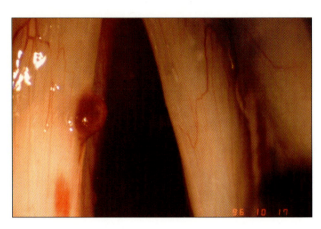

Fig 4–24. (10×) Figure 4–23 at higher magnification. A prominent varix is seen leading to the mid-vocal fold on the right.

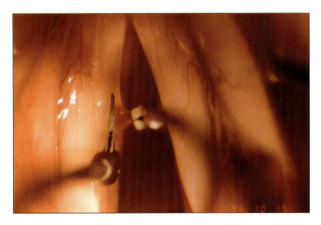

Fig 4–25. (7×) The polyp is retracted with a microcup forceps and an upturned scissors is utilized to perform an epithelial cordotomy.

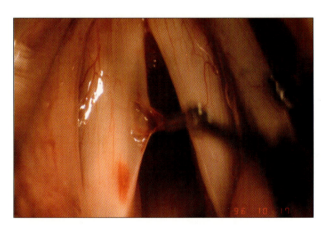

Fig 4–26. (7×) An alligator forceps is utilized to excise the contents of the subepithelial vascular mass.

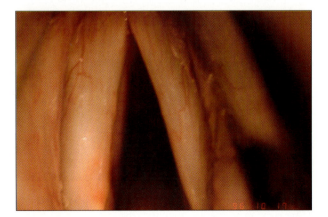

Fig 4–27. (7×) The lesion has been excised and the subepithelial blood from the contusion was drained through a small needle cordotomy.

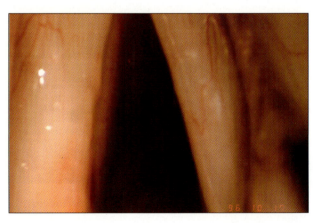

Fig 4–28. (10×) Figure 4–27 at higher magnification. There has been minimal disturbance of any normal vocal fold tissue.

Case 4E

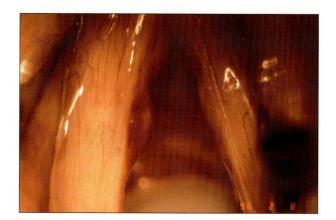

Fig 4–29. (7×) There is a spheroid hemorrhagic mass arising from the medial surface of the left vocal fold. There is a sessile swelling on the contralateral side. There is prominent diffuse microvascular injection. This patient is a rock singer.

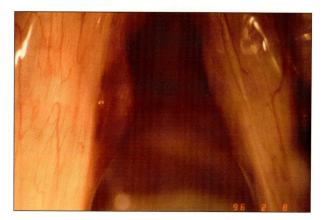

Fig 4–30. (10×) Figure 4–29 at higher magnification.

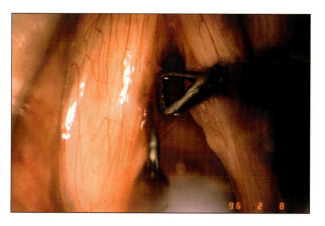

Fig 4–31. (7×) The epithelial mass is retracted and a cordotomy is performed with an upturned scissors.

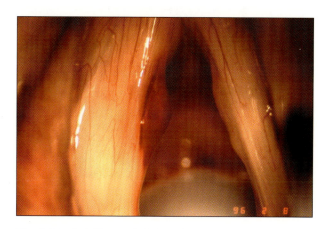

Fig 4–32. (7×) The epithelial cordotomy has been done.

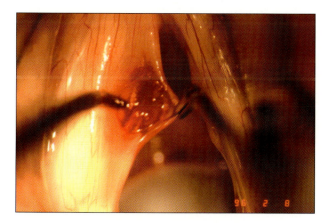

Fig 4–33. (7×) The microflap is developed and the subepithelial fibrovascular polyp is mobilized from the underlying normal SLP and the overlying basement membrane of the epithelium. It can then be excised by means of a variety of forceps.

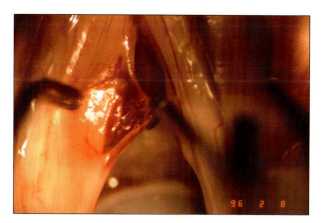

Fig 4–34. (7×) The fibrovascular tissue has been removed with maximum preservation of the normal layered microstructure.

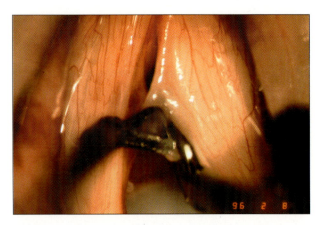

Fig 4–35. (7×) The contralateral vocal fold revealed swelling. It was retracted and a cordotomy was performed in a similar fashion. The mildly swollen tissue was suctioned gently from the epithelial basement membrane to create a more normal contour of the vocal edge.

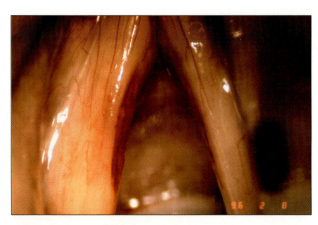

Fig 4–36. (7×) Both lesions have been excised. There is excellent coaptation of the epithelial edges and the vocal folds are smooth and straight.

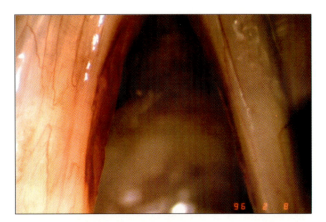

Fig 4–37. (10×) Figure 4–36 at higher magnification.

Case 4F

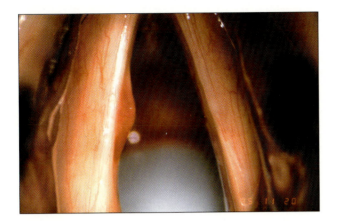

Fig 4–38. (7×) A sessile fibrovascular mass is seen arising from the medial surface of the left vocal fold.

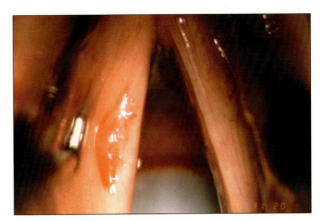

Fig 4–39. (7×) The vocal fold is retracted so that the medial surface lesion is better visualized.

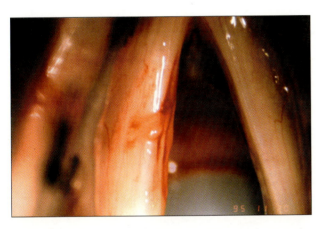

Fig 4–40. (7×) After performing an epithelial cordotomy, the fibrovascular contents are dissected from the normal layered microstructure and can be seen as it is withdrawn through the cordotomy site.

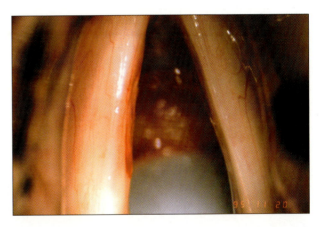

Fig 4–41. (7×) Subsequent to excision, the vocal fold is smooth and well contoured.

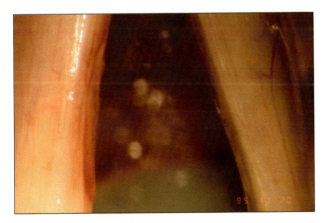

Fig 4–42. (10×) Figure 4–41 at higher magnification.

Case 4G

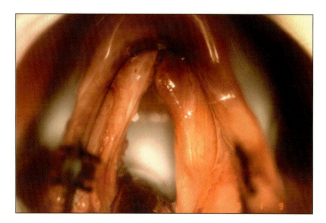

Fig 4–43. (4×) This is a Latin singer with a fibrovascular polyp on the right fold and a contralateral nodule. The lesions are not well exposed without external counterpressure.

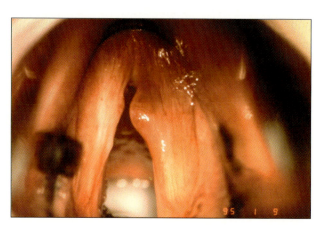

Fig 4–44. (4×) With external counterpressure, the lesions are better exposed and better visualized.

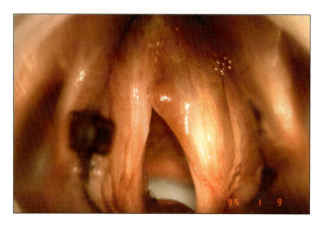

Fig 4–45. (4×) A subepithelial infusion is performed. The polyp is lifted which reveals that there is a significant amount of normal SLP underlying it.

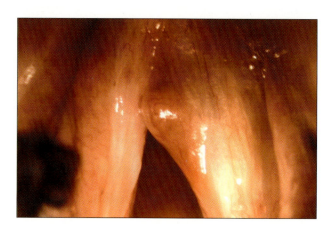

Fig 4–46. (7×) Figure 4–45 at higher magnification.

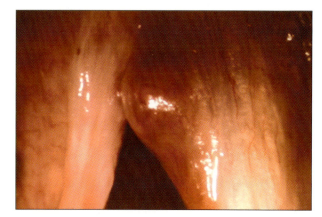

Fig 4–47. (10×) Figure 4–46 at even higher magnification. Bubbles are seen underlying the epithelium from the turbulence of the infusion.

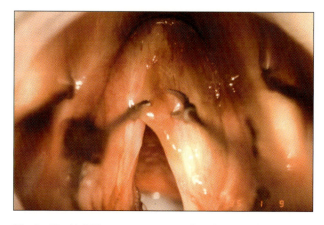

Fig 4–48. (4×) The mass is retracted and a curved microscissors is used to perform an epithelial cordotomy.

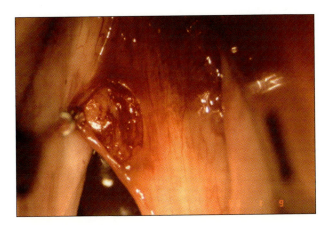

Fig 4–49. (7×) The contents of the fibrovascular polyp have been dissected from the layered microstructure and excised. The epithelial microflap is retracted to reveal the cavity that the fibrovascular tissue had been situated in.

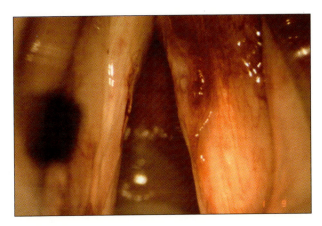

Fig 4–50. (7×) The microflap has been redraped and there is excellent coaptation of the epithelial edges. The vocal fold is now normally contoured. The contralateral lesion has been excised.

Case 4H

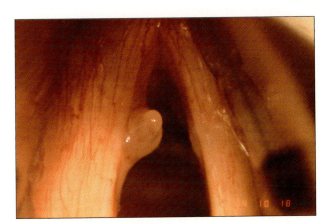

Fig 4–51. (7×) A multilobulated hemorrhagic polyp is seen on the left vocal fold. There is a sessile nodule seen on the contralateral fold.

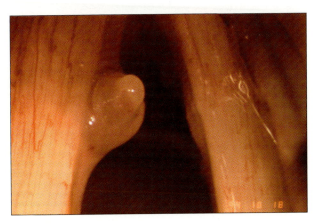

Fig 4–52. (10×) Figure 4–51 at higher magnification.

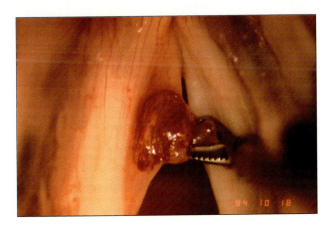

Fig 4–53. (7×) A subepithelial infusion was not done in this case. An epithelial cordotomy has been performed and the fibrovascular mass has been dissected from the underlying normal SLP. The contents of the polyp were extremely adherent to the basement membrane, and therefore, it could not be completely preserved. A significant portion of the caudal base of the flap was preserved.

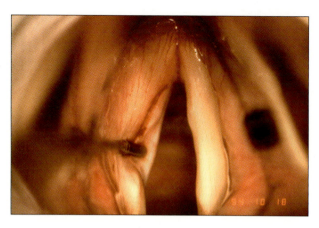

Fig 4–54. (4×) The medial surface of the vocal fold is visualized by retracting it with a dissector.

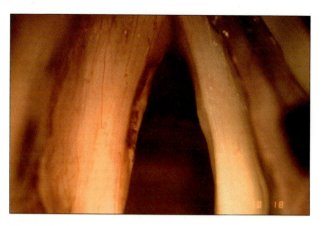

Fig 4–55. (7×) There is a small epithelial defect, which healed in a brief period of time. Subsequently, the right-sided nodule was excised.

Case 4I

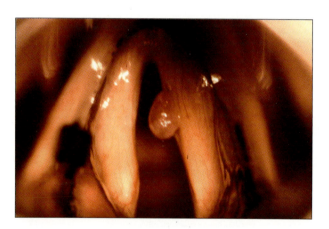

Fig 4–56. (4×) A fibrovascular polyp is seen arising from the surface of the right mid-medial vocal fold.

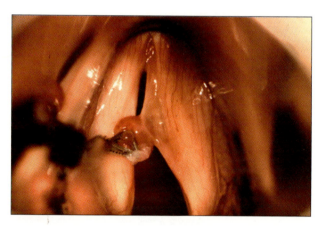

Fig 4–57. (4×) The polyp is retracted revealing that it is pedunculated with a fairly narrow base.

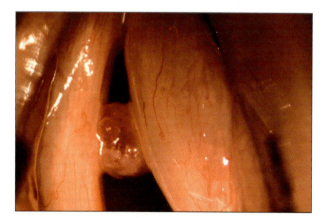

Fig 4–58. (7×) A subepithelial infusion is performed to enhance hemostasis, as well as to facilitate the excision.

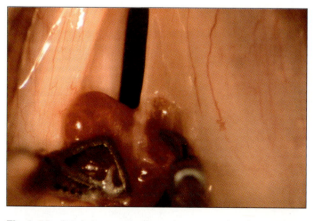

Fig 4–59. (10×) A curved microscissors is utilized to perform an initial epithelial cordotomy. Additionally, two prominent varices are also noted adjacent to the polyp.

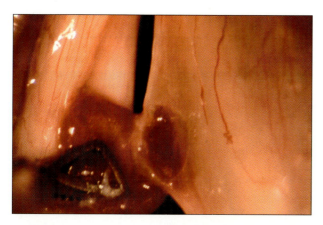

Fig 4–60. (10×) The tissue difference between the polyp and the underlying normal SLP can be seen as well as palpated.

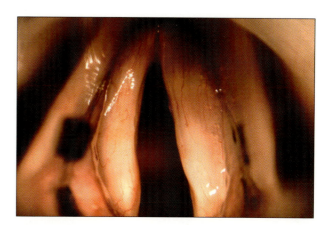

Fig 4–61. (4×) The image subsequent to excision.

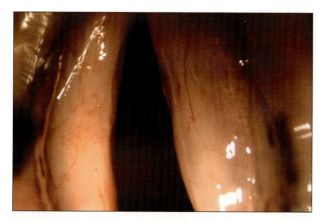

Fig 4–62. (7×) Figure 4–61 at higher magnification.

Case 4J

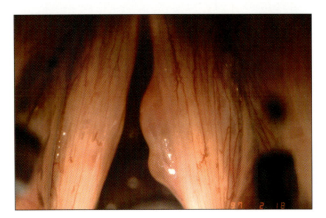

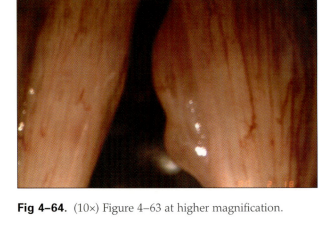

Fig 4–63. (7×) This patient was a severe vocal abuser. There is a sessile fibrovascular polyp emanating from the medial surface of the right vocal fold. There is an excessive amount of vascular injection within the SLP of both vocal folds. There are multiple associated varices and ectasias.

Fig 4–64. (10×) Figure 4–63 at higher magnification.

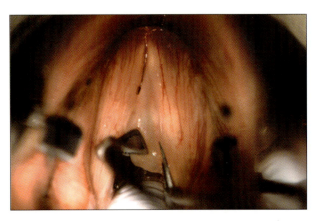

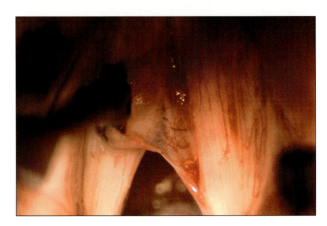

Fig 4–65. (4×) The mass is retracted and a superior-surface epithelial cordotomy is performed. A subepithelial infusion was not used. The contents of the mass revealed a gelatinous polyp.

Fig 4–66. (7×) The epithelial microflap is being retracted. A subepithelial resection of the polyp contents was performed with forceps and microscissors.

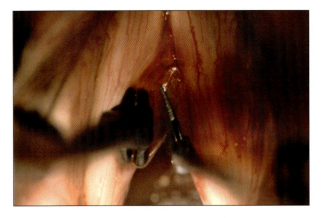

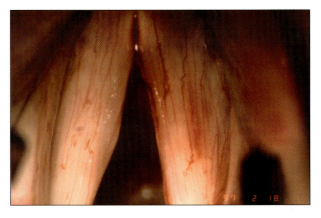

Fig 4–67. (7×) There is excessive residual epithelium. Therefore, it is excised using a straight triangular forceps and an upturned scissors.

Fig 4–68. (7×) There is excellent apposition of the epithelial edges and the vocal fold is smooth and straight.

Case 4K

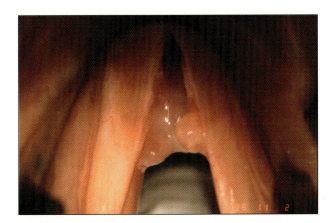

Fig 4–69. (7×) Bilateral multilobulated hemorrhagic polyps are noted.

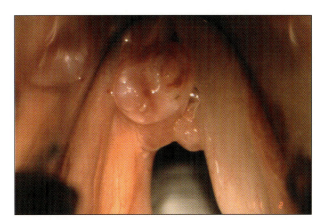

Fig 4–70. (7×) The polyps have been positioned above the level of the glottal aperture demonstrating their more extensive nature than can be appreciated on the previous image. A subepithelial infusion has been performed on the right.

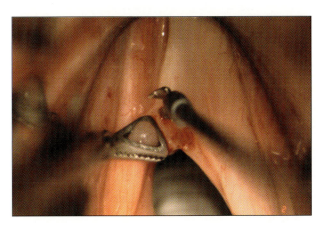

Fig 4–71. (7×) The right polyp is retracted and a curved microscissors is used to perform an epithelial cordotomy.

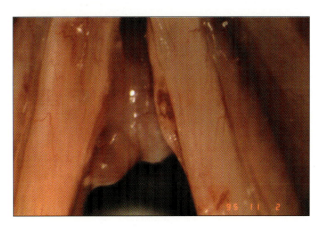

Fig 4–72. (7×) The right polyp has been excised, which allows for improved visualization of the left one.

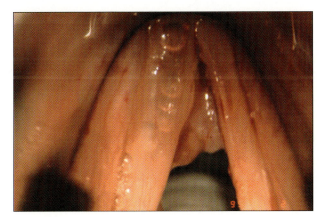

Fig 4–73. (7×) A subepithelial infusion has now been performed on the left. The bubbles can be seen as a result of the turbulent infusion.

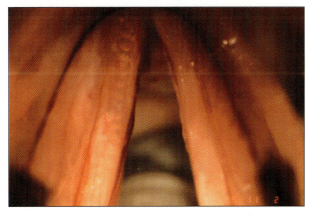

Fig 4–74. (7×) Both lesions have been resected and the vocal folds are smooth and straight.

Case 4L

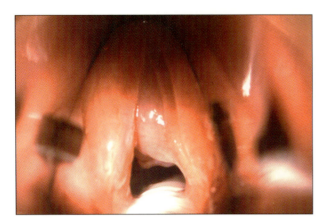

Fig 4–75. (4×) A large hemorrhagic polyp arising from the medial and subcordal surface of the right vocal fold.

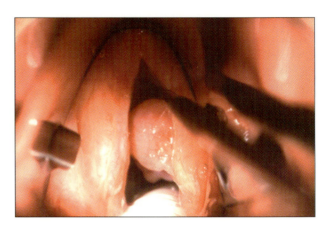

Fig 4–76. (4×) The polyp is retracted so that the dimensions of the base can better be seen. The base does not extend to the anterior glottal commissure.

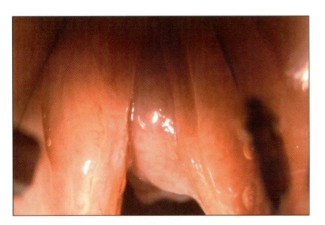

Fig 4–77. (7×) Figure 4–76 at higher magnification.

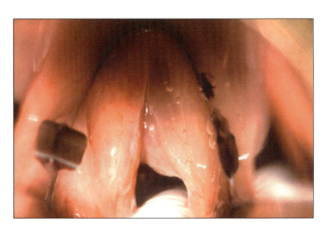

Fig 4–78. (4×) A subepithelial infusion is performed.

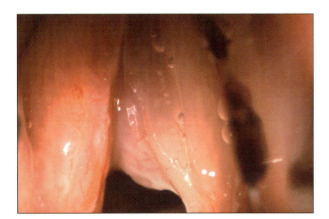

Fig 4–79. (7×) Figure 4–78 at higher magnification.

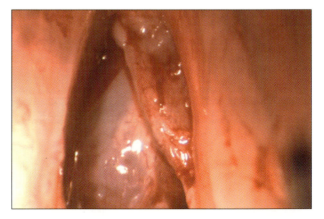

Fig 4–80. (10×) An epithelial cordotomy is made with cold instruments.

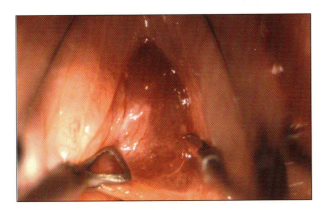

Fig 4–81. (7×) A microscissors is used to dissect the normal SLP from the normal fibrovascular mass.

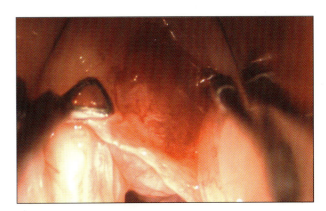

Fig 4–82. (7×) The dissection is advanced to better define the base of the polyp.

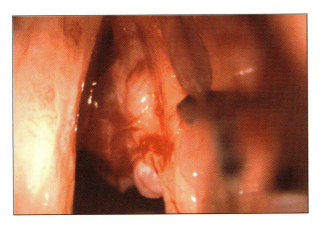

Fig 4–83. (7×) The base of the polyp is inverted subglottically to identify its inferior margin.

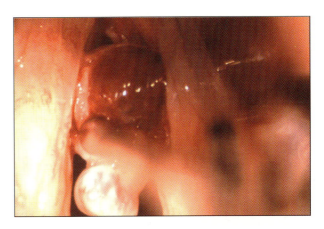

Fig 4–84. (7×) The base of the polyp is now well seen.

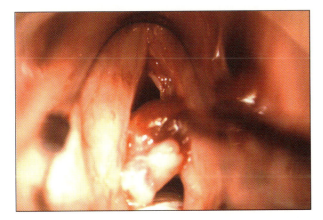

Fig 4–85. (4×) The polyp is excised by means of a microscissors.

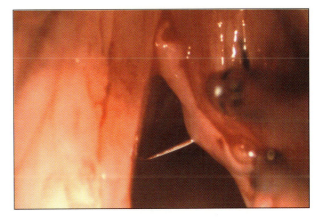

Fig 4–86. (10×) An inferior microflap is preserved for coaptation of the epithelial edges due to the size of the lesion and the defect. The epithelial edges are sutured to facilitate more rapid healing.

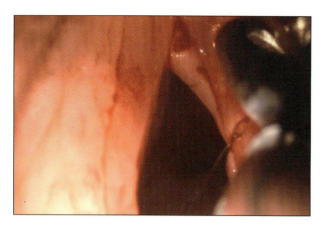

Fig 4–87. (10×) An endoscopic knot tier is seen on the right side of the image.

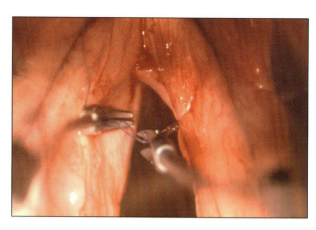

Fig 4–88. (7×) The suture is retracted with an alligator forceps and trimmed.

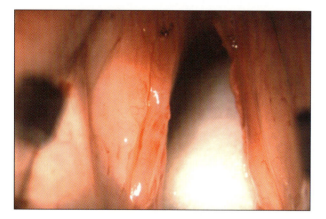

Fig 4–89. (7×) The epithelial edges are redraped now that a suture has been placed to maintain its basic favorable position.

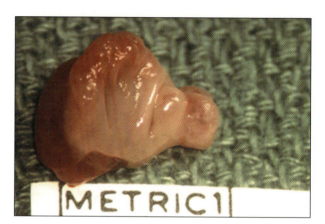

Fig 4–90. The excised specimen.

Case 4M

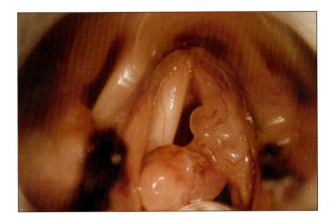

Fig 4–91. (4×) An extremely large hemorrhagic polyp.

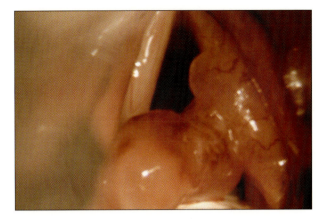

Fig 4–92. (7×) Figure 4–91 at higher magnification.

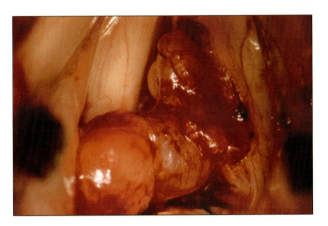

Fig 4–93. (7×) A subepithelial infusion was performed. The lesion was quite vascular, so that the initial incision was made by means of a microspot CO_2 laser. There was a large feeding vessel posteriorly.

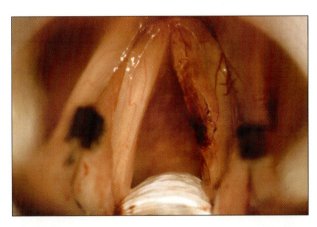

Fig 4–94. (4×) The lesion has been excised. The eschar from the CO_2 laser can be seen posteriorly where the feeding vessel was situated.

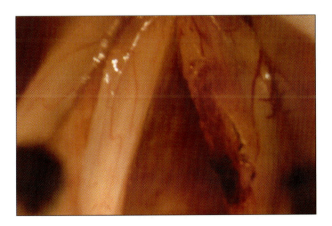

Fig 4–95. (7×) Higher magnification of Figure 4–94. Because of the patient's chronic hyperfunction, the SLP was naturally distended. Therefore, subsequent to the polyp excision, there was a normal amount of SLP left to allow for good mucosal wave vibration after epithelialization of the small defect.

Case 4N

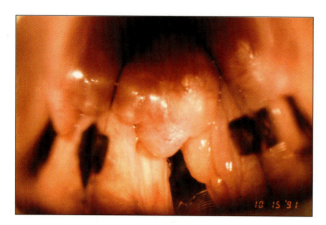

Fig 4–96. (4×) A large, highly vascular hemorrhagic polyp.

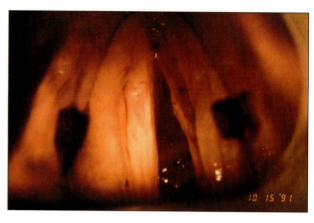

Fig 4–97. (4×) Because of the lesion's size, it could not be retracted easily. Because of this, as well as its vascularity, the CO_2 laser was used to excise the mass.

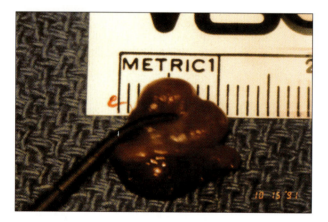

Fig 4–98. (4×) The excised specimen.

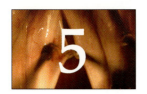

5

Nodules

Vocal fold nodules may present visually and acoustically in a varied manner. There are divergent opinions as to the value of phonomicrosurgical intervention. It is likely that the different philosophies about the efficacy of a surgical intervention are based in part on confusion in the literature as to what constitutes vocal nodules. There is little disagreement that the majority of these lesions are the result of vocal abuse or inappropriate vocal use. Therefore, irrespective of the decision to excise vocal nodules, virtually all of these individuals will benefit from vocal therapy.

Strobovideolaryngoscopy is critical when assessing nodules. High-pitch assessment is necessary to analyze the mechanical effect that fibrovascular nodules have on vocal fold vibration. The nodules may be even better defined if the high-frequency phonatory task is also done with low subglottal pressures so that the patient becomes diplophonic or aphonic with an aperiodic mucosal wave or the acoustic signal ceases. In this setting, stretching the vocal fold physiologically thins any residual SLP that is left under the fibrovascular nodule so that the voice becomes disordered. This type of evaluation also exhibits evidence that surface nodular excrescences frequently have significant unrecognized involvement of the SLP that might be clinically undetected during stroboscopic examination at a normal pitch frequency. This iceberg effect is found intraoperatively when an epithelial cordotomy is performed.

In most cases, it is advantageous to employ surgery as a secondary management. The philosophy regarding surgical intervention is highly individualized to patients and surgeons as well as associated involved professionals, such as speech-language pathologists and voice teachers who spend the greatest amount of time with the patient. An initial trial of vocal therapy should reduce hyperfunctional behavior and reduce the generalized edema of the SLP that typically accompanies these lesions. Even if the nodules do not resolve and disappear visually, the patient may be satisfied with the quality and stamina of his or her voice so that sur-

gical intervention is not necessary. If further improvement is desired by the patient, and clear nodules are seen, phonomicrosurgical excision may further enhance vocal quality. The prior vocal therapy will benefit the patient during the postoperative rehabilitative process to prevent injury and recurrence.

The philosophy that nodules should not be resected despite their continued presence after adequate vocal rehabilitation arose from unsatisfactory surgical outcomes. In many cases, the trauma induced by the procedure was more deleterious to vocal fold vibration than the lesion itself. This was especially so when the CO_2 laser without a microspot was used injudiciously and/or small nodules were avulsed or stripped. During the last decade, as the instrumentation and techniques have improved, the author has been more frequently resecting nodules that were refractory to vocal rehabilitation.

Similar to the aforementioned techniques for excising vocal polyps, phonomicrosurgical resection of vocal nodules can be performed by means of an epithelial microflap with subepithelial resection or by amputation. Observations from the postresection results of a cohort of musical theater performers revealed that the voice result is enhanced by a subepithelial resection of the fibrovascular SLP.[110] However, currently this approach is limited by suboptimal hand instrumentation. Cold instruments provide improved precision considering the small size of these lesions and the need for palpation during the procedure.[77] The use of the subepithelial infusion technique must be used selectively.[104,105] Nodules that are less well defined visually and by palpation may become obscured by the infusion-induced distension of the SLP.

The patients who are not typical surgical candidates will present with what has been termed "nodular swelling." Anatomically these vocal folds have fusiform swelling of the SLP, which is usually bilateral and symmetric, and in the mid-musculo-membranous region. A discrete mass is not seen on telescopic laryngo-stroboscopy. Prioritization of vocal activities and vocal therapy should adequately treat these individuals.

Case 5A

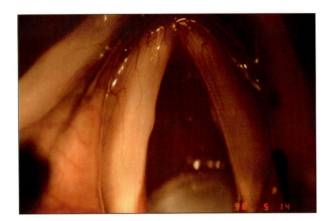

Fig 5–1. (7×) Small bilateral fibrous nodules in a classical singer.

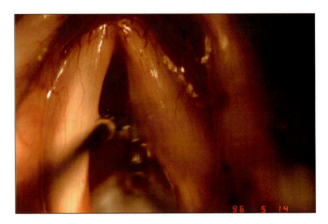

Fig 5–2. (7×) The right nodule is retracted with a mini-microcup forceps and amputated with a mini-microscissors.

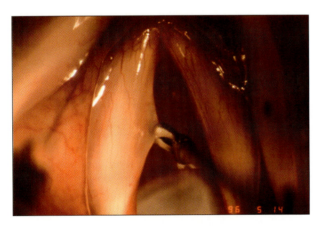

Fig 5–3. (7×) The left nodule is retracted and the residual pliability of the superficial lamina propria can be seen.

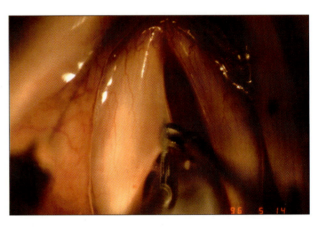

Fig 5–4. (7×) The left nodule is retracted with a mini-microcup forceps and amputated with a mini-microscissors.

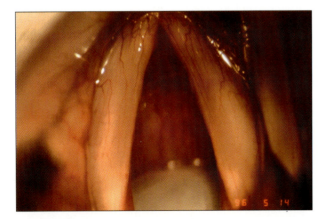

Fig 5–5. (7×) The vocal folds are smooth and straight with minimal disturbance of the layered microstructure.

Case 5B

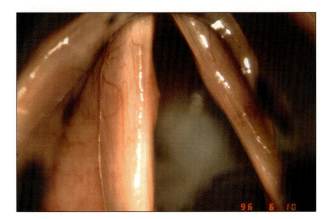

Fig 5–6. (7×) Bilateral sessile nodules in a musical theater performer. The surgical field is now rotated and the anterior commissure is not seen without external counterpressure.

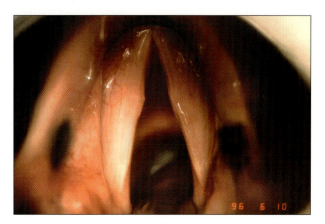

Fig 5–7. (4×) With external counterpressure, rotation is achieved and the nodules are in the center of the surgical field.

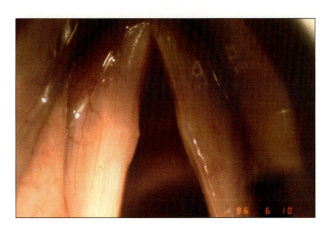

Fig 5–8. (7×) Figure 5–7 at higher magnification.

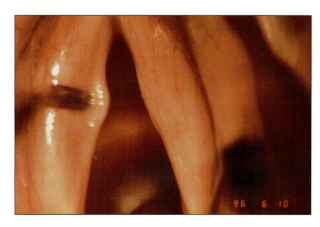

Fig 5–9. (7×) A dissector is used to define the depth of the fibrous nodule.

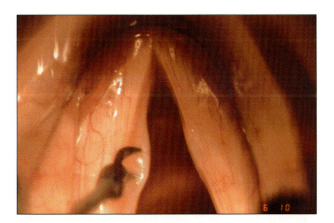

Fig 5–10. (7×) A curved microscissors is used to perform an epithelial cordotomy at the edge of the left lesion.

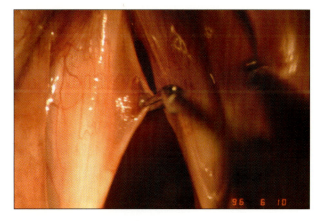

Fig 5–11. (7×) A microalligator forceps is used to retract the microflap after the fibrous component has been dissected from the basement membrane.

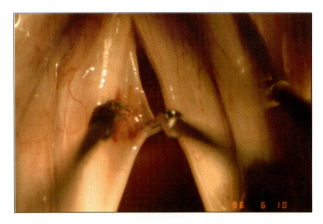

Fig 5–12. (7×) The microscissors is utilized to mobilize the fibrous contents of the nodule for excision.

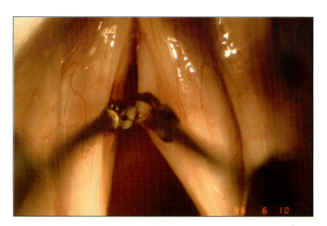

Fig 5–13. (7×) The right-sided lesion is much smaller. The instruments are not small and precise enough to perform a subepithelial resection. Therefore, a cup forceps is used to retract the nodule and the overlying epithelium for amputation.

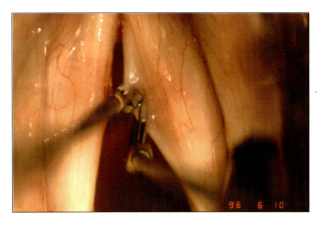

Fig 5–14. (7×) To avoid removing too much tissue, the nodule is removed in two passes.

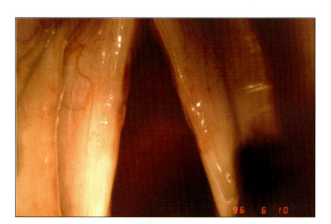

Fig 5–15. (7×) The vocal folds are now smooth and straight.

Case 5C

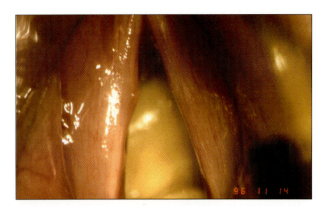

Fig 5–16. (7×) This is a classical female vocalist in whom bilateral vocal nodules are noted. There is a small fibrous nodule on the right vocal fold that could only be visualized when the tissues were retracted or when visualizing the patient while singing at an extremely high frequency during stroboscopy.

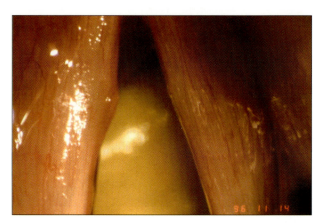

Fig 5–17. (10×) Figure 5–16 at higher magnification. The yellow endotracheal tube cuff can be seen distally.

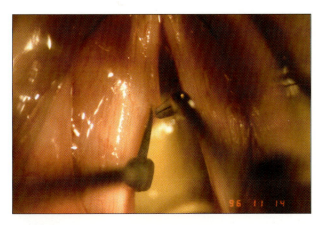

Fig 5–18. (7×) A microalligator forceps is used to retract the left nodule and an upturned microscissors is used to incise the epithelium.

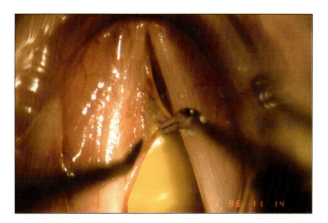

Fig 5–19. (7×) An epithelial microflap is developed by means of a sharp dissector. This allows for mobilization of the contents of the nodule.

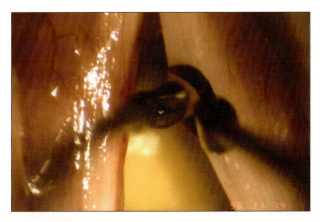

Fig 5–20. (10×) The right nodule is retracted with a mini-microcup forceps and amputated with a mini-microscissors.

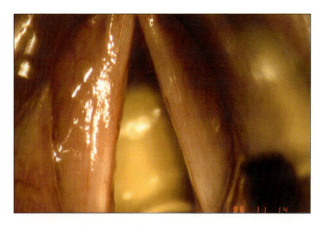

Fig 5–21. (7×) The vocal folds are seen subsequent to the bilateral excisions.

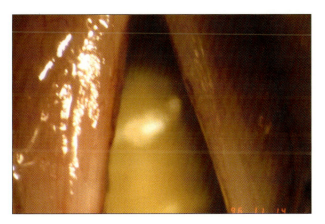

Fig 5–22. (10×) Figure 5–21 at higher magnification.

Case 5D

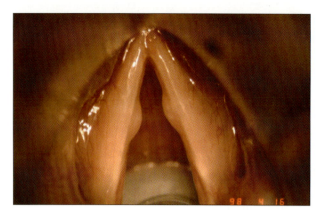

Fig 5–23. (4×) Bilateral sessile spheroid masses are seen in a 7-year-old boy. He has been extremely hoarse since infancy and has been in voice therapy for 4 years without substantive improvement.

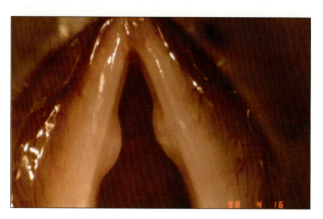

Fig 5–24. (7×) Figure 5–23 at higher magnification. Palpation was suggestive of a fibrous mass rather than cysts.

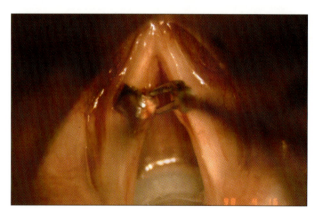

Fig 5–25. (4×) An epithelial cordotomy was performed and a cup forceps is being utilized to resect the fibrous nodule without the epithelium. The alligator forceps is being utilized to push the fibrous contents of the nodule within the jaws of the forceps without including the overlying epithelium.

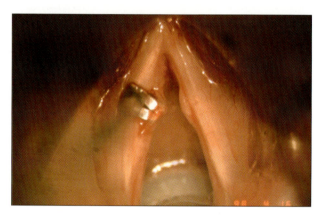

Fig 5–26. (4×) The contents of the nodule being withdrawn with the cup forceps.

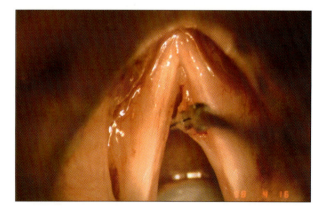

Fig 5–27. (4×) The prior procedure has been performed on the right. The alligator forceps is seen underneath the microflap on the right.

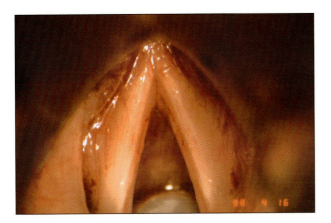

Fig 5–28. (4×) Both nodules have been excised with no loss of epithelium or normal SLP.

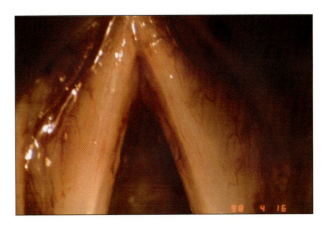

Fig 5–29. (7×) Figure 5–28 at higher magnification. Note the excellent coaptation of the epithelial edges.

Case 5E

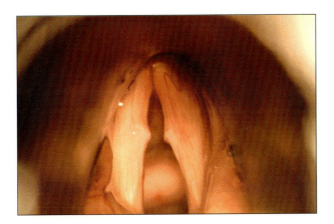

Fig 5–30. (4×) Bilateral sessile nodules are noted in this radio disk jockey.

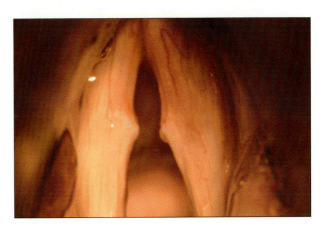

Fig 5–31. (7×) Figure 5–30 at higher magnification.

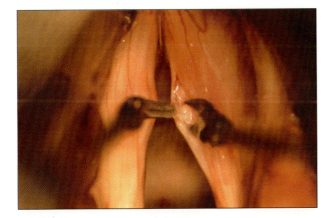

Fig 5–32. (7×) An epithelial cordotomy has been done on the right. The microflap is retracted with a mini-micro alligator forceps and a mini-microscissors is used to dissect the fibrous tissue from the underlying SLP and overlying epithelial basement membrane.

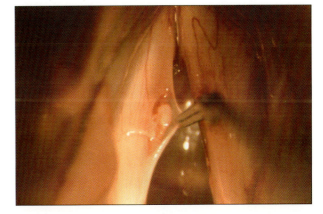

Fig 5–33. (7×) The prior procedure is performed on the left and an alligator forceps is used to retract the microflap.

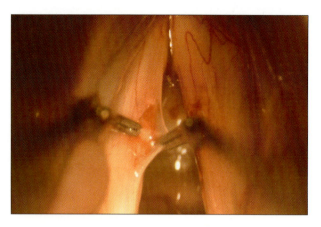

Fig 5–34. (7×) A second alligator forceps is used to remove the fibrous tissue.

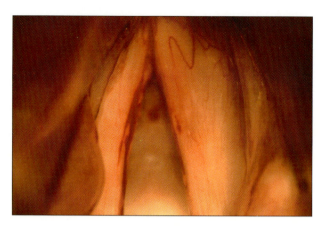

Fig 5–35. (7×) The vocal folds are now smooth and straight. A small amount of blood is seen in the incision.

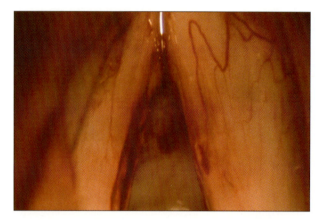

Fig 5–36. (10×) Figure 5–35 at higher magnification.

Case 5F

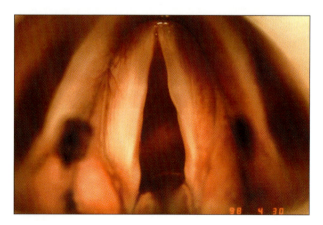

Fig 5–37. (4×) Bilateral sessile nodules are noted in a classical singer.

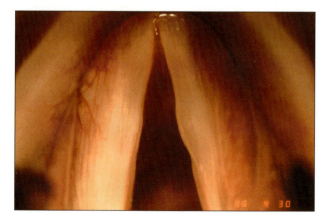

Fig 5–38. (7×) Figure 5–37 at higher magnification.

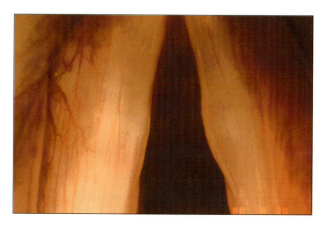

Fig 5–39. (10×) Figure 5–38 at even higher magnification.

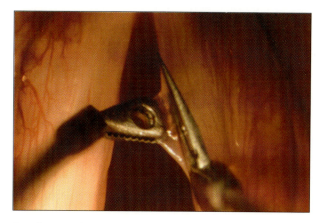

Fig 5–40. (10×) A forceps is utilized to retract the nodule and an epithelial cordotomy is performed.

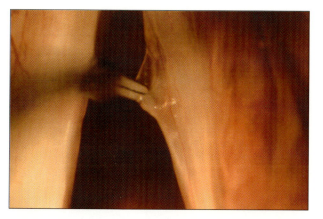

Fig 5–41. (10×) The fibrovascular contents of the nodule are removed by means of an alligator forceps.

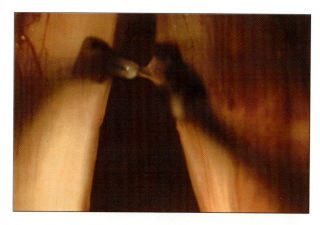

Fig 5–42. (10×) The subepithelial fibrovascular contents have been withdrawn and a curved microscissors is utilized to amputate that tissue.

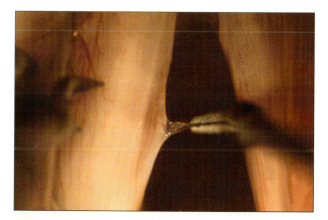

Fig 5–43. (10×) The prior procedure has been performed on the left and the fibrovascular nodule contents are withdrawn.

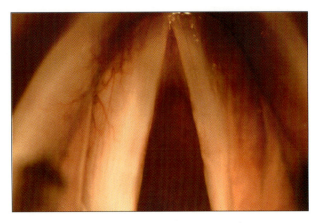

Fig 5–44. (7×) The postexcision appearance of the vocal folds revealing that the incisions are nearly imperceptible.

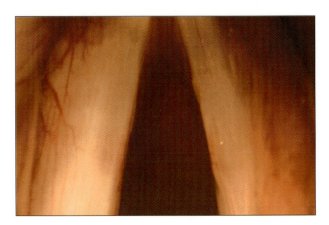

Fig 5–45. (10×) Figure 5–44 at higher magnification.

Case 5G

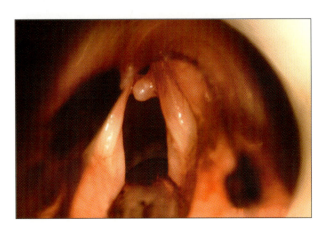

Fig 5–46. (4×) Without external counterpressure, a fibrous mass is noted at what appears to be the right anterior glottis.

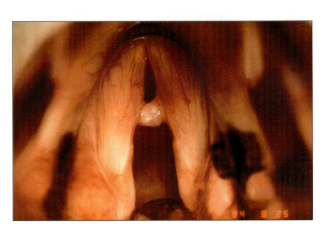

Fig 5–47. (4×) After external laryngeal counterpressure, it can be seen that there are bilateral fibrous nodules in the mid-musculomembranous region. There are prominent subepithelial varices as well.

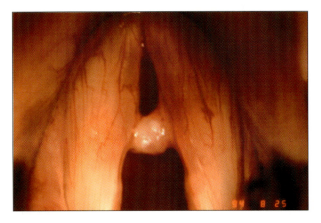

Fig 5–48. (7×) Figure 5–47 at higher magnification.

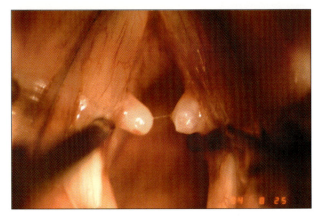

Fig 5–49. (7×) Bilateral dissectors are placed to better delineate the contours of these lesions and their base.

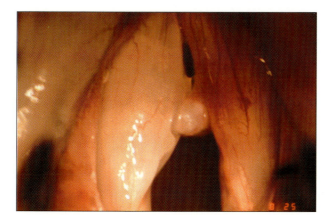

Fig 5–50. (7×) A subepithelial infusion of saline and adrenaline is performed to enhance the precision of the excision.

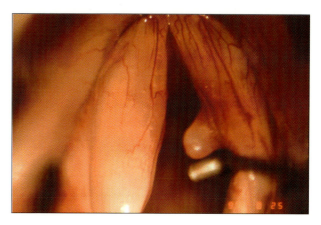

Fig 5–51. (7×) The left-sided lesion has been amputated. The right vocal fold is being retracted by a blunt angled probe.

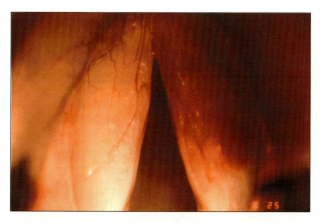

Fig 5–52. (7×) The right lesion has now been amputated. There was a large feeding vessel at its base. The mild bleeding was controlled with topical saline and adrenaline on a cottonoid.

Case 5H

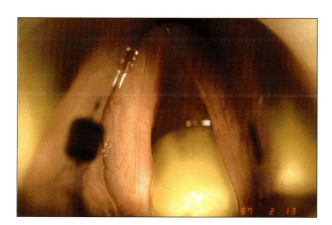

Fig 5–53. (4×) Bilateral fibrous nodules that are barely perceptible because of their tangential position on the medial surface of the vocal fold. They were well seen on stroboscopy. This patient is a classical singer with difficulties in her upper register.

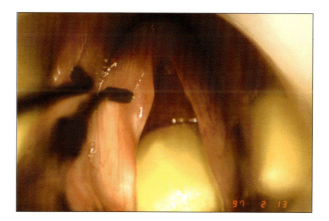

Fig 5–54. (4×) A dissector is used to define the fibrous nodule on the medial-subcordal surface, which is associated with an ectasia.

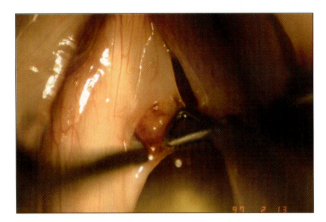

Fig 5–55. (7×) An epithelial cordotomy is performed and the contents of the fibrous mass are mobilized with a sharp dissector.

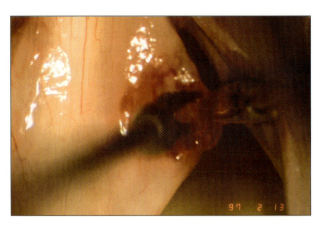

Fig 5–56. (10×) The fibrovascular tissue is somewhat adherent to the basement membrane. It is being retracted with a cup forceps, which has been placed inside of the microflap for retraction of the subepithelial tissue. A curved microscissors is used to separate the fibrovascular tissue from the basement membrane of the microflap. Note the magnitude of retraction necessary for adequate exposure. The cup forceps, which was leaning on the right vocal fold, created a minor temporary contour-depression in the right vocal fold.

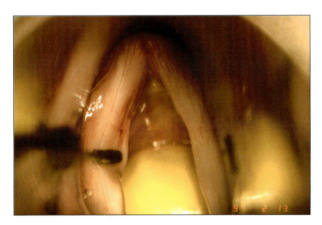

Fig 5–57. (4×) A dissector is used to retract the left vocal fold for optimal visualization of the medial surface, which reveals excellent coaptation of the epithelial edges.

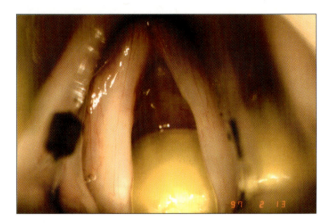

Fig 5–58. (4×) The appearance of the vocal folds without retraction.

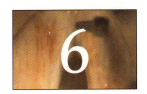

Varices and Ectasias

Varices and ectasias of the vocal folds are the result of microvascular trauma within the SLP. The majority of the patients with a history of recurrent vocal hemorrhage, who require phonomicrosurgical intervention, are female vocalists. Many patients will undergo resection of these vascular malformations while the surgeon is excising separate vocal fold pathology, which was the indication for the surgery. Recently, Zeitels and Sataloff compiled a series of patients who underwent phonomicrosurgical resection of varices and ectasias.[93,110] The greatest number of lesions were noted on the superior surface of the middle musculo-membranous vocal fold, which has been termed the *striking zone*.

These superior-surface lesions were generally situated where the lateral extent of mucosal wave excursion would reverse direction.[93] This suggested that these vascular injuries were the result of a deceleration force similar to a whiplash injury. We believe that the momentum of the SLP in the mucosal wave, as well as the intralumenal blood of the microvasculature, is restricted by the elastic recoil of the tissues and the basement membrane of the overlying epithelium. This leads to subepithelial vascular trauma, which is easily visible through the normal translucent epithelium. The cushioning effect of the SLP prevents vessel rupture deeper within Reinke's compartment. The superficial location of these vascular malformations, just under the basement membrane, facilitates surgical accessibility without significant trauma to the underlying SLP.

In the Harvard Jefferson study,[93] a new technique was designed to resect the vascular lesion by means of cold instruments and multiple epithelial cordotomies. The approach is analogous to a vein stripping of the superficial venous system from the lower extremity to redistribute the aberrant vascularity. It was advantageous to redistribute the susceptible central vascular-malformations of the vocal folds out of the striking zone where they were much more likely to hemorrhage.

The procedure was highly successful in preventing recurrent hemorrhage. When cold instruments were used to perform multiple epithelial cordotomies to access the lesions, there was no postoperative deterioration in vocal function or mucosal wave flexibility. This was true despite the fact that many epithelial incisions were made on the medial vocal fold surface and virtually all patients were singers. The location of the epithelial incision(s) (lateral or medial) had no bearing on mucosal wave propagation. This finding invalidated the concept that a lateral microflap was advantageous for resecting medial surface lesions. Final epithelial pliability was directly related to disturbance of the SLP. The study also revealed that patients healed more slowly after CO_2 laser ablation than after cold-instrument resection. Several patients developed epithelial stiffness subsequent to laser ablation.

At present, a study is underway utilizing a pulsed dye laser to coagulate the offending microvasculature without disturbing the overlying epithelium or creating heat within the SLP, which could result in fibrosis. The initial promising results may replace hand dissection of vessels since this is technically very difficult. Ultimately, the pulsed-dye laser might even be used in a clinic setting and without general anesthesia since the delivery system is a narrow fiber through a cannula.

Case 6A

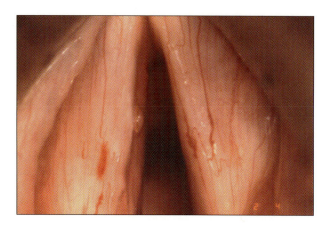

Fig 6–1. (7×) A classical singer with recurrent vocal hemorrhage in both vocal folds. Multiple varices and ectasias can be seen. (From Hochman I, Sataloff RT, Hillman RE, Zeitels SM. *Ann Otol Rhinol Laryngol.* 1998;108:10–16 with permission.)

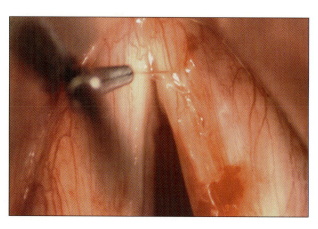

Fig 6–2. (10×) After performing an epithelial cordotomy, one of the varices is grasped with alligator forceps and resected from the SLP. (From Hochman I, Sataloff RT, Hillman RE, Zeitels SM. *Ann Otol Rhinol Laryngol.* 1998;108:10–16 with permission.)

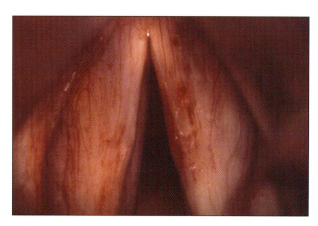

Fig 6–3. (4×) The majority of the varices and ectasias have been resected with cold instruments such as sharp picks and microscissors. Multiple epithelial cordotomies are performed to access the vascular malformations. (From Hochman I, Sataloff RT, Hillman RE, Zeitels SM. *Ann Otol Rhinol Laryngol.* 1998;108:10–16 with permission.)

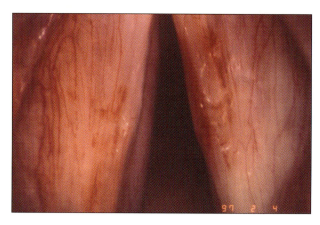

Fig 6–4. (10×) Figure 6–3 at higher magnification. (From Hochman I, Sataloff RT, Hillman RE, Zeitels SM. *Ann Otol Rhinol Laryngol.* 1998;108:10–16 with permission.)

Case 6B

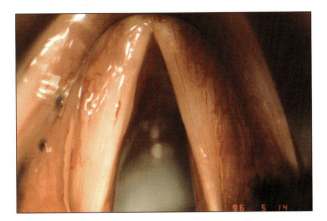

Fig 6–5. (7×) A classical vocalist with a prominent varix on the superior surface of the musculo-membranous vocal fold. There is a nodule noted on the medial surface.

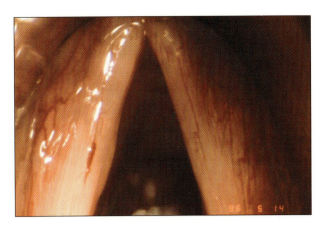

Fig 6–6. (10×) Figure 6–5 at higher magnification.

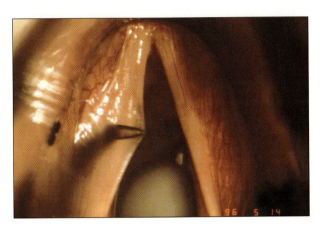

Fig 6–7. (7×) An epithelial cordotomy is performed with a sharp pick and the varix is dissected.

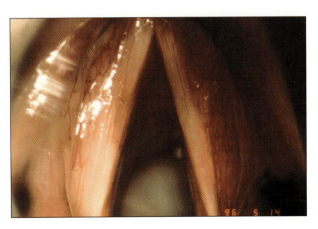

Fig 6–8. (7×) The final image after both the varix and the nodule are resected.

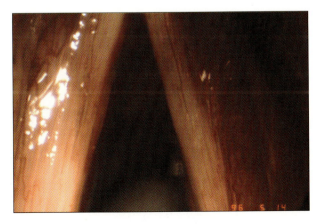

Fig 6–9. (10×) Figure 6–8 at higher magnification.

Case 6C

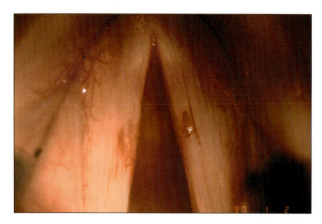

Fig 6–10. (7×) A musical theater performer with multiple varices and ectasias.

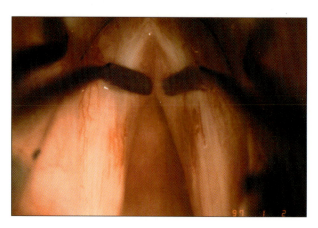

Fig 6–11. (7×) Dissectors are placed bilaterally to better visualize the medial surface of the vocal folds.

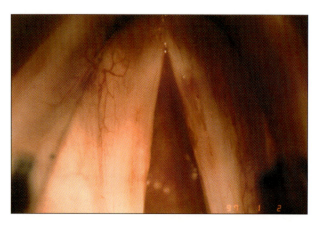

Fig 6–12. (7×) The image after the vascular lesions have been resected by means of multiple epithelial cordotomies.

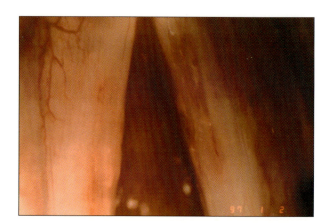

Fig 6–13. (10×) Higher magnification of Figure 6–12.

Case 6D

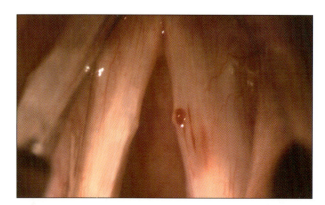

Fig 6–14. (7×) A pop music performer with a fibrous vocal nodule on the left. There is an ectatic vascular nodule on the right with a number of associated varices.

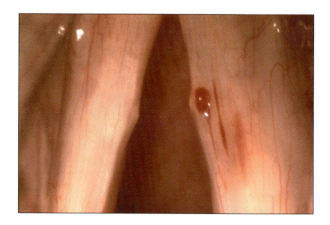

Fig 6–15. (10×) Figure 6–14 at higher magnification.

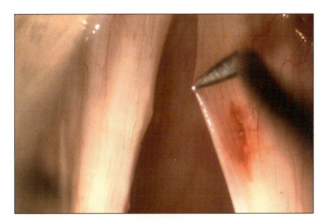

Fig 6–16. (10×) The ectatic nodule is dissected with a sharp pick.

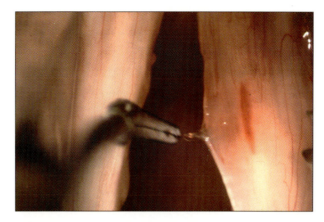

Fig 6–17. (10×) The lesion is retracted with an alligator forceps.

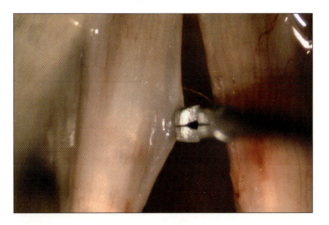

Fig 6–18. (10×) The fibrous nodule is retracted with a cup forceps.

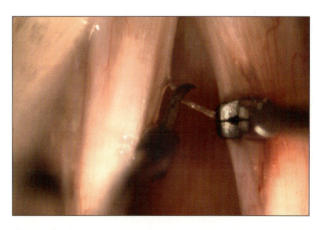

Fig 6–19. (10×) There is a varix associated with that nodule, which is then resected with the microscissors.

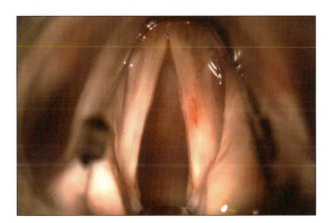

Fig 6–20. (4×) The final image after resection of the lesions.

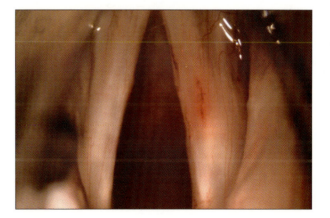

Fig 6–21. (7×) Figure 6–20 at higher magnification.

Case 6E

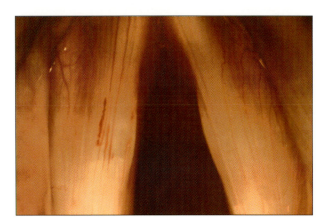

Fig 6–22. (10×) A rock performer with multiple varices on the superior surface of the left musculo-membranous vocal fold. There are bilateral sessile nodules.

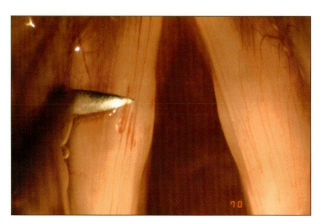

Fig 6–23. (10×) A sharp pick is used to perform an epithelial cordotomy to dissect the varices. (From Hochman I, Sataloff RT, Hillman RE, Zeitels SM. *Ann Otol Rhinol Laryngol.* 1998;108: 10–16 with permission.)

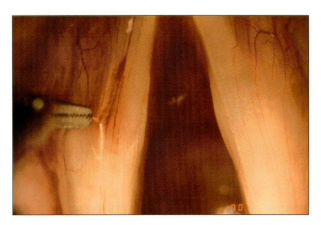

Fig 6–24. (10×) One of the varices is removed with an alligator forceps.

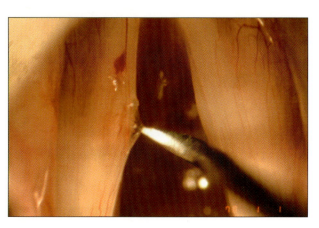

Fig 6–25. (10×) The sessile nodule on the left is dissected with a sharp pick.

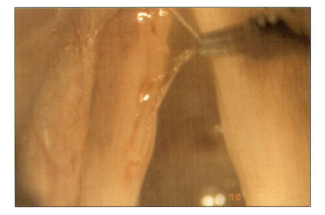

Fig 6–26. (10×) A varix associated with the nodule is also dissected with the sharp pick. The varix on the superior surface of the left vocal fold is completely resected and retracted with an alligator forceps.

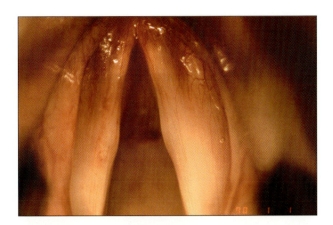

Fig 6–27. (7×) The image subsequent to resection of the varices and prior to resection of the nodules.

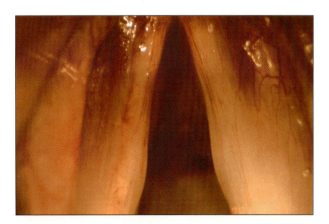

Fig 6–28. (10×) Figure 6–27 at higher magnification.

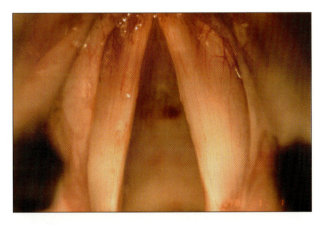

Fig 6–29. (7×) The image subsequent to resection of the varices and nodules.

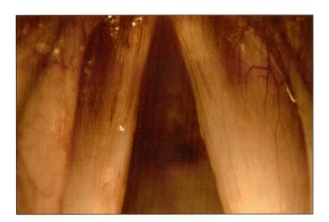

Fig 6–30. (10×) Figure 6–29 at higher magnification.

Case 6F

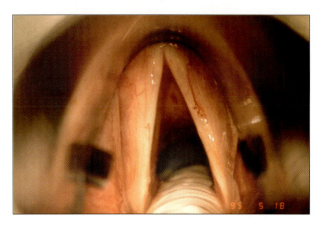

Fig 6–31. (4×) A classical vocalist with a network of connected varices and ectasias on the superior surface of the right vocal fold. (From Hochman I, Sataloff RT, Hillman RE, Zeitels SM. *Ann Otol Rhinol Laryngol.* 1998;108:10–16 with permission.)

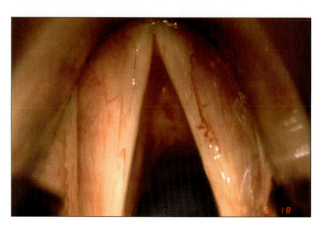

Fig 6–32. (7×) Figure 6–31 at higher magnification. (From Hochman I, Sataloff RT, Hillman RE, Zeitels SM. *Ann Otol Rhinol Laryngol.* 1998;108:10–16 with permission.)

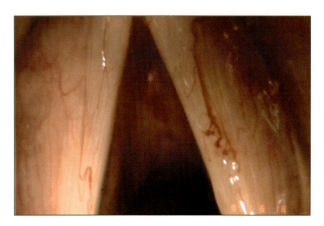

Fig 6–33. (10×) Figure 6–31 again at even higher magnification. (From Hochman I, Sataloff RT, Hillman RE, Zeitels SM. *Ann Otol Rhinol Laryngol.* 1998;108:10–16 with permission.)

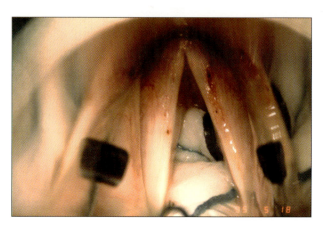

Fig 6–34. (4×) The lesions have been ablated with the microspot CO_2 laser.

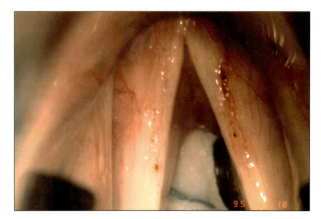

Fig 6–35. (7×) Figure 6–34 at higher magnification. (From Hochman I, Sataloff RT, Hillman RE, Zeitels SM. *Ann Otol Rhinol Laryngol.* 1998;108:10–16 with permission.)

Case 6G

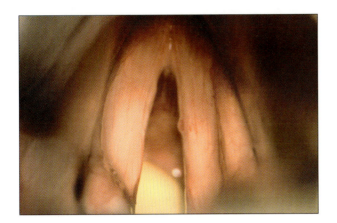

Fig 6–36. (4×) An ectatic nodule with associated varices is noted on the right

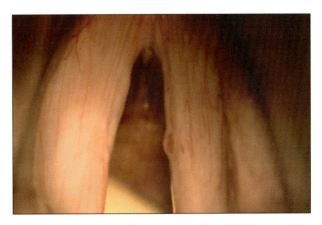

Fig 6–37. (7×) Figure 6–36 is noted at higher magnification.

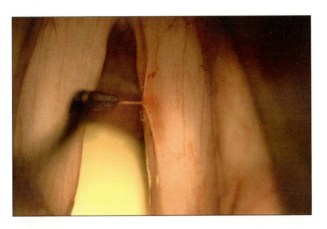

Fig 6–38. (7×) The nodule has been resected and one of the varices is retracted.

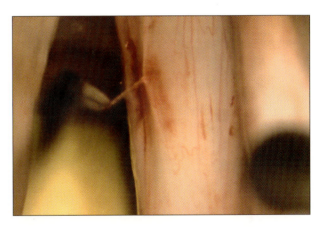

Fig 6–39. (10×) Figure 6–38 at higher magnification. The blood within the small vessel cannot be seen since it is on stretch.

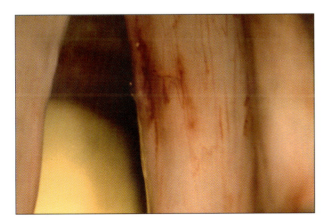

Fig 6–40. (10×) The varix has been laid down so that the blood within the vessel wall can be observed coursing perpendicular to the long axis of the vocal fold

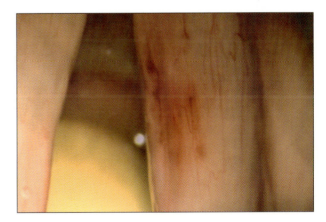

Fig 6–41. (10×) The vascular lesions have been resected.

Case 6H

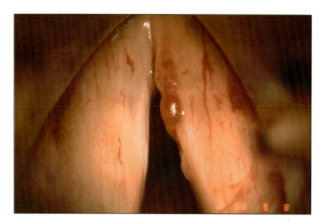

Fig 6–42. (7×) An auctioneer with progressive severe hoarseness. There are multiple subepithelial vascular lesions that include a spectrum of ectasias, varices, and a polyp. (Courtesy of Endocraft LLC.)

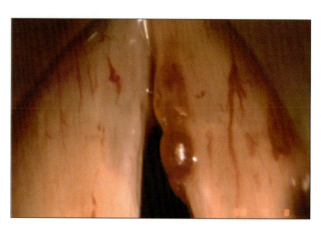

Fig 6–43. (10×) Figure 6–42 is noted at higher magnification. (Courtesy of Endocraft LLC.)

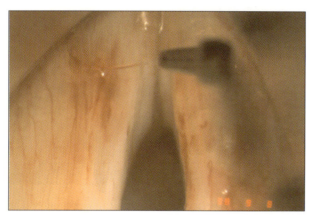

Fig 6–44. (10×) The right-sided lesions have been resected by means of a subepithelial resection approach. A varix is withdrawn from the left fold after performing an epithelial cordotomy. (Courtesy of Endocraft LLC.)

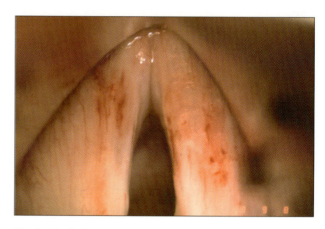

Fig 6–45. (7×) All of the lesions have been resected. (Courtesy of Endocraft LLC.)

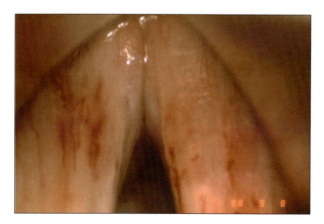

Fig 6–46. (10×) Figure 6–45 is noted at higher magnification. (Courtesy of Endocraft LLC.)

Case 6I

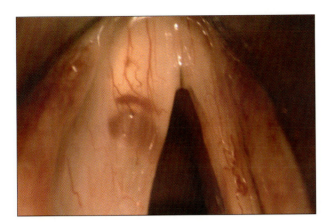

Fig 6–47. (10×) A persistent erythematous blush was noted along with stiffness on stroboscopy in a musical theater performer. A hematoma was suspected with feeding vessels seen anteriorly. (Courtesy of Endocraft LLC.)

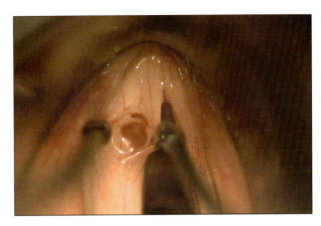

Fig 6–48. (4×) An epithelial cordotomy was done and after retracting the microflaps, an ectatic well-defined fibrovascular mass was noted. (Courtesy of Endocraft LLC.)

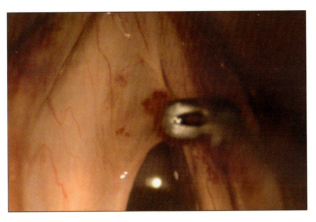

Fig 6–49. (10×) The mass was grasped with a cup forceps and retracted. The underlying normal SLP is well seen. (Courtesy of Endocraft LLC.)

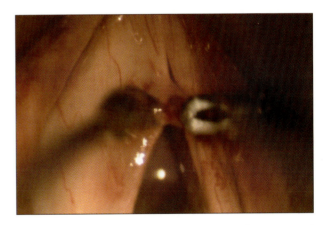

Fig 6–50. (10×) The fibrovascular mass is sharply dissected from the SLP by means of a microscissors. (Courtesy of Endocraft LLC.)

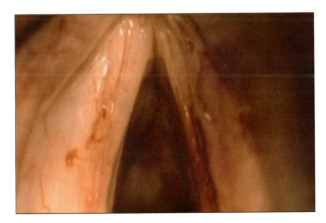

Fig 6–51. (7×) The mass has been completely resected with maximal preservation of the epithelium and the SLP. (Courtesy of Endocraft LLC.)

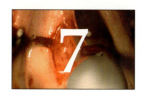

Cysts

Subepithelial cysts arise in the SLP and present in a variety of sizes. They may be attached to the vocal ligament and/or the epithelial basement membrane. Small cysts may also be freely suspended within the SLP. Small cysts may be confused with nodules if visual examination is performed without stroboscopy. Stroboscopic examination typically reveals a characteristic asymmetric disordered oscillation of the mucosa because of the well circumscribed stiffness in the area of the cyst. If the cyst protrudes from the medial surface of the glottal edge, a nodule may be observed on the contra-lateral vocal fold. Asymmetric spheroid masses on the medial surface of the vocal fold should alert the clinician that there may be a cyst on one side.

It is presumed that most subepithelial cysts probably arise from obstructed ducts within the SLP since they contain mucus. Cysts may also be composed of an epithelial rest (similar to a cholesteatoma). On occasion, small ovoid subepithelial masses that are thought preoperatively to be a cyst within the SLP are found at microlaryngoscopy to be fibrous masses. These masses are usually firmer to palpation and may be the result of an old microvascular injury or a rheumatoid lesion. The subepithelial infusion technique[104,105] is extremely helpful during the phonomicrosurgical resection of well-defined cysts and firm masses within the SLP. Similar to small nodules, the infusion can obscure the boundaries of small mucous cysts and lead to unnecessary dissection and trauma of normal SLP.

Masses within the SLP, with few exceptions, should be resected with cold instruments.[77] It is not uncommon for the mucous cysts to rupture, especially toward the end of the dissection, while grasping the fragile wall for retraction. The surgeon must be careful to retrieve the entirety of the cyst wall without undue trauma to the underlying normal SLP. Keratin cysts can usually be resected en bloc without difficulty. Regardless, great care should be taken to minimally disturb any normal SLP and epithelium. This approach will optimize postoperative mucosal-wave oscillation and vocal quality. Although the wave usually improves, *typically* it does not return to normal if the cyst has already replaced a substantial amount of normal SLP, which will not regenerate. The need for extremely fine delicate tangential-dissection precludes effective use of the CO_2 laser.

Case 7A

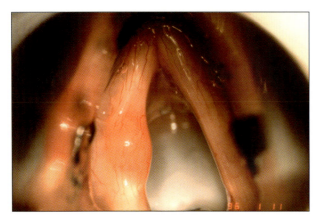

Fig 7–1. (4×) A spheroid mass, which has an erythematous hue, is seen on the superior and medial surface of the left vocal fold.

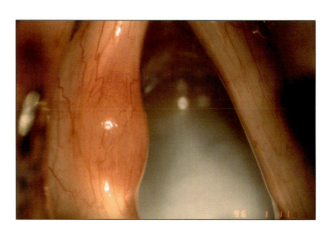

Fig 7–2. (7×) Figure 7–1 at higher magnification.

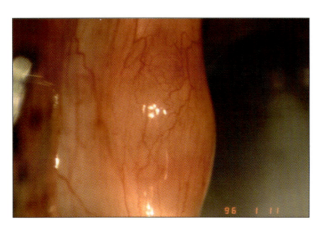

Fig 7–3. (10×) Figure 7–1 at even higher magnification. Note that light reflex at the center of the lesion and note the distribution of the microvascular overlying the lesion.

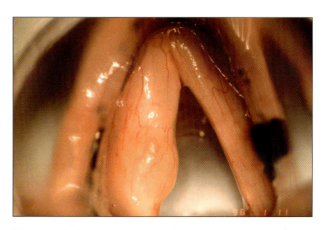

Fig 7–4. (4×) A subepithelial infusion is done on the left.

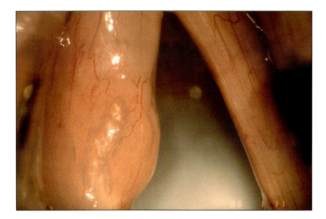

Fig 7–5. (7×) Figure 7–4 at higher magnification.

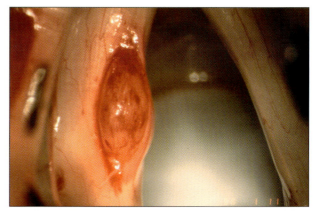

Fig 7–6. (7×) An epithelial cordotomy is done overlying the lesion and a subepithelial mucoid cyst is noted.

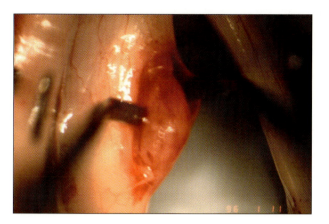

Fig 7–7. (7×) Curved dissectors are used to mobilize the cyst from its attachments.

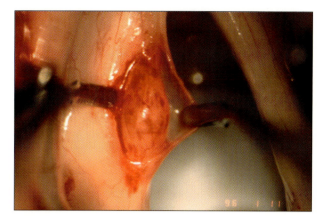

Fig 7–8. (7×) A curved left dissector is utilized to demonstrate the thin translucent epithelium that was overlying the cyst.

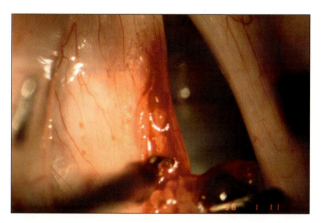

Fig 7–9. (7×) The cyst is grasped with an angled forceps and withdrawn from the SLP. The final resection is performed by excising the base with a curved microscissors.

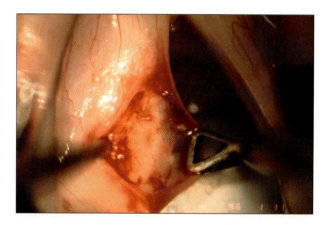

Fig 7–10. (7×) The edges of the microflaps are retracted for visualization of the cavity where the cyst had been situated. There was maximal preservation of normal SLP and epithelium.

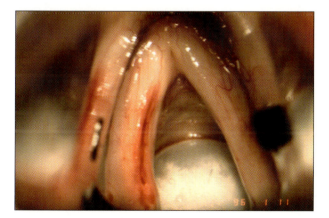

Fig 7–11. (4×) Note the normally contoured vocal fold and minimal trauma outside the perimeter of the location of the mass.

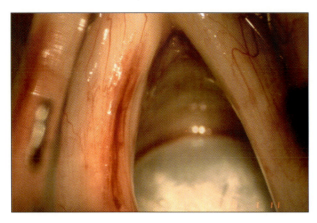

Fig 7–12. (7×) There is excellent coaptation of the epithelial edges. There was a significant amount of normal SLP underlying the cyst, so that the vocal fold contour was only minimally affected by resection of the mass.

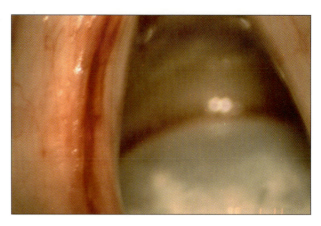

Fig 7–13. (10×) Figure 7–12 at higher magnification.

Case 7B

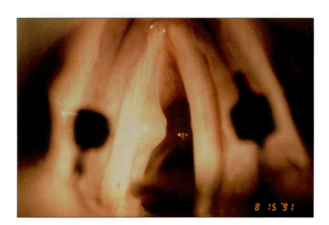

Fig 7–14. (4×) A subepithelial cyst is noted on the left vocal fold.

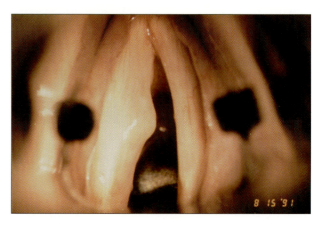

Fig 7–15. (4×) A subepithelial infusion has been performed.

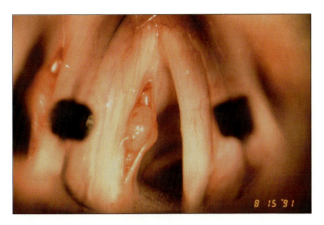

Fig 7–16. (4×) An epithelial cordotomy has been performed, which reveals the underlying cyst.

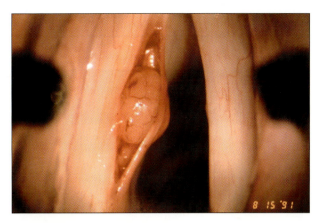

Fig 7–17. (7×) Figure 7–16 at higher magnification. This case was performed more than 8 years ago. The epithelial cordotomy and the amount of dissection within the normal SLP is more extensive here than what would be done today.

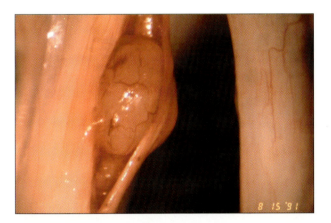

Fig 7–18. (10×) Figure 7–16 at even higher magnification. Note the intact microvasculature on the cyst wall.

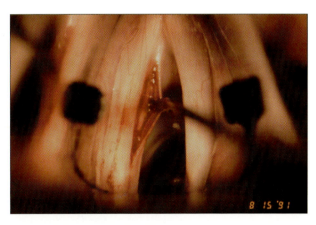

Fig 7–19. (4×) The epithelial microflap is retracted for visualization.

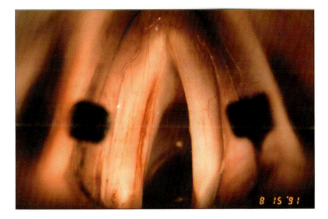

Fig 7–20. (4×) There is excellent apposition of the epithelial edge and the vocal fold is well contoured.

Case 7C

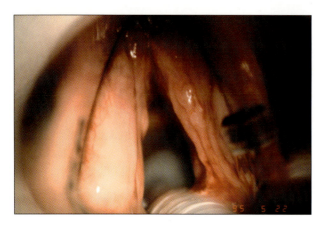

Fig 7–21. (4×) A small subepithelial mass is seen on the medial surface of the left vocal fold. This patient was a heavy smoker and had chronic reflux. He was also a vocal abuser.

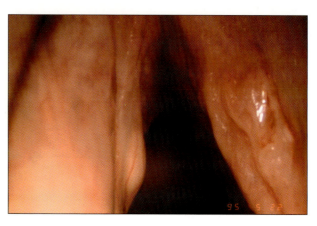

Fig 7–22. (10×) Figure 7–21 at higher magnification. Note the extensive irregularities of the right vocal fold, which ultimately represented keratosis with atypia in a sulcus vocalis.

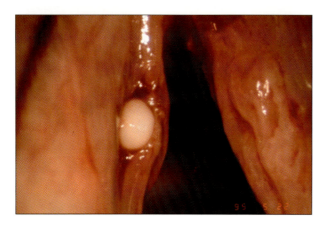

Fig 7–23. (10×) An epithelial cordotomy was done on the left and a keratin cyst was noted.

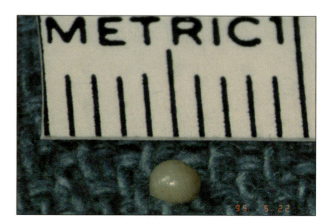

Fig 7–24. The resected cyst.

Case 7D

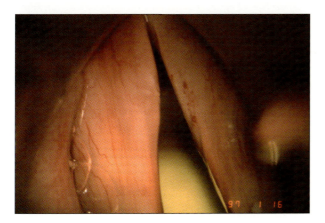

Fig 7–25. (7×) There is a sessile swelling of the left vocal fold. On the contralateral side, there is a sulcus deformity. (Courtesy of Endocraft LLC.)

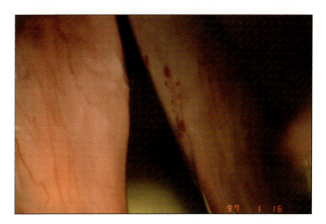

Fig 7–26. (10×) Figure 7–25 at higher magnification. There is an ill-defined subepithelial mass on the left, which was easier to appreciate during stroboscopy. There are multiple ectasias in the region of the sulcus which are well seen at this higher magnification, but were not well visualized during stroboscopy due to their tangential position. (Courtesy of Endocraft LLC.)

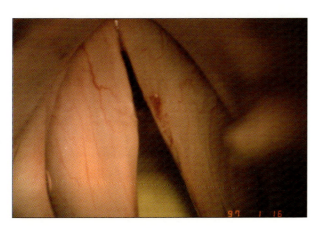

Fig 7–27. (7×) A subepithelial infusion is performed on the left. (Courtesy of Endocraft LLC.)

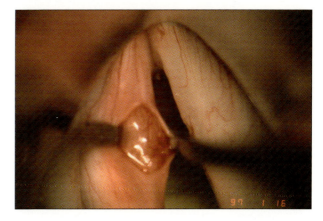

Fig 7–28. (7×) An epithelial cordotomy is performed and a subepithelial mucoid cyst is noted. This suggests that the sulcus deformity on the right may very well have originated as a cyst on that side as well. (Courtesy of Endocraft LLC.)

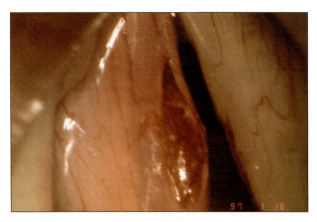

Fig 7–29. (10×) Once dissection has begun on the cyst, it begins to protrude through the epithelial cordotomy. (Courtesy of Endocraft LLC.)

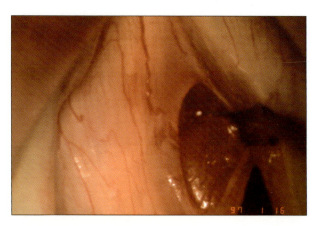

Fig 7–30. (10×) Dissection continues by separating the cyst attachments to the basement membrane of the epithelial microflap. (Courtesy of Endocraft LLC.)

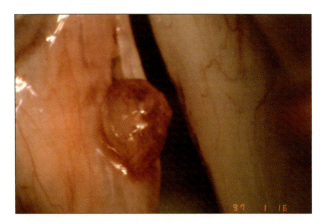

Fig 7–31. (10×) The cyst continues to be withdrawn through the cordotomy. (Courtesy of Endocraft LLC.)

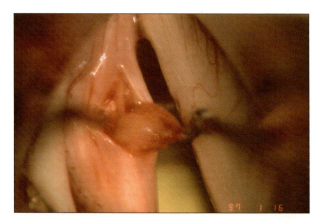

Fig 7–32. (7×) The cyst is retracted with an alligator forceps and the dissector is utilized to separate it from the underlying normal superficial lamina propria. (Courtesy of Endocraft LLC.)

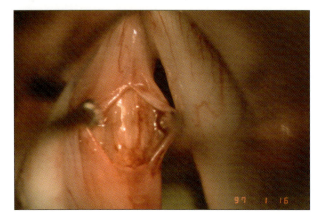

Fig 7–33. (7×) The epithelial microflaps are retracted to visualize the cavity that the cyst was situated in. Note the intact microvasculature of the residual normal SLP. (Courtesy of Endocraft LLC.)

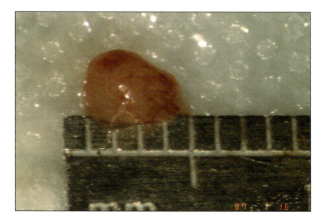

Fig 7–34. The resected mass. (Courtesy of Endocraft LLC.)

Case 7E

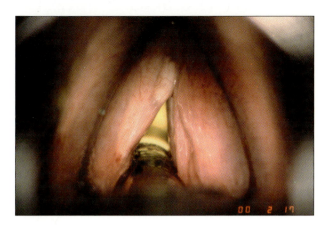

Fig 7–35. (4×) A white subepithelial mass is noted in the left anterior medial surface of a 30-year-old businessman. (Courtesy of Endocraft LLC.)

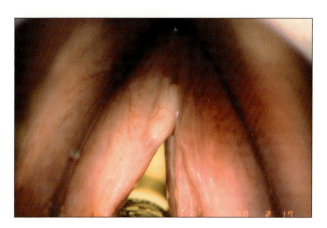

Fig 7–36. (7×) Figure 7–35 at higher magnification. (Courtesy of Endocraft LLC.)

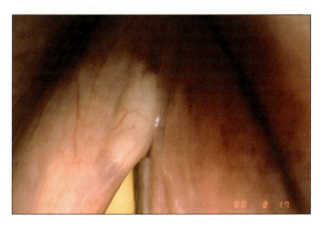

Fig 7–37. (10×) Figure 7–35 at highest magnification. (Courtesy of Endocraft LLC.)

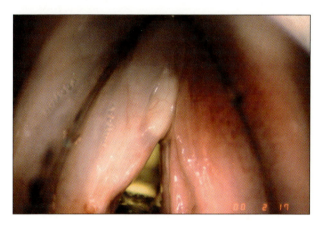

Fig 7–38. (7×) A subepithelial infusion has been performed. (Courtesy of Endocraft LLC.)

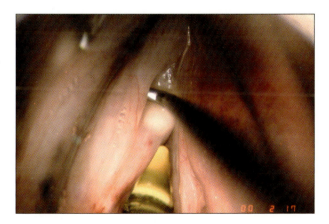

Fig 7–39. (7×) The infusion reveals that there is a sulcus at the superior edge of the cyst. A blunt right-angle probe has been placed in the sulcus. (Courtesy of Endocraft LLC.)

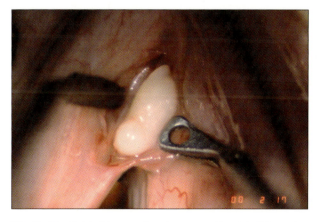

Fig 7–40. (10×) After performing a small epithelial cordotomy, a keratin cyst is noted. It is mobilized primarily with a dissector. (Courtesy of Endocraft LLC.)

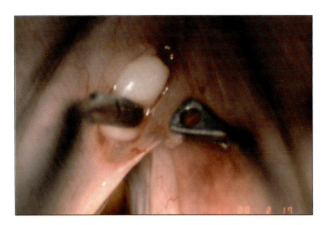

Fig 7–41. (10×) The cyst is dissected from the basement membrane of the epithelium. (Courtesy of Endocraft LLC.)

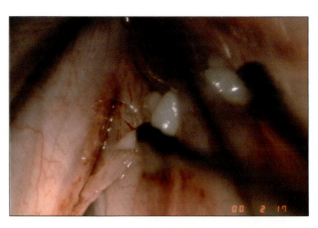

Fig 7–42. (10×) The cyst is retracted with and alligator forceps and the last attachment to the epithelium is seen. (Courtesy of Endocraft LLC.)

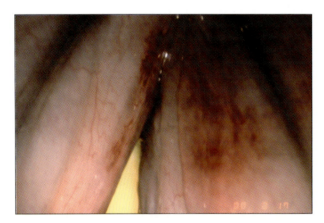

Fig 7–43. (10×) The microflap is repositioned and there is excellent apposition of the epithelial edges. (Courtesy of Endocraft LLC.)

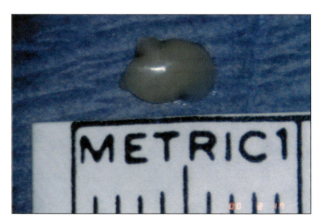

Fig 7–44. The resected keratin cyst with an intact capsule. (Courtesy of Endocraft LLC.)

Case 7F

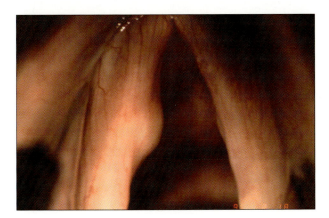

Fig 7–45. (7×) A subepithelial cyst is seen on the left vocal fold and a contralateral nodule noted.

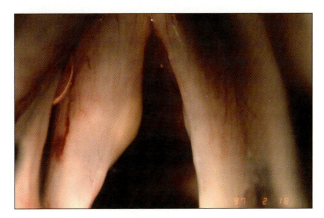

Fig 7–46. (7×) A subepithelial infusion is performed. The puncture site can be seen laterally. There is excellent vaso-constriction of the microvasculature.

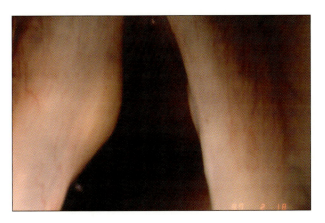

Fig 7–47. (10×) Figure 7–46 at higher magnification. The vasoconstriction has allowed for visual delineation of the mucus-containing yellow cyst.

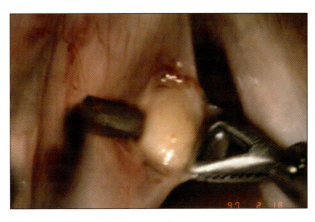

Fig 7–48. (10×) The flaps are being retracted. During the completion of the dissection of the cyst, the cyst began to leak.

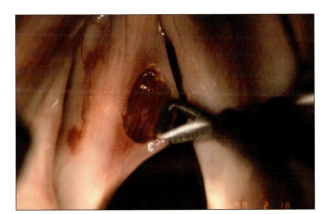

Fig 7–49. (7×) Because most of the dissection had been completed, it was easy to grasp the cyst and withdraw it from the cavity to complete its resection. Retraction of the micro-flap shows there is no residual cyst noted and there is normal SLP still left at the base of the cyst cavity.

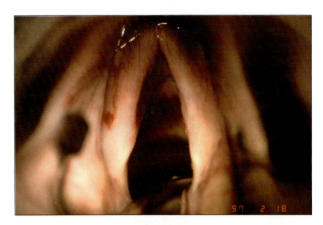

Fig 7–50. (4×) The postresection appearance of the vocal fold with an improved contour.

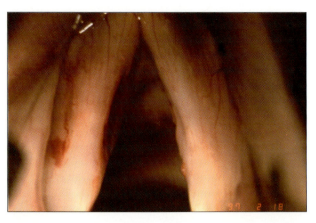

Fig 7–51. (7×) Figure 7–50 at higher magnification. There is a slight excavation in the region of the cyst because of the size of the cyst, as well as the fact that the rest of the fold was still edematous from the infusion. This area ultimately healed with a normal contour. The nodule on the right has been resected.

Case 7G

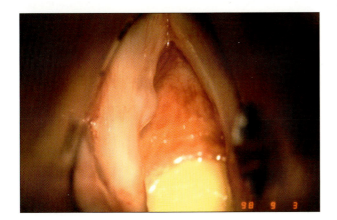

Fig 7–52. (4×) A spheroid mass is noted on the medial surface of the left fold.

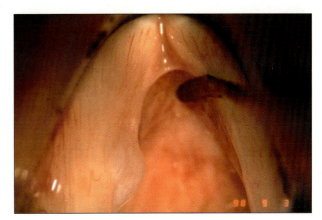

Fig 7–53. (7×) Figure 7–52 at higher magnification; A dissector has been positioned to demonstrate a congenital anterior microweb.

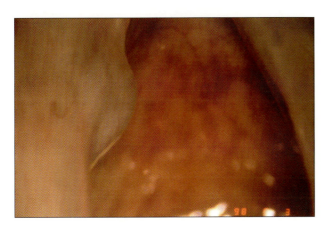

Fig 7–54. (10×) The mass is seen at the highest magnification.

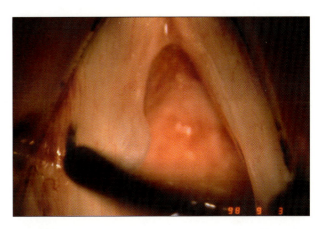

Fig 7–55. (7×) An infusion needle has been placed lateral to the lesion.

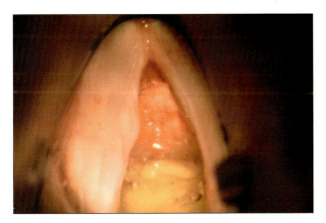

Fig 7–56. (4×) The subepithelial infusion of saline and epinephrine has been placed.

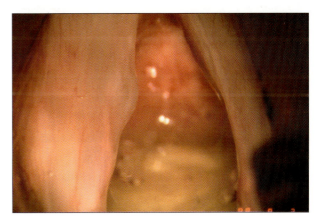

Fig 7–57. (7×) The infusion is seen at higher magnification.

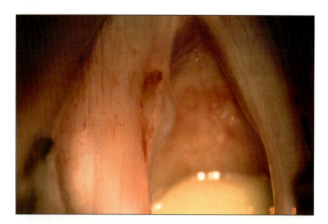

Fig 7–58. (7×) An epithelial cordotomy has been placed at the superior edge of the lesion.

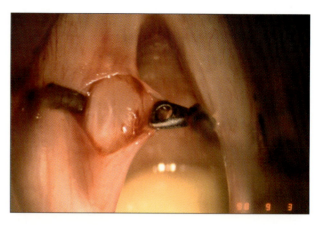

Fig 7–59. (7×) Exposure of the cyst is achieved by means of a dissector and angled forceps.

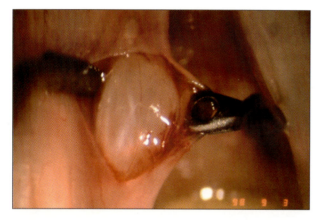

Fig 7–60. (10×) The wall of the cyst is better seen at higher magnification.

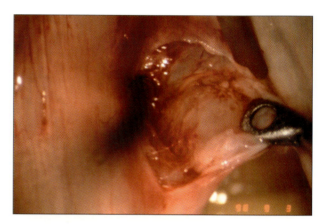

Fig 7–61. (10×) The cyst is retracted, while its deep attachments will be separated by means of a microscissors.

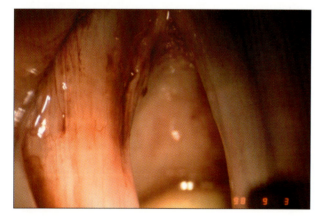

Fig 7–62. (7×) The postresection result demonstrating a smooth vocal fold edge and excellent coaptation of the epithelial edges.

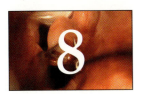

Granulomas

ARYTENOID GRANULOMAS

The majority of granulomas are found in the arytenoid region (Figure 8–1) but may occur in other areas where there has been traumatic disruption of mucosa. These lesions typically arise in patients who have laryngo-pharyngeal reflux (LPR). Reflux creates an environment of generalized mucositis, and the traumatic disruption of glottal epithelium predisposes patients to a hypertrophic inflammatory reaction.

There are classical descriptions of posterior glottal granulomas that occur after an endotracheal intubation. In this instance, the posteriorly situated endotracheal tube has disrupted the periarytenoid epithelium. These patients frequently have simultaneous endotracheal and nasogastric tubes and the latter predisposes to extra-esophageal reflux. In many cases the nasogastric tube is still in place and there is ongoing arytenoid trauma secondary to coughing and vocal hyperfunction.

The typical outpatient posterior glottal granuloma is the result of vocally induced trauma in a reflux environment. These patients demonstrate vocal hyperfunction that causes high-impact collision forces of the arytenoids during phonation.[158] Videolaryngoscopy reveals hyperfunction of the lateral cricoarytenoid musculature that results in hyper-rotation of the arytenoids (Figure 8–2) and abnormal concussion, leading to ongoing epithelial trauma. It is common to find granulomas that show a bilobed configuration, which reflects the conformation of the contralateral arytenoid from the closure pattern of the arytenoids during phonation.

These patients require vocal therapy as an adjunct to their treatment, which includes antireflux management and possible microlaryngeal resection. The importance of reducing vocal hyperfunction, a predisposing traumatic behavior, cannot be overstated. Abusive vocal behavior is usually the culprit with recurrent recalcitrant arytenoid-granulomas. If the hyperfunctional activity of the lateral cricoarytenoid muscles is still observed, low-dose botulinum toxin[159] can be used to chemically unload this closure pattern. Administration of 1.5–2.5 international units bilaterally is a good initial dose. Small and medium sized lesions (<4 mm) may be managed by outpatient injections. With larger lesions, the injection can be placed at the time of the endoscopic excision of the granuloma by placing the needle through the ventricle along the anterior face of the arytenoid until the cricoid cartilage can be palpated. The BOTOX is therefore directed toward the lateral cricoarytenoid muscle rather than the thyroarytenoid muscle. This will help minimize the vocal insufficiency and hypophonia that the patient must be prepared for.

Arytenoid granulomas, which do not occur subsequent to instrumentation of the larynx, frequently occur in vocal overusers. Therefore, embarking on BOTOX injections must be done with great care, since these individuals must be apprised of resulting hypophonia. Essentially, the BOTOX is chemically altering the patient's adductory biomechanics so that the interarytenoid muscle assumes a more dominant role, which is less traumatic to the medial arytenoid mucosa.

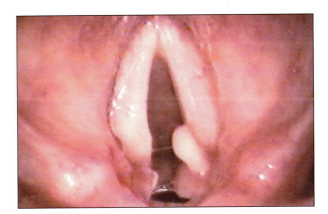

Fig 8–2. A clinic image showing hyperfunctional closure of the arytenoids. The bilobular nature of the granuloma on the right results from the pattern of contact from the left arytenoid.

Fig 8–1. Jackson's drawings of classical arytenoid granulomas and contact ulcers. (From Jackson Cl, Jackson C.: *The Larynx and Its Diseases*; 1937:151–162 with permission.)

Phonomicrosurgical resection should be performed when behavior modification and medication have not led to a resolution and/or there is concern about a neoplastic process. Granulomas are frequently exophytic with a surprisingly narrow base. When they are small or medium in size, they may not impair glottal closure. However, large granulomas will result in a substantial glottal chink in the musculo-membranous region, which leads to further glottal insufficiency during laryngeal sound production and increased vocal hyperfunction.

On rare occasions, granulomas will require excision due to airway compromise, especially in older patients or those with impaired arytenoid mobility. The use of the laser or cold instruments alone is individualized based on the surgeon preference and the anatomical characteristics of the lesion.[77] The critical surgical principle is to remove the mass without disturbing the arytenoid perichondrium. Injecting the base of the granuloma with a small amount of an aqueous based steroid such as depomedrol may help to prevent recurrence but has not been done routinely after the introduction of BOTOX management.

POSTSURGICAL GRANULOMAS

Infrequently, a granuloma will form in the site of the resection of a benign vocal edge lesion. Most often this occurs secondary to vocal overuse precluding epithelialization in patients who have significant LPR. Voice rest and control of the LPR will usually obviate the need for re-excision. Inhaled steroids can also be helpful. Granulation and granulomas are actually quite common after cancer resections in the glottis and supraglottis as the tissue defect is healing. Similar noninvasive measures should be incorporated with watchful waiting as it is not unusual for epithelialization to be completed in 6–8 weeks. In this setting, patience is a virtue.

TEFLON GRANULOMAS

Teflon granulomas are less commonly encountered due to the diminishing role of Teflon injection for the treatment of glottal incompetence and the commensurate popularity of laryngoplastic phonosurgery.[160–162] Large Teflon granulomas can impair the airway as well as the voice. Safe management of the airway is the primary goal and voice enhancement is second. Although endoscopic laser excision has been the gold standard for almost 20 years, Netterville et al[163,164] recently described transcervical excision under local anesthesia by means of a thyroplasty approach. This procedure shows significant promise and may replace many of the endoscopic procedures because the transcervical approach facilitates a more effective resection and simultaneous phonatory feedback.

The vocal dysfunction is secondary to a number of factors. First and foremost, the rigid spheroid mass of a large granuloma does not vibrate. During glottal closure the rigid mass typically impairs vibration of the contralateral (potentially) normal vocal fold. This is caused by compression of the normal delicate pliable musculo-membranous tissue and the aberrant conformation of the subglottal airstream. The rigid Teflon mass, which is often present for years, will frequently lead to scarring and/or a sulcus deformity of the contralateral vocal fold.

Endoscopic phonomicrosurgical goals include using the CO_2 laser to develop a more appropriately contoured vocal fold, including the subglottic region. Although initially the epithelium was not preserved, during the last 7 years, an epithelial microflap is maintained and often sutured in place after cyto-reducing the granuloma. During the last 4 years, axillary fat is retrieved and placed under the microflap to improve the viscoelastic properties of the vocal fold.

Case 8A

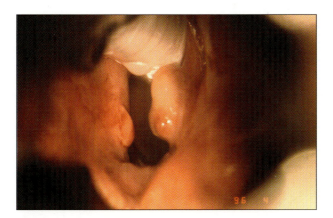

Fig 8–3. (4×) Bilateral granulomas are seen. The endotracheal tube is positioned anterior to the laryngoscope. (Courtesy of Endocraft LLC.)

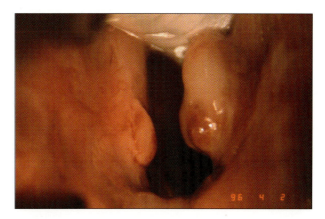

Fig 8–4. (7×) Figure 8–3 at higher magnification. (Courtesy of Endocraft LLC.)

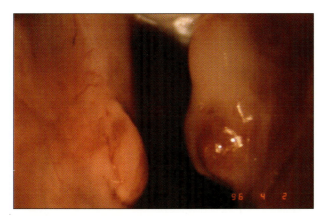

Fig 8–5. (10×) Figure 8–3 at even higher magnification. (Courtesy of Endocraft LLC.)

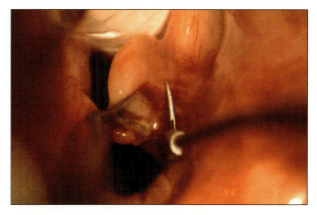

Fig 8–6. (7×) Subsequent to a subepithelial infusion, the granuloma is retracted and an upturned microscissors is used to resect the lesion without disturbing the arytenoid perichondrium. (Courtesy of Endocraft LLC.)

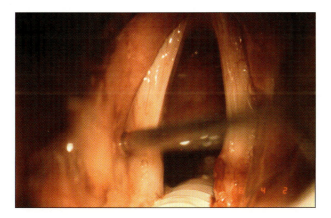

Fig 8–7. (7×) The laryngoscope is repositioned and a needle has been placed just anterior to the left arytenoid in the ventricle for placement of botulinum toxin into the lateral cricoarytenoid muscle. The location is determined by palpation of the cricoid cartilage through the ventricle. (Courtesy of Endocraft LLC.)

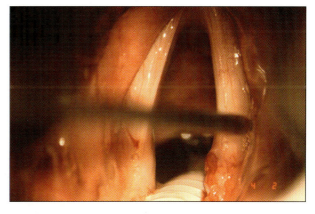

Fig 8–8. (7×) The prior procedure is performed on the right. (Courtesy of Endocraft LLC.)

Case 8B

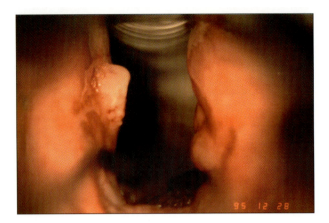

Fig 8–9. (7×) A classic granuloma and contact ulcer are seen. The endotracheal tube is anterior to the laryngoscope. A dissector is situated to delineate the posterior aspect of the left arytenoid.

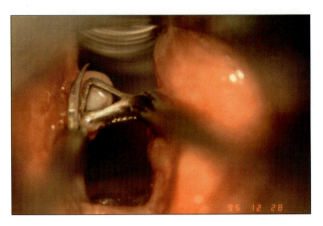

Fig 8–10. (7×) The ulcer/granuloma is grasped with an angled forceps and a microscissors is used to excise it. Care is taken not to disturb the arytenoid perichondrium.

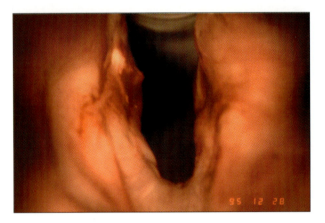

Fig 8–11. (7×) A small area of granulation is resected on the right side as well. Note the interarytenoid hyperplasia consistent with the chronic reflex.

Case 8C

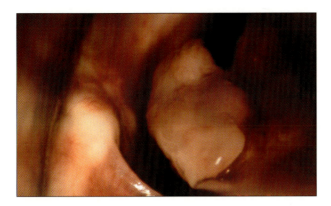

Fig 8–12. (7×) A large granuloma emanating from the right arytenoid.

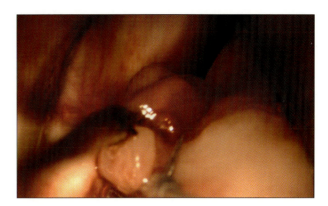

Fig 8–13. (7×) The granuloma is retracted and a microscissors is used to resect the lesion without disturbing the underlying arytenoid perichondrium.

Case 8D

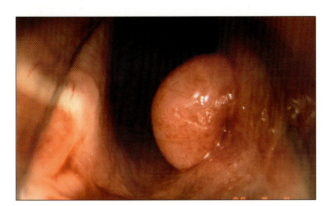

Fig 8–14. (7×) This 55-year-old patient is a general surgeon who had undergone multiple previous resections of this granuloma in Europe with subsequent recurrence. A unilateral spheroid mass is seen on the right.

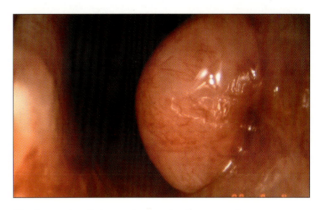

Fig 8–15. (10×) Figure 8–14 at higher magnification.

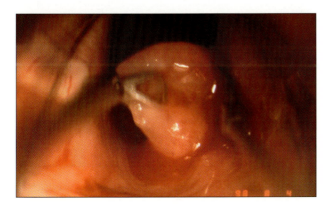

Fig 8–16. (7×) The lesion is grasped with an angled forceps and resected with a microscissors.

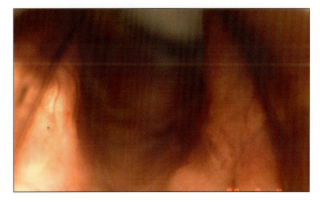

Fig 8–17. (7×) Care was taken not to disturb any normal tissues and to minimize the epithelial disruption. Subsequent to this, BOTOX was placed into the lateral cricoarytenoid muscles bilaterally and the granulomas have not recurred.

Case 8E

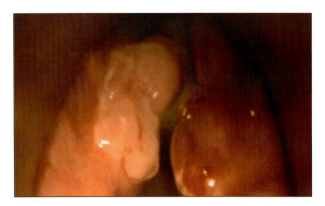

Fig 8–18. (7×) Classic arytenoid granulomas demonstrating the "cup and saucer" deformities.

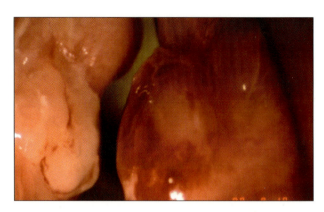

Fig 8–19. (10×) Figure 8–18 at higher magnification.

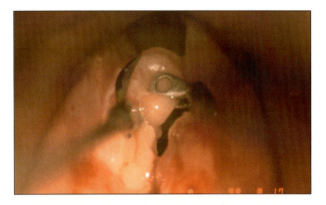

Fig 8–20. (7×) A portion of the left granuloma is grasped and resected with microscissors.

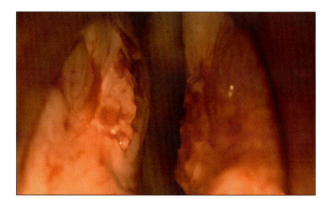

Fig 8–21. (10×) Both granulomas have been trimmed to the normal contour of the medial arytenoid without disturbing the perichondrium. BOTOX was injected into this patient as well.

Case 8F

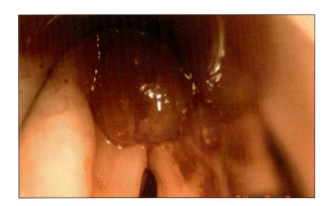

Fig 8–22. (7×) This patient had previously undergone resection of a T1 glottic carcinoma that was in continuity with the anterior glottal commissure. Approximately 1 month later, he developed a granuloma anteriorly. Despite conservative management, which included treatment for reflux, voice rest, and a steroid inhaler, the lesion did not regress.

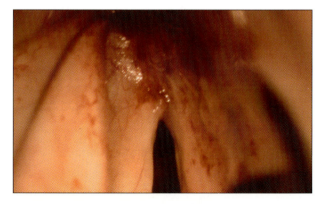

Fig 8–23. (7×) The lesion had a narrow base and was excised without difficulty. There was no evidence of malignancy in the specimen and he healed uneventfully.

Case 8G

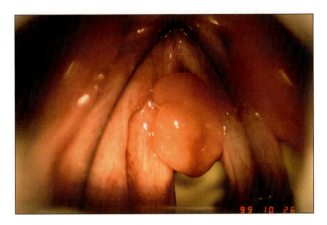

Fig 8-24. (4×) A large granuloma is seen in the mid left fold subsequent to subepithelial fat implantation for sulcus vocalis. (Courtesy of Endocraft LLC.)

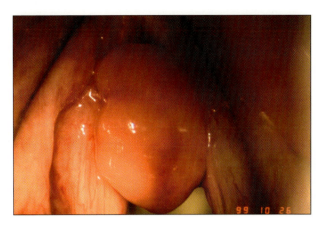

Fig 8-25. (7×) Figure 8–24 at higher magnification. (Courtesy of Endocraft LLC.)

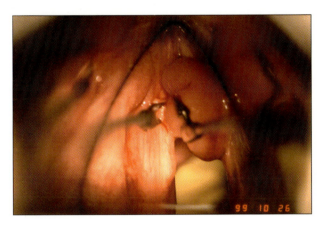

Fig 8-26. (4×) The granuloma is retracted with open alligator forceps to expose the narrow-pedicle base to allow for microscissors amputation. (Courtesy of Endocraft LLC.)

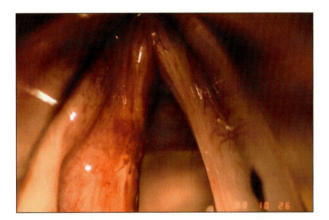

Fig 8-27. (7×) The vocal fold is now smooth and straight with minimal disturbance of epithelium. (Courtesy of Endocraft LLC.)

Case 8H

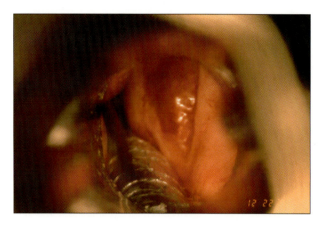

Fig 8–28. (4×) This patient presented with severe stridor and a large right Teflon granuloma. The exposure was quite difficult and a Dedo laryngoscope is in place. The current prototype glottiscopes portrayed in throughout most of this text were not available at the time of this surgery.

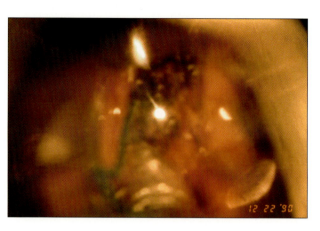

Fig 8–29. (4×) The granuloma is being cytoreduced with the CO_2 laser. The photograph is taken through the laser plume to delineate the flare, which is indicative of combusting Teflon.

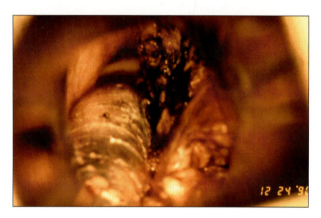

Fig 8–30. (4×) There is an eschar from the cytoreduction of the Teflon granuloma revealed and there is an improved glottal aperture.

Case 8I

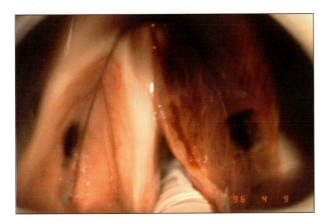

Fig 8–31. (4×) This patient had severe dysphonia and a large Teflon granuloma on the right. Prior to presentation, she had undergone previous microlaryngoscopic resections.

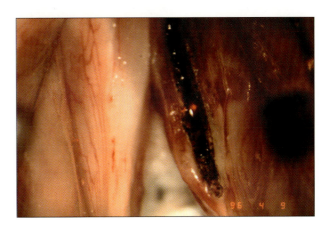

Fig 8–32. (7×) An epithelial incision is made with the microspot CO_2 laser.

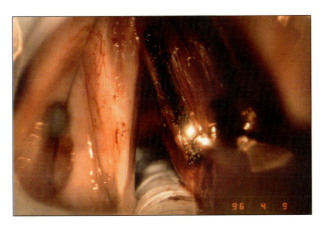

Fig 8–33. (4×) The photograph is taken during impact to display the characteristic flare from combusting Teflon.

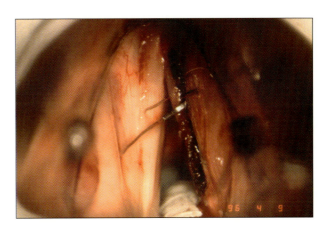

Fig 8–34. (4×) Subsequent to cytoreduction of the granuloma, a suture is placed to achieve primary closure of the wound. The epithelium has been preserved medially.

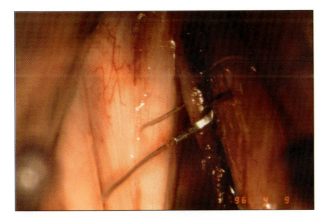

Fig 8–35. (7×) Figure 8–34 at higher magnification.

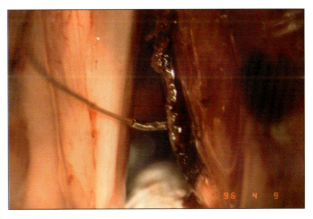

Fig 8–36. (7×) A second suture is placed.

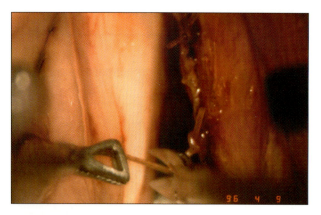

Fig 8–37. (7×) The suture is cut with a microscissors.

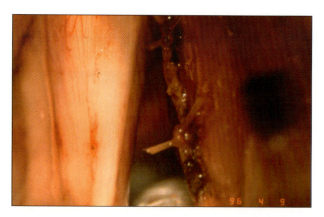

Fig 8–38. (7×) The final appearance of the glottal aperture subsequent to the procedure. The patient healed well and her voice was dramatically improved. She has not required further surgery.

Case 8J

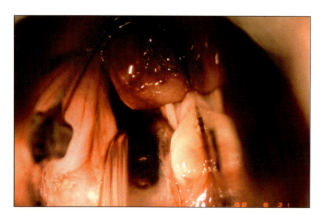

Fig 8–39. (4×) A spheroid mass was noted after a patient underwent a transcervical (laryngoplasty) resection of a Teflon granuloma and placement of a strap-muscle flap. A small tear in the ventricular surface of the vocal fold allowed for a reactive granuloma to form.

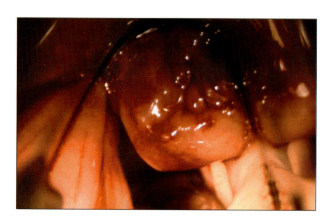

Fig 8–40. (7×) Figure 8–39 at higher magnification.

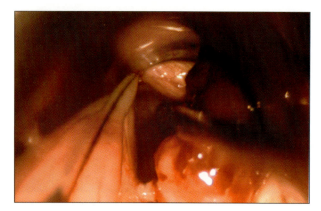

Fig 8–41. (7×) A suction is used to retract the mass, which was mobile and arising from a narrow pedicle.

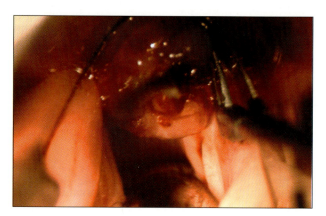

Fig 8–42. (7×) The mass was retracted with an alligator forceps and amputated with a microscissors. No Teflon was noted in the specimen.

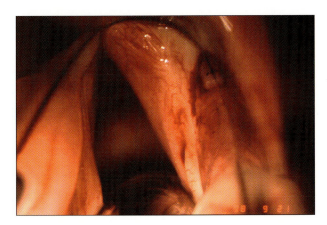

Fig 8–43. (7×) The patient's voice improved and there was no recurrence.

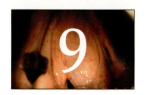

Polypoid Corditis / Reinke's Edema

Polypoid corditis presents as extensive swelling of the SLP (Reinke's space). The swelling is usually situated on the superior surface of the musculo-membranous vocal fold. This entity is another manifestation of vocal fold pathology that is of multifactorial genesis. Zeitels et al[109] have recently demonstrated that these patients typically smoke extensively, have laryngo-pharyngeal reflux, and demonstrate vocal hyperfunction. The swelling probably occurs from the increased aerodynamic pressures that drive vocal fold mucosal oscillation in a general environment of glottal mucositis, which is secondary to smoking and reflux. The swelling is typically bilateral but often asymmetric in volume.

Individuals with polypoid corditis have an abnormally low-pitched voices (females: <150, males: <100 Hz) because the mass-loaded folds oscillate at an inordinately low frequency. Females present more frequently than men and undergo phonomicrosurgical management more frequently because of the greater discrepancy from their normal fundamental frequency (180–230 Hz). Control of the medical factors with surgery will usually elevate female voices to about 150 Hz, the normal fundamental frequency for female smokers.[109]

These individuals should discontinue smoking, have their reflux controlled, and should undergo preoperative vocal therapy before undergoing a procedure. The technique for the procedure is based on raising a thin epithelial microflap after incising the mucosa near the vestibular fold. A microscissors is used for the initial incision unless there is prominent subepithelial vascular injection, in which case the CO_2 laser can be advantageous. The gelatinous hypertrophied SLP should then be carefully contoured and reduced to a more normal volume. This can be done by suctioning or by direct removal. Great care must be taken not to overreduce the SLP, which results in an inordinately stiff vocal system.[109] **The vocal ligament should never be visualized directly, because this would indicate that all of the SLP has been removed.** Overreduction of the SLP and associated epithelial stiffness can result in a severely strained harsh voice since these individuals already employ high subglottal pressures to drive their floppy mass-loaded folds. Vocally, it is preferable to leave a larger fold than to create a visually pleasing smaller fold.

Once the SLP has been reduced, the epithelium is redraped and trimmed appropriately. The author has ascribed to the philosophy that both vocal folds can be resected in one procedure if the incisions are confined to the superior surface of the vocal folds. This approach was noted to be efficacious[109] and not associated with complications.[109,122] If there is keratotic or dysplastic epithelium, it should be excised and sent to pathology for histopathological analysis. After an initial period of vocal rest (10–14 days) patients receive vocal therapy and must be monitored closely. Preventing recurrence depends on modification of the predisposing factors, especially smoking.

Case 9A

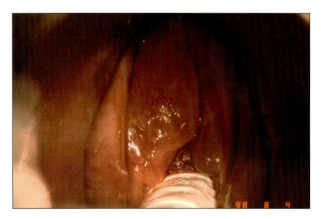

Fig 9–1. (4×) This female presented with severe polypoid corditis "Reinke's edema." She had obstructive laryngeal sleep apnea, as well as a fundamental frequency of approximately 80 Hz. (Courtesy of Endocraft LLC.)

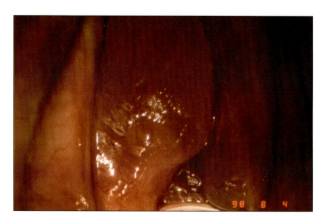

Fig 9–2. (7×) Figure 9–1 at higher magnification. Note, there is no discernible glottal aperture. (Courtesy of Endocraft LLC.)

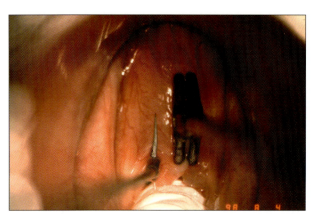

Fig 9–3. (4×) A straight triangular flap forceps is utilized to grasp the lesion and retract it, so that the epithelium is on tension. Then, an upturned microscissors is utilized to begin a superior-surface epithelial cordotomy. (Courtesy of Endocraft LLC.)

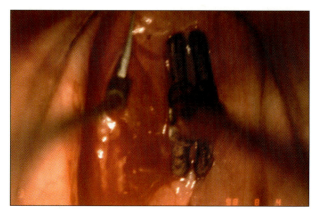

Fig 9–4. (7×) The microscissors is utilized to advance the epithelial incision anteriorly. (Courtesy of Endocraft LLC.)

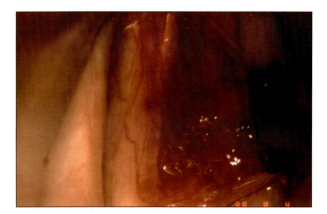

Fig 9–5. (7×) The epithelial microflap is then retracted to reveal the myxoid tissue of the SLP. (Courtesy of Endocraft LLC.)

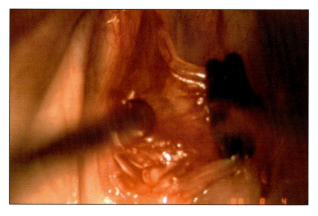

Fig 9–6. (7×) A micro-suction is used to remove the relatively acellular swollen tissue for more normal contouring. (Courtesy of Endocraft LLC.)

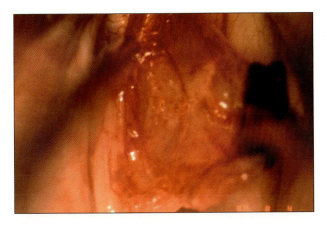

Fig 9–7. (7×) Suctioning the redundant SLP is maintained along the basement membrane surface to avoid over-reduction of this tissue, which can lead to severe hoarseness. (Courtesy of Endocraft LLC.)

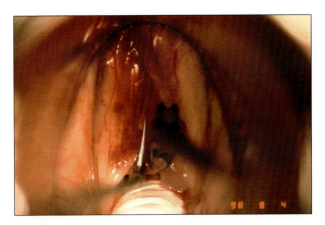

Fig 9–8. (4×) An upturned scissors is utilized to trim the redundant epithelium. (Courtesy of Endocraft LLC.)

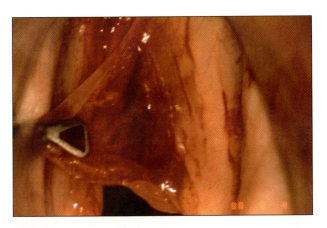

Fig 9–9. (7×) The prior procedure is being performed on the right. Note the translucent epithelium. (Courtesy of Endocraft LLC.)

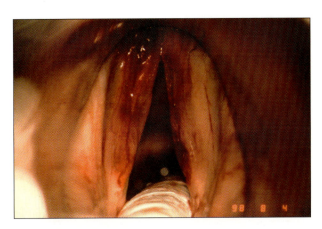

Fig 9–10. (4×) The resection has been completed. Note the tremendous improvement from the initial state. (Courtesy of Endocraft LLC.)

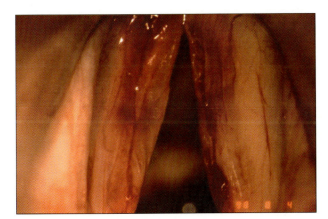

Fig 9–11. (7×) Figure 9–10 at higher magnification. There is excellent apposition of the epithelial edges and the vocal folds are more appropriately contoured. (Courtesy of Endocraft LLC.)

Case 9B

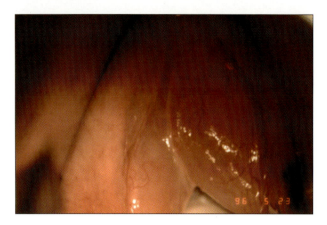

Fig 9–12. (7×) Severe polypoid corditis with almost no discernible glottal aperture.

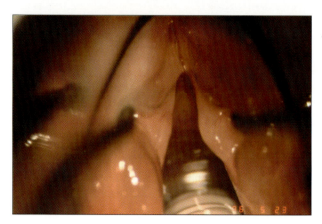

Fig 9–13. (7×) The majority of the swollen tissue is on the superior surface of the vocal fold, and this can be appreciated when the redundant tissue is retracted laterally.

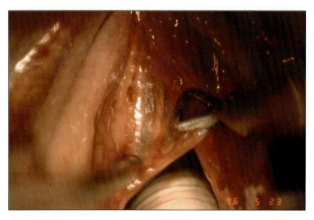

Fig 9–14. (7×) After an epithelial cordotomy has been done on the left, the suction is utilized along the basement membrane of the microflap to more appropriately contour the vocal fold.

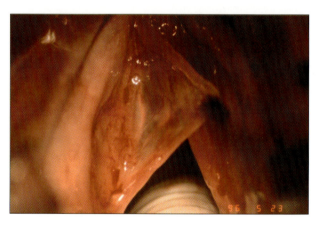

Fig 9–15. (7×) The epithelial microflap is retracted to help determine how much redundant mucosa should be resected.

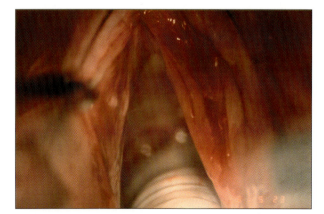

Fig 9–16. (7×) The microflap is also redraped to help make the determination of the magnitude of the epithelial excision.

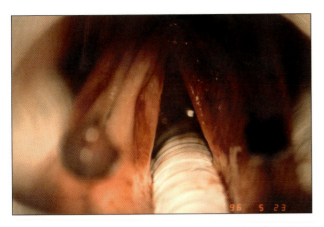

Fig 9–17. (4×) The resection has been completed on both sides.

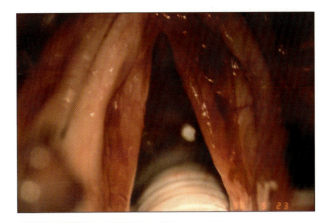

Fig 9–18. (7×) Figure 9–17 at higher magnification.

Case 9C

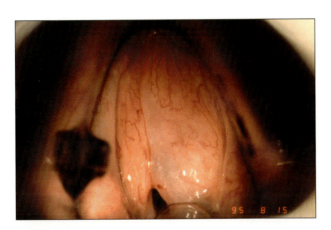

Fig 9–19. (4×) Massive polypoid corditis significantly worse on the right than on the left. This patient was a 39-year-old female who frequently runs marathons, but who smokes excessively. She also functioned as a telephone operator at a hospital.

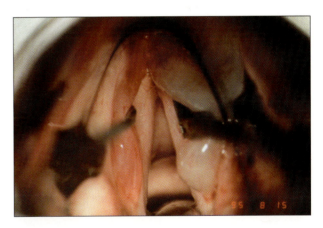

Fig 9–20. (4×) As is typically the case, the swelling was situated on the superior surface of the cord. This can be seen well when the redundant tissues are retracted laterally.

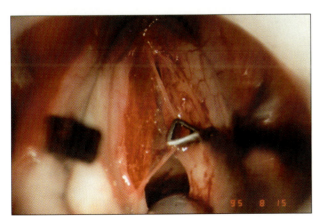

Fig 9–21. (4×) The epithelial microflap has been raised and the redundant myxoid tissue of the left SLP has been removed.

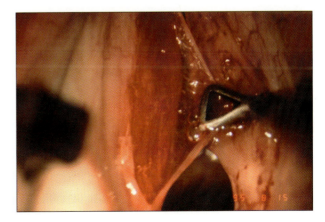

Fig 9–22. (7×) Figure 9–21 at higher magnification. Note the translucent epithelium.

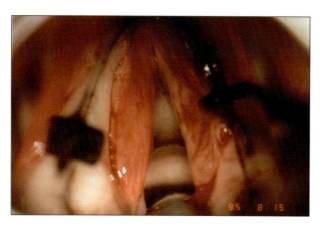

Fig 9–23. (4×) Subsequent to subepithelial resection of the myxoid tissue on the right, the epithelial microflap is draped laterally to help determine the magnitude for excision of the redundant epithelium.

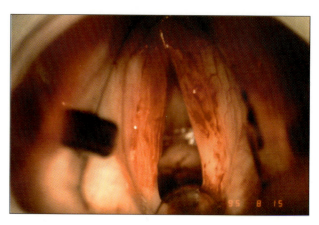

Fig 9–24. (4×) The postexcisional image shows excellent contours of the vocal folds compared to the initial presurgical state.

Case 9D

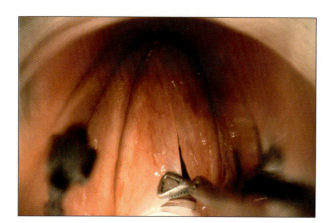

Fig 9–25. (4×) Moderate bilateral Reinke's edema. The left vocal fold is retracted with a forceps to facilitate the superior surface epithelial cordotomy.

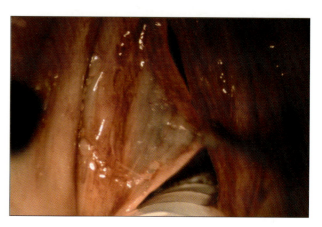

Fig 9–26. (7×) The epithelial microflap is retracted and most of the myxoid tissue has been removed by means of suctioning and cup forceps with sharp dissection as necessary.

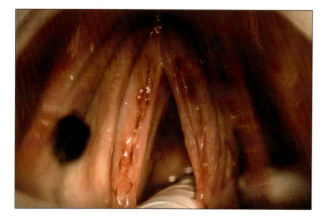

Fig 9–27. (4×) The postsurgical image with the vocal folds more appropriately contoured. There is excellent coaptation of the epithelial edges.

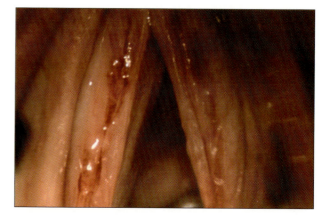

Fig 9–28. (7×) Figure 9–27 at higher magnification.

Case 9E

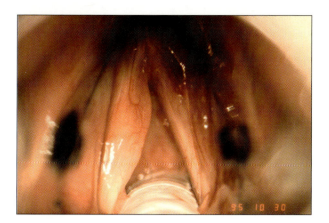

Fig 9–29. (4×) This patient had undergone stripping of her vocal folds many years prior to this presentation for polypoid corditis.

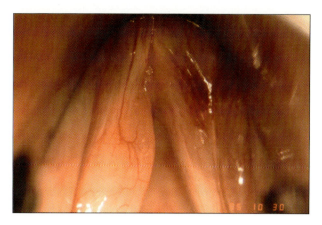

Fig 9–30. (7×) Figure 9–29 at higher magnification. Note the unusual contours, especially on the right. This resulted from recurrence of the edema in an environment of prior scarring.

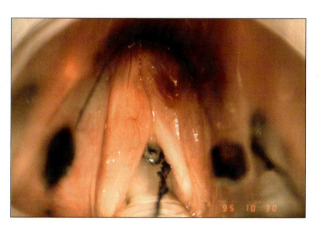

Fig 9–31. (4×) A cottonoid with saline is placed subglottically for use with the microspot CO_2 laser.

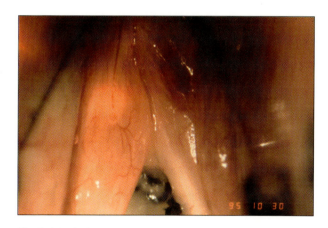

Fig 9–32. (7×) Figure 9–31 at higher magnification.

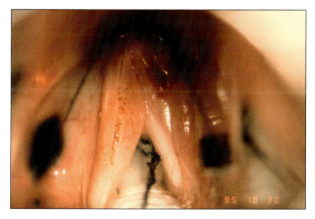

Fig 9–33. (4×) An epithelial cordotomy is performed on the left with a 0.3 mm microspot with a repeated pulse mode and 1.75 watts of power.

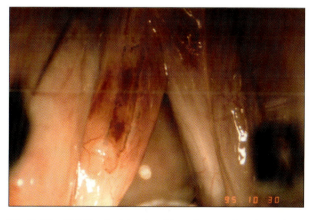

Fig 9–34. (7×) The incision is widened to suction the redundant superficial lamina propria.

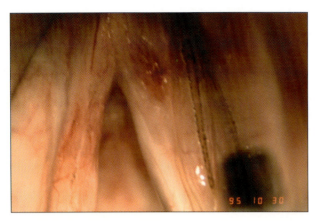

Fig 9–35. (7×) The redundant myxoid tissue has been aspirated from the left vocal fold and it is more appropriately contoured. It can be seen that there is an iatrogenic sulcus deformity through much of the right vocal fold. On its superior surface, there is significant redundant polypoid change. Therefore, the laser was used to perform an epithelial incision on this side.

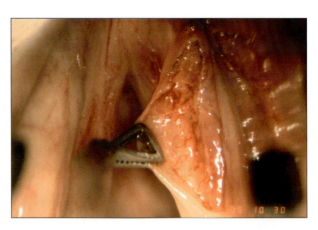

Fig 9–36. (7×) The microflap was raised to provide access for cytoreduction of the myxoid tissue.

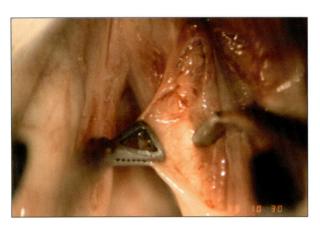

Fig 9–37. (7×) A curved dissector is used to mobilize the myxoid tissue from the basement membrane of the epithelium. It is then resected by means of a angled forceps and a microscissors.

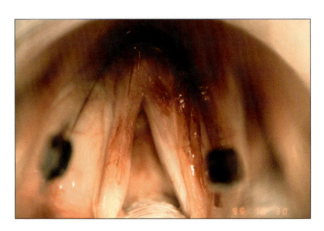

Fig 9–38. (4×) The postsurgical image with improved vocal fold contours.

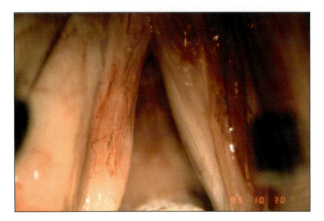

Fig 9–39. (7×) Figure 9–38 at higher magnification.

Case 9F

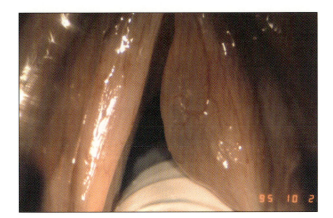

Fig 9–40. (7×) An unusual case of unilateral polypoid corditis.

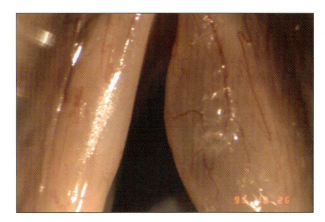

Fig 9–41. (10×) Figure 9–40 at higher magnification.

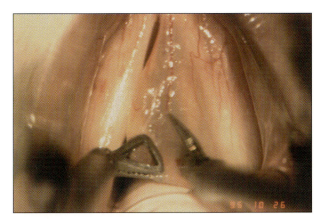

Fig 9–42. (7×) The lesion is retracted and an upturned scissors is utilized to perform a superior surface epithelial cordotomy.

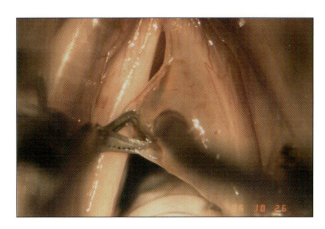

Fig 9–43. (7×) Suction is used to aspirate the redundant myxoid tissue for improved contouring.

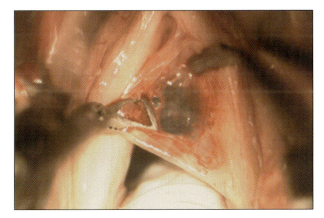

Fig 9–44. (7×) Subsequently, a curved microdissector is utilized to enhance the resection of the redundant superficial lamina propria tissue. The translucent epithelium is well seen.

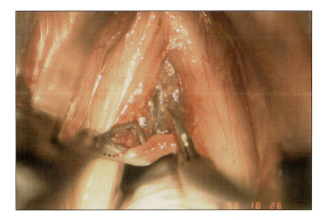

Fig 9–45. (7×) The epithelial microflap is retracted for excision of the redundant epithelium.

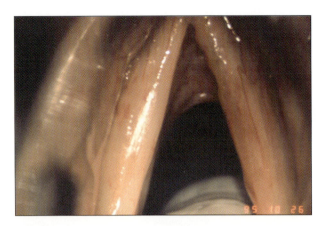

Fig 9–46. (7×) The postsurgical image delineating the significant improvement in vocal fold contour.

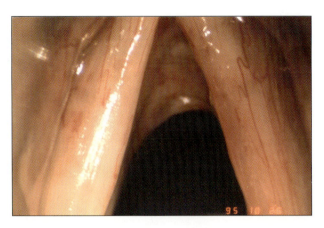

Fig 9–47. (10×) Figure 9–46 at higher magnification. The epithelial cordotomy is barely perceptible.

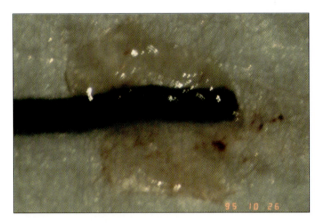

Fig 9–48. The epithelium has been placed on a cottonoid. Again, note its translucent nature.

Case 9G

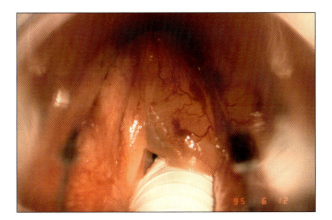

Fig 9–49. (4×) Severe asymmetric polypoid corditis. The right side is significantly larger than the left. Note the prominent subepithelial vascularity.

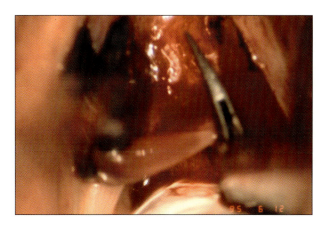

Fig 9–50. (10×) Despite the use of the microspot CO_2 laser during the epithelial incision and during part of the dissection, there was significant bleeding, which obscured precise visualization during the procedure. In this image, a microscissors is used to resect the redundant epithelium.

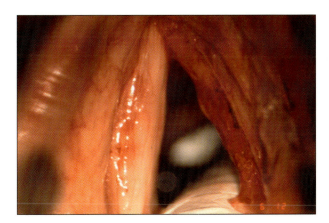

Fig 9–51. (7×) When the epithelial resection was completed, an excessive amount was removed, so that there was not good coaptation of the epithelial edges. The carbonized eschar can be seen in the midpoint of the epithelial incision. Despite the fact that the voice quality was ultimately fine, it did take longer to heal because of the need for secondary epithelialization. The voice result was ultimately unhampered because an excessive amount of SLP was not removed.

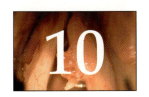

Papillomatosis

Patients, who have respiratory papillomatosis of the glottis usually present with hoarseness. Most commonly, the glottal disease is confined to the musculo-membranous region, although it is not unusual to find extension into the arytenoid, ventricle, and subglottis. The patients presented in this chapter are adults and their lesions tend to be more plaquelike than the juvenile variety. Because the disease is confined to the epithelium, great care should be taken to maximally preserve the underlying SLP. In all cases of initial presentation and in most recurrent cases, the subepithelial infusion technique with cold instrument dissection is best suited for this goal. An en bloc resection by means of a microflap can frequently be accomplished. Every attempt to perform a narrow margin excision should be made, even if this requires serial procedures (to preserve the integrity of the anterior commissure). Preliminary findings by Zeitels and Sataloff[165] suggest that resecting the disease inhibits recurrence in those who present initially and in 30% of chronic patients.

Patients with recurrent papillomatosis are tremendously challenging. When aggressive recurrent disease is encountered, the surgeon and patient must delicately balance airway safety, the effects of multiple general anesthesias, and quality of life issues, such as employment disturbance, vocal dysfunction, and procedural disability. This often requires extensive communication to ensure that the patient's and surgeon's goals are mutually aligned.

The author's preference is to use cold instruments in the majority of cases, especially on initial presentation when there is no prior scarring of the SLP. In recurrent cases, the microspot CO_2 laser is equally effective. At present, we are exploring the use of a pulsed-dye laser with these lesions as well, due to the subepithelial vascularity that accompanies these lesions. Again, preliminary observations suggest that this technology is advantageous, especially in the anterior commissure since the papilloma can be treated without completely resecting the epithelium. Although microsurgical removal is helpful in the management of this disease at present, at some point surgery will probably be replaced by one of the alternative medical treatment modalities that are currently being explored.

Case 10A

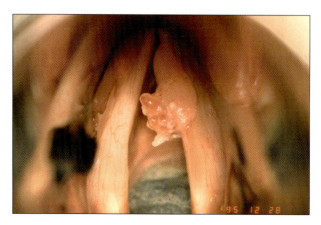

Fig 10–1. (4×) An exophytic single focus of papilloma on the right vocal fold.

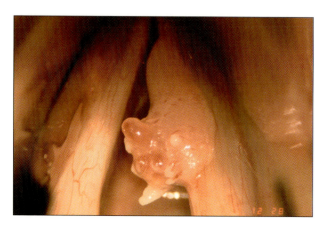

Fig 10–2. (7×) Figure 10–1 at higher magnification.

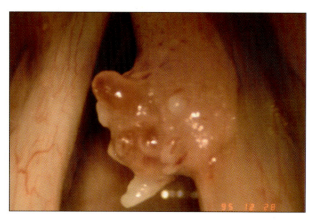

Fig 10–3. (10×) Figure 10–1 at even higher magnification.

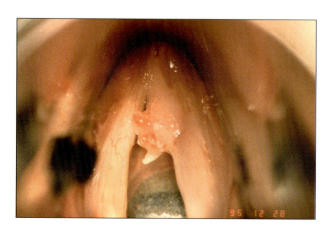

Fig 10–4. (4×) Subepithelial infusion of saline and 1/10,000 epinephrine has been placed into the SLP in the right vocal fold.

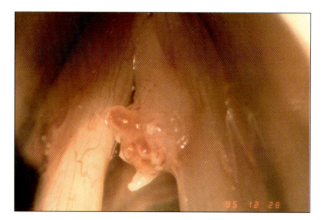

Fig 10–5. (7×) Figure 10–4 at higher magnification. Note the lateral edge of the lesion has been medialized.

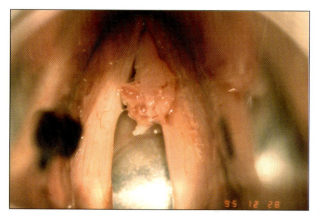

Fig 10–6. (4×) A perimeter incision has been made around the lateral aspect of the lesion.

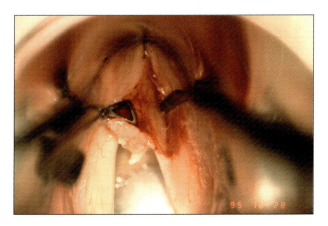

Fig 10–7. (4×) The lesion is retracted as a microflap and a dissector is used to sweep the superficial lamina propria from the basement membrane back to the patient. Note the minimal bleeding secondary to the infusion.

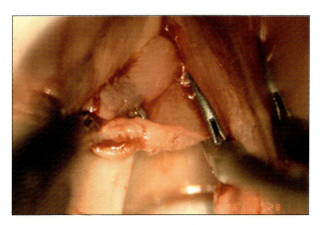

Fig 10–8. (7×) The microflap containing the lesion is retracted and an upturned scissors is used to complete the excision.

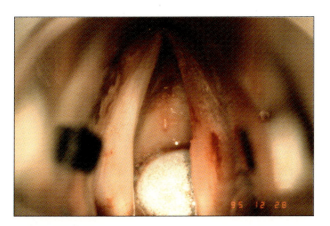

Fig 10–9. (4×) The lesion has been completely resected.

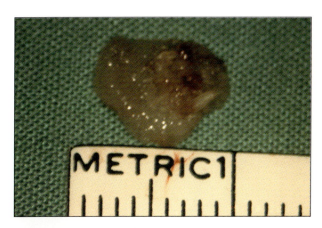

Fig 10–10. The specimen is resected en bloc and sent to the pathologist on a carrier for whole mount sectioning.

Case 10B

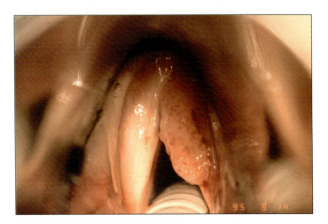

Fig 10–11. (4×) The diffuse single focus of papilloma covering the superior and medial surface of the right musculomembranous vocal fold.

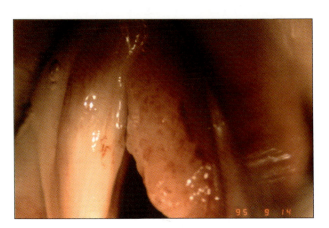

Fig 10–12. (7×) Figure 10–11 at higher magnification.

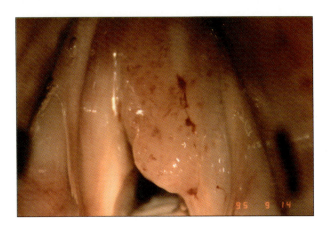

Fig 10–13. (7×) A subepithelial infusion of saline epinephrine has been performed. Note the smaller glottal aperture.

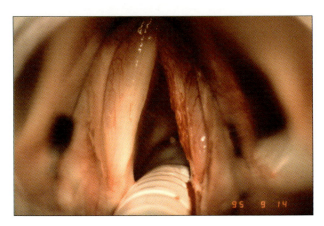

Fig 10–14. (4×) The lesion has been resected in its entirety with maximal preservation of the underlying superficial lamina propria.

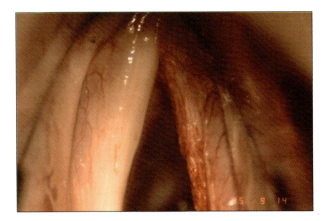

Fig 10–15. (7×) Figure 10–14 at higher magnification. Note the intact microvasculature of the SLP.

Case 10C

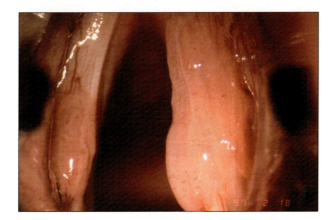

Fig 10–16. (7×) Bilateral papillomatous lesions of the vocal folds. The lesion on the right is much larger and covers most of the medial and superior surface of the vocal fold.

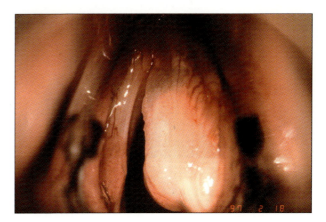

Fig 10–17. (4×) A subepithelial infusion of saline and adrenaline has been performed. Note the narrowing of the glottal aperture and the vasoconstriction of the microvasculature.

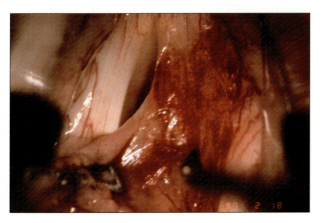

Fig 10–18. (7×) The microflap encompassing the papillomatous mass is retracted and a curved dissector is being utilized to sweep the normal superficial lamina propria back to the patient.

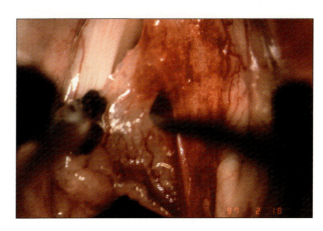

Fig 10–19. (7×) There is further dissection of the superficial lamina propria more anteriorly.

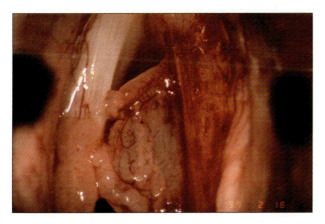

Fig 10–20. (7×) The microflap is well seen and no residual papilloma is seen on the surface of the right vocal fold.

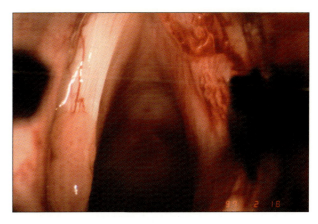

Fig 10–21. (7×) A triangular microflap forceps is utilized to retract the microflap laterally to determine the caudal extent of the disease.

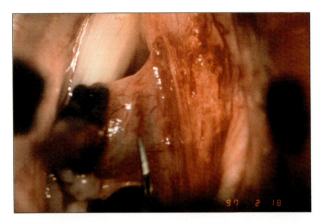

Fig 10–22. (7×) The microflap is retracted and an upturned scissors can now be used to resect the papillomatous mass en bloc and with clear margins.

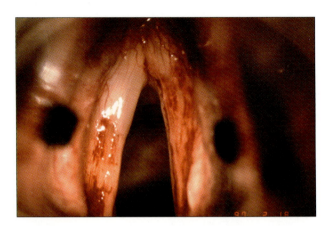

Fig 10–23. (4×) Both lesions have been resected.

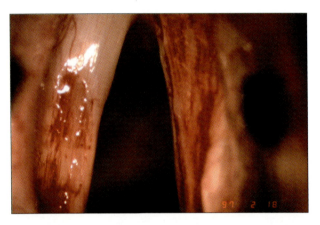

Fig 10–24. (7×) Higher magnification of Figure 10–23 showing maximal preservation of the normal superficial lamina propria with its microvasculature.

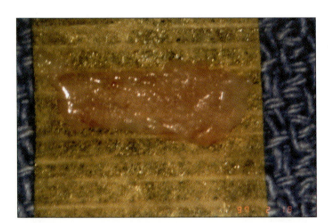

Fig 10–25. The specimen is mounted on a carrier for whole mount sectioning.

Case 10D

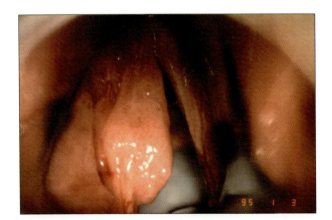

Fig 10–26. (4×) A large papillomatous lesion encompassing most of the surface of the left vocal fold.

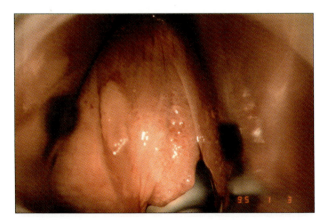

Fig 10–27. (4×) A subepithelial infusion has been performed. This medializes the edge of the lesion, so that it can be resected with a clear margin. It also brings a focus of papilloma that was in the ventricle into view for resection.

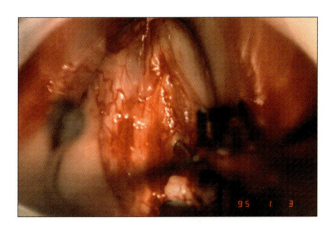

Fig 10–28. (4×) A straight triangular forceps is used to retract the microflap and a curved dissector is used to sweep the normal SLP back to the patient.

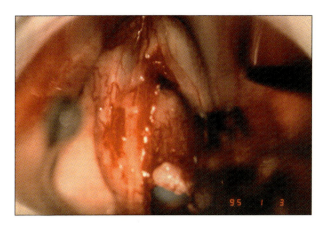

Fig 10–29. (4×) Further dissection of the microflap is performed anteriorly.

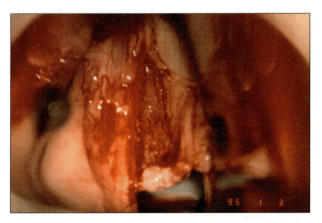

Fig 10–30. (4×) The microflap is still attached at its caudal margin.

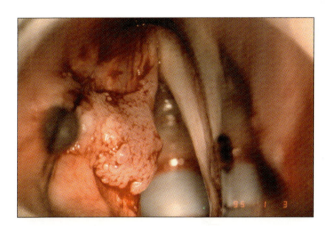

Fig 10–31. (4×) The microflap is retracted so that the caudal edge of the disease can be determined.

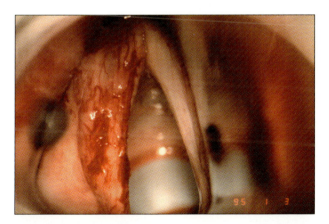

Fig 10–32. (4×) The disease has been resected with maximal preservation of normal epithelium and normal SLP.

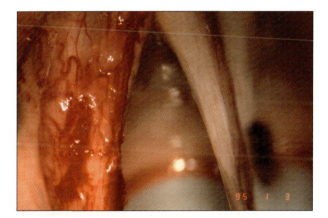

Fig 10–33. (7×) Figure 10–32 at higher magnification. Note the intact residual microvasculature of the SLP.

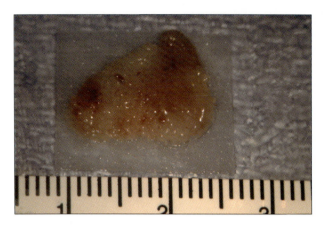

Fig 10–34. The lesion is mounted on a carrier for whole mount sectioning.

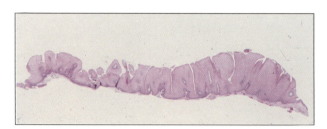

Fig 10–35. (5×) H&E of the resected specimen. Note that there is almost no superficial lamina propria adjacent to the basement membrane and a clear margin with normal epithelium at the edge of the papillomatous lesion.

Case 10E

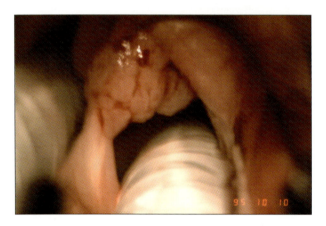

Fig 10–36. (7×) An anterior papillomatous mass that is not well seen.

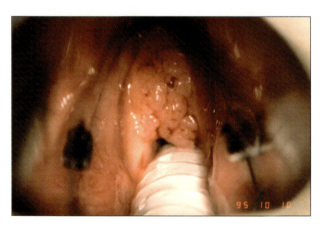

Fig 10–37. (4×) After external counterpressure with 1-inch silk tape and a laryngeal cushion, the lesion is well visualized.

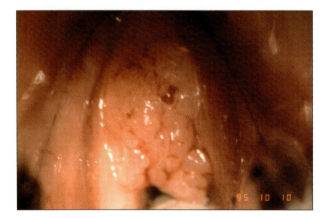

Fig 10–38. (7×) Higher magnification of Figure 10–37.

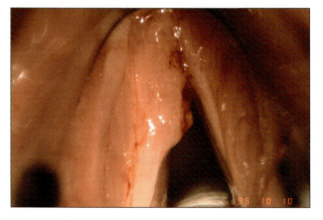

Fig 10–39. (7×) A portion of the mass is amputated to facilitate a more precise excision near the base. The CO_2 laser with the microspot is utilized for this purpose.

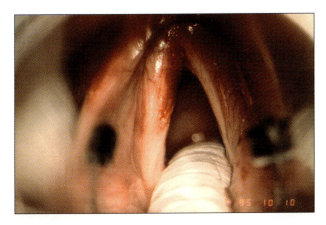

Fig 10–40. (4×) The left-sided lesion has been resected by means of cold instruments.

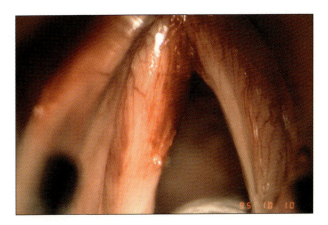

Fig 10–41. (7×) Figure 10–40 at higher magnification.

Case 10F

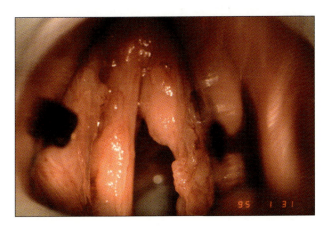

Fig 10–42. (4×) There is diffuse foci of papilloma on both musculo-membranous vocal folds and vestibular folds.

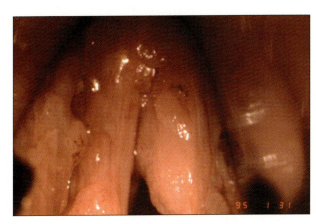

Fig 10–43. (7×) A subepithelial infusion has been performed into the right vocal fold.

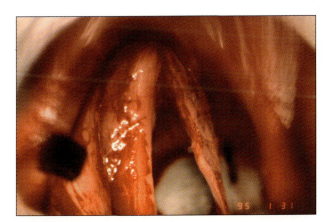

Fig 10–44. (4×) Most of the disease has been resected. To avoid webbing, epithelium is left intact with some disease anteriorly on the left.

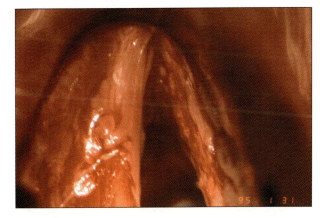

Fig 10–45. (7×) Figure 10–44 at higher magnification.

Case 10G

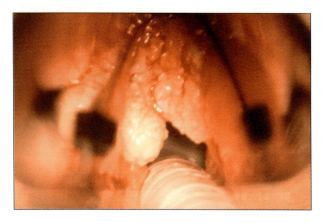

Fig 10–46. (4×) Diffuse severe papilloma covering most of both musculo-membranous vocal folds.

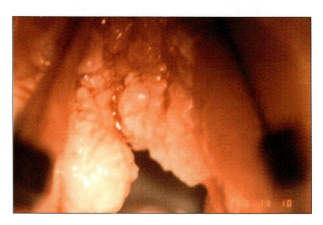

Fig 10–47. (10×) Figure 10–46 at higher magnification.

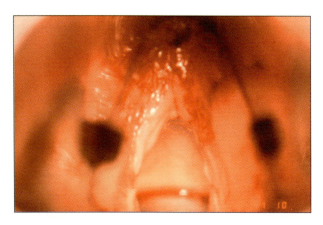

Fig 10–48. (4×) Most of the disease has been resected. Epithelium has been left intact on the left anteriorly and medially to avoid webbing.

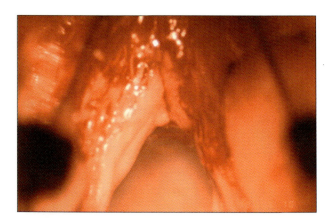

Fig 10–49. (7×) Figure 10–48 at higher magnification. The residual disease must be resected at a second stage procedure.

Case 10H

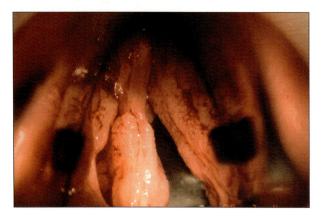

Fig 10–50. (4×) Diffuse papilloma on the true vocal folds and vestibular folds.

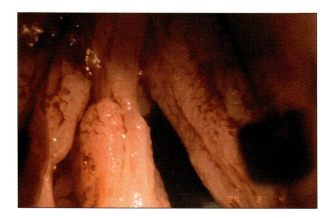

Fig 10–51. (7×) Figure 10–50 at higher magnification.

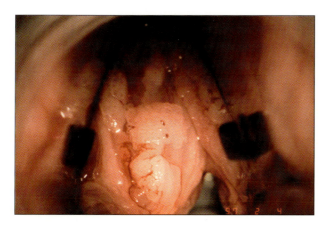

Fig 10–52. (4×) A subepithelial infusion of saline and adrenaline has been performed on the left.

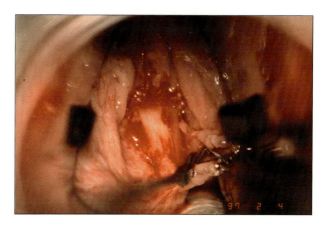

Fig 10–53. (4×) The largest focus on the left is being resected as a microflap.

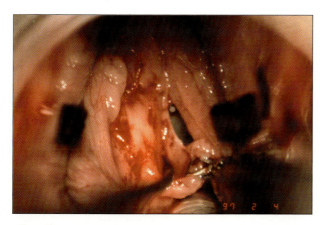

Fig 10–54. (4×) The microflap is retracted and a dissector is used to preserve the SLP.

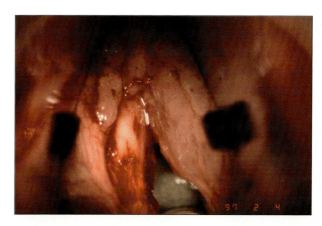

Fig 10–55. (4×) The large focus on the left has been removed and a subepithelial infusion has been performed on the right.

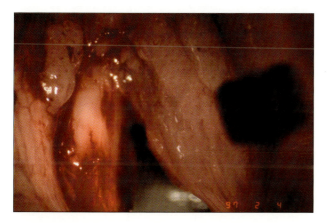

Fig 10–56. (7×) Figure 10–55 at higher magnification.

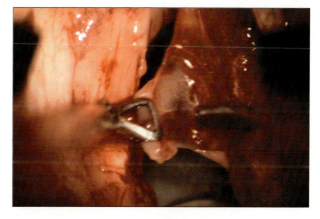

Fig 10–57. (7×) The superficial lamina propria is being dissected from the basement membrane from the right papillomatous microflap.

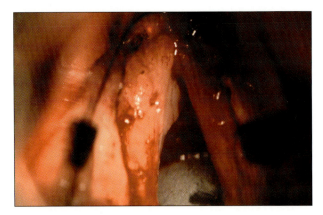

Fig 10–58. (4×) Virtually all of the papillomatous epithelium on the right vocal fold has been removed with maximal preservation of the SLP. Much of the left-sided disease has been removed as well. Cold instruments were utilized.

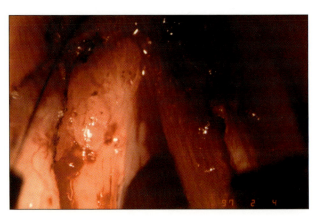

Fig 10–59. (7×) Figure 10–58 at higher magnification. The microspot CO_2 laser was utilized to resect the vestibular fold lesions. Residual disease was resected at a second stage.

Case 10I

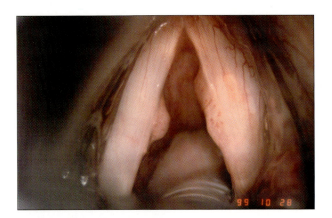

Fig 10–60. (4×) Bilateral sessile papillomatous masses are seen on the medial surface of both vocal folds. (Courtesy of Endocraft LLC.)

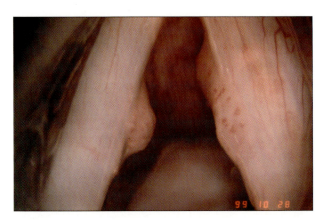

Fig 10–61. (7×) Figure 10–60 seen at higher magnification. (Courtesy of Endocraft LLC.)

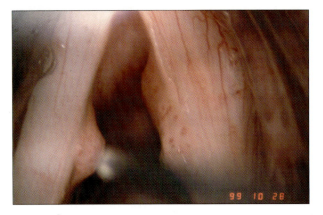

Fig 10–62. (7×) The fiber of a pulsed-dye laser is directed at the left lesion to coagulate the subepithelial microvasculature. (Courtesy of Endocraft LLC.)

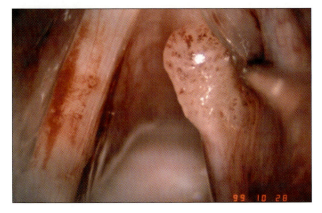

Fig 10–63. (7×) The left-sided lesion has been resected. The microvasculature of the right lesion has been coagulated by the laser, which is well seen as the fold is retracted. (Courtesy of Endocraft LLC.)

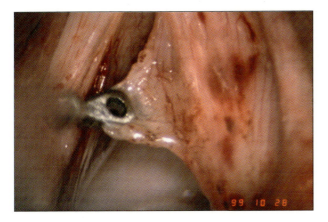

Fig 10–64. (7×) The diseased epithelium can be resected as a precise microflap because the microvasculature of the SLP is coagulated. Some subepithelial ecchymosis can be seen in the right vocal fold. (Courtesy of Endocraft LLC.)

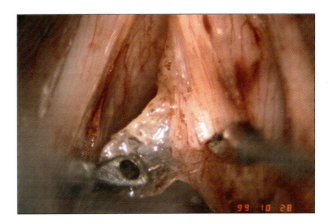

Fig 10–65. (7×) The epithelial microflap is further dissected with a microscissors, also with minimal bleeding. (Courtesy of Endocraft LLC.)

Case 10J

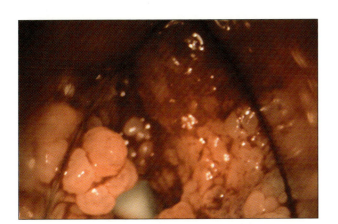

Fig 10–66. (4×) Massive papillomatous changes are seen in the glottal introitus. (Courtesy of Endocraft LLC.)

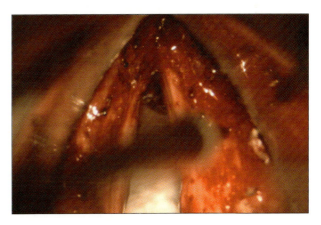

Fig 10–67. (4×) The pulsed-dye laser is used to ablate the microvasculature to enhance the precision of the cold instrument resection of the disease. (Courtesy of Endocraft LLC.)

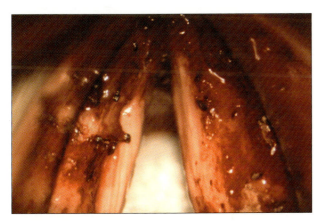

Fig 10–68. (4×) Most of the disease has been resected. (Courtesy of Endocraft LLC.)

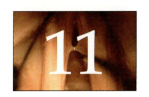

11

Sulcus, Scar, Synechia, and Web

SULCUS DEFORMITIES AND EPITHELIAL SCARRING

Vocal fold sulcus deformities refer to areas of nonvibratory epithelium, which are often adherent to the underlying laminae propria. It may take the form of a circular pit or pocket, a linear depression, or a more broad-based plaque-like area (sulcus vergeture). The consistent characteristic of these lesions is the loss of normal superficial lamina propria, which results in decreased epithelial pliability and reduced mucosal wave vibration. With larger sulcus deformities, the clinician will be able to observe the vibratory stiffness of the epithelium. Smaller pocket sulcus deformities are often noted intraoperatively when the patient is undergoing phonomicrosurgery for a more observable lesion.

A clinical clue that a sulcus may be present is the finding of asymmetric swelling of a vocal fold that appears situated primarily on the medial or subcordal surface. In this instance, the intact SLP at the caudal margin of the sulcus becomes swollen in association with chronic hoarseness and commensurate hyperfunction. A sulcus vergeture will often show a flattened medial surface with diffuse swelling at the perimeter where SLP is still present. This often leads to a bowed excavated contour along the medial surface of the vocal fold edge, which is exacerbated by hyperkinetic attempts to close the musculo-membranous glottal gap by means of lateral cricoarytenoid hyperfunction.

Boucheyer[145] has suggested that some pocket sulcus deformities occur as a result of a ruptured cyst. This is consistent with the author's observations in which several cases were encountered in which surgery ensued because of a unilateral cyst and under high magnification a small sulcus was noted on the contralateral side. However, recently an epidermoid cyst was noted simultaneously with a sulcus suggesting a coincident relationship rather than a causal one (see Figure 7–39).

Treatment of sulcus deformities varies based on the severity of the anatomical deformity and the vocal deficit. Voice therapy is an integral component of management because patients must learn strategies to optimize their vocal function by reducing excessive hyperfunctional strain, which has diminished advantages in a stiff vocal system. Typically, the patient must relax the vocal musculature and accept more monotone speech with limitations of maximal range tasks.

In pocket sulci, phonomicrosurgical intervention is based on excision of the epithelial segment, which is adherent to the vocal ligament, while preserving all residual normal

superficial lamina propria. As to be expected, the vocal outcome subsequent to the resection of confined smaller pocket sulci is superior to large vergeture deformities. In the former, one can often achieve primary apposition of the normal SLP and excellent coaptation of the normal epithelium. At times these goals are facilitated by suture placement.

Sulcus vergeture deformities behave similarly to broad-based epithelial scarring as can be seen subsequent to poorly controlled mucosal stripping. The author has had no success in vocally improving patients after raising a microflap and laying it back down or by incising the microflap. Presumably this is because the anatomical deficit is the loss of SLP. Therefore augmentation of this layer has been done by raising a microflap, suturing it in place, and then placing lysed axillary fat within the cavity. This has resulted in some improvement in vocal function acoustically, aerodynamically, and stroboscopically; however the procedure is technically very difficult. Furthermore, the fat does not have the viscoelasticity of normal SLP and undergoes variable resorption.

Spontaneous epithelial scarring from vocal abuse and iatrogenic scarring from laryngeal trauma (ie, prolonged intubation and other laryngeal surgery) simulate a sulcus vergeture and are quite common. This has led to significant surgical research in this area so that the ideal substance to augment lost SLP should be identified in the near future.[166,167]

Many presbyphonic patients have extensive sulcus vergeture deformities of the medial vocal fold surface. The bowed concave contour of the medial edge may not be the result of underlying muscular atrophy but rather tissue (SLP) loss with compensatory lateral cricoarytenoid hyperfunction. Therefore, this is often a hyperkinetic/hyperfunctional disorder, rather than a hypokinetic one with muscle atrophy.

SYNECHIA

Synechia are typically the result of prior laryngeal surgery or trauma and can usually be corrected by resection, with minimal difficulty unless accompanied by a dense scar and/or stenosis.

WEB

Small anterior mucosal microwebs are commonly encountered in adults and typically do not require intervention. If they are discovered intraoperatively, they can be carefully incised; however, it is not clear whether this results in a substantive improvement in vocal function. Fibrous anterior glottal webs in adults typically occur as a result of prior microsurgery of the vocal folds, unlike congenital webs in the pediatric population. These adult webs are typically accompanied by loss of underlying vocal fold length and underlying SLP. When it becomes profound, the airway can be restricted and these webs must be repaired endoscopically or transcervically. To prevent recurrence, a stent, keel, or prosthesis must usually be placed until epithelialization occurs.

The author has not found that lengthening foreshortened vocal folds that accompany a moderate to small acquired anterior web improves vocal quality, despite the successful use of elegant epithelial flaps. With acquired webs, the foreshortened vocal fold usually signifies that underlying SLP is missing and that the lengthened reconstructed area continues to be nonvibratory. Furthermore, more surgery may increase the size of the nonvibratory segment in an attempt to lengthen the vocal fold. Therefore, excision and reconstruction of anterior webs for vocal indications are not encouraged unless there is a plan to reconstruct the lost SLP. The patient must be fully apprised that phonosurgical reconstruction of an anterior commissure web will require staged procedures similar to repairing a burn wound.

Case 11A

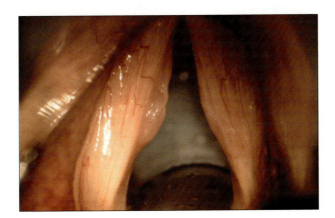

Fig 11–1. (7×) There is diffuse vascular injection bilaterally. A sessile polypoid swelling is seen emanating from the medial surface of the left vocal fold. A similar finding is noted on the right; however, it is less prominent. The swelling begins discretely on the medial surface and extends to the subcordal surface.

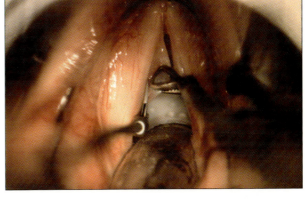

Fig 11–2. (4×) The patient is noted to have a left sulcus deformity. The swelling that is seen on the medial and subcordal surface is the result of chronic hyperfunction and dilation of the normal superficial lamina propria, as the momentum of the vibration is restricted by the epithelial adherence on the superior and upper medial surface of the vocal fold. An upturned scissors is utilized to perform an epithelial cordotomy.

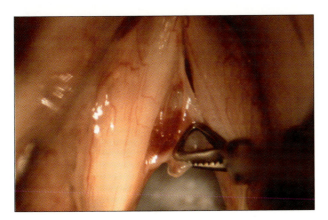

Fig 11–3. (7×) The epithelial microflap is retracted and the redundant myxoid tissue and epithelium are delineated.

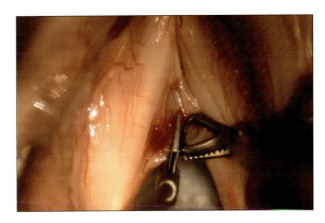

Fig 11–4. (7×) The redundant epithelium is excised by means of an upturned microscissors.

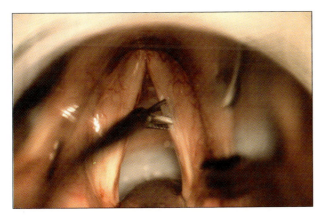

Fig 11–5. (4×) An angle triangular forceps is placed in the right-sided sulcus.

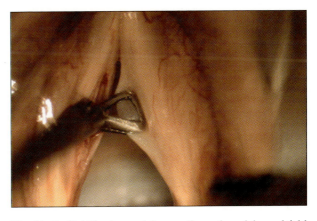

Fig 11–6. (7×) The base of the swollen subcordal vocal fold is retracted.

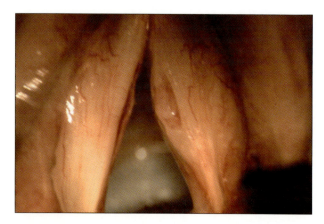

Fig 11–7. (7×) A subepithelial infusion is done to enhance the precision of the sulcus resection. It does an excellent job of delineating this pocket sulcus deformity. The base of the sulcus, which is attached to the vocal ligament, is seen as a deep depression. The distended normal superficial lamina propria exaggerates the appearance of the deformity.

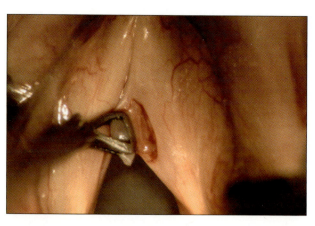

Fig 11–8. (7×) An epithelial incision is made at the edge of the sulcus superiorly. This allows for sharp dissection of the epithelial sulcus with maximum preservation of the residual normal SLP.

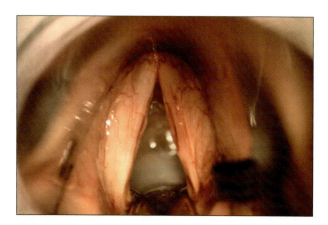

Fig 11–9. (4×) Both sulcus deformities have been resected.

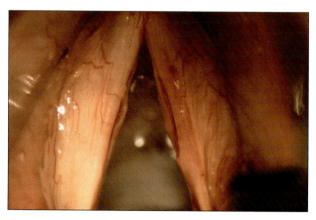

Fig 11–10. (7×) There is excellent coaptation of the epithelial edges considering the nature of the initial deformity. He healed well and had a dramatic improvement in voice quality.

Case 11B

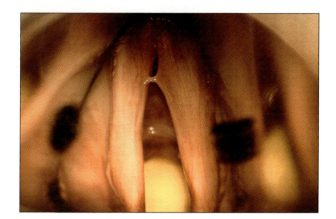

Fig 11–11. (4×) This is a 75-year-old minister with a history of long-term hoarseness. He had never had a previous intubation or vocal fold microsurgery. He is a vocal overuser. A synechia is noted anteriorly between the musculomembranous vocal folds.

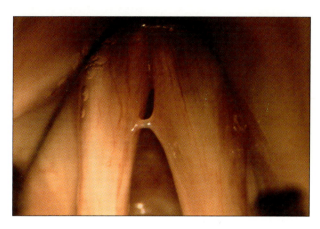

Fig 11–12. (7×) Figure 11–11 at higher magnification.

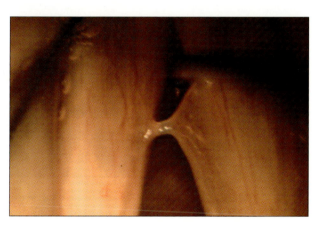

Fig 11–13. (10×) The right vocal fold is retracted anteriorly to better delineate the synechia.

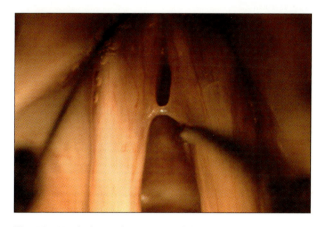

Fig 11–14. (7×) Another image of the prior lesion.

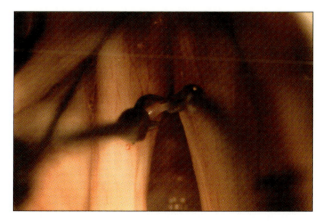

Fig 11–15. (7×) The synechia is grasped with a microalligator forceps and a microscissors is used to amputate the epithelial attachment on the left.

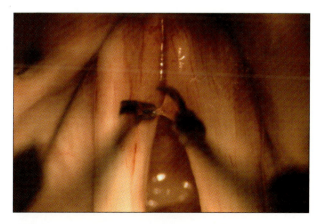

Fig 11–16. (7×) Subsequent to this, a similar excision is performed on the contralateral side.

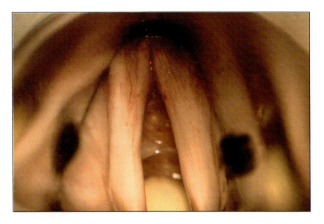

Fig 11–17. (4×) The postoperative image subsequent to excision of the synechia.

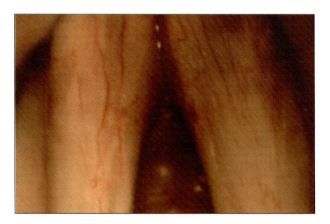

Fig 11–18. (10×) Figure 11–17 at higher magnification.

Case 11C

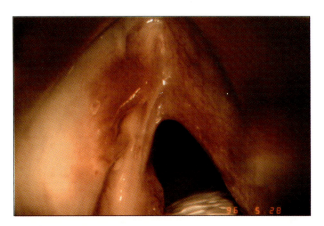

Fig 11–19. (7×) This patient has undergone multiple procedures for papillomatosis of the vestibular folds and the true vocal folds. Diffuse scarring is noted in both regions. Most prominent is a synechia between the left vestibular fold and the superior surface of the left true fold, which could potentially obscure papillomatous changes in the ventricle. A focus of papilloma is seen medial to the left arytenoid.

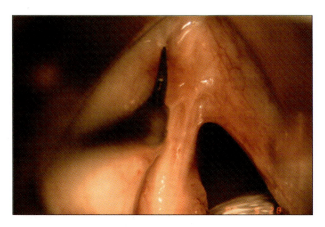

Fig 11–20. (7×) An upturned scissors is utilized to incise the synechia along the vestibular fold.

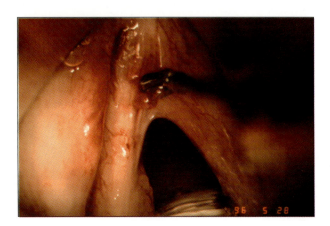

Fig 11–21. (7×) The residual soft tissue from the synechia is grasped with a cup forceps and excised. It was not felt that incising the anterior glottal web would improve his vocal quality or enhance the management of his papillomatous disease, so it was not disturbed. The focus of papilloma along the left arytenoid was subsequently resected.

Case 11D

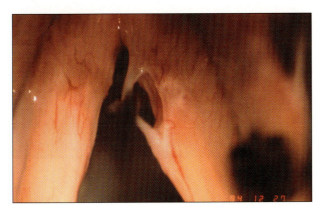

Fig 11–22. (7×) This patient underwent vocal fold surgery 15 years previously; however, there were no records as to the nature of the problem. At this time, a synechia (epithelial bridge) is noted along the right vocal fold, which is being retracted by a curved dissector. A sulcus deformity is also noted on the left.

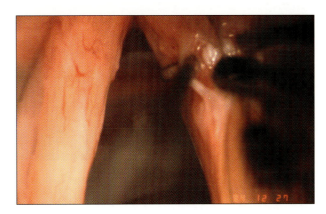

Fig 11–23. (7×) Retraction of the edge of the epithelium reveals a residual sulcus deformity on the right as well, with keratin at its base.

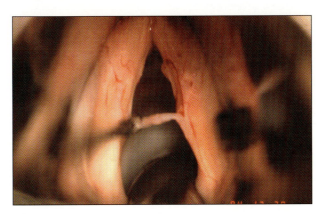

Fig 11–24. (4×) The synechia is excised with a microscissors.

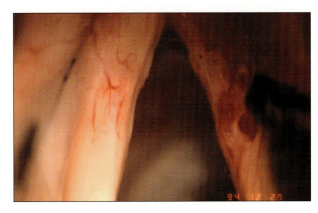

Fig 11–25. (7×) A dissector is used to better define the sulcus. The sites of attachment of the synechia are used to complete an epithelial excision for resection of the sulcus.

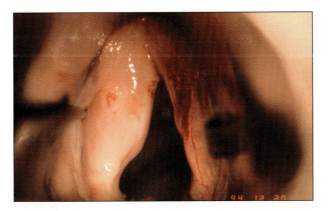

Fig 11–26. (4×) The sulcus on the right has been resected. A subepithelial infusion is being performed on the left. The needle is seen at the lateral aspect of the vocal fold near the vestibular fold.

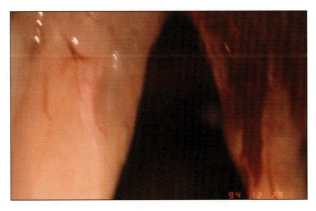

Fig 11–27. (10×) The infusion allows for excellent visualization of the sulcus deformity on the left.

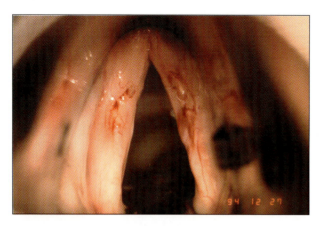

Fig 11–28. (4×) The sulcus deformities of both vocal folds have been resected with maximal preservation of normal epithelium and normal SLP.

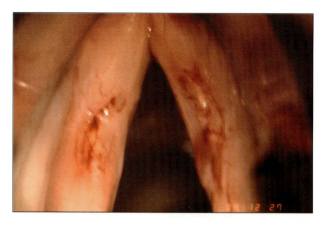

Fig 11–29. (7×) Figure 11–28 at higher magnification.

Case 11E

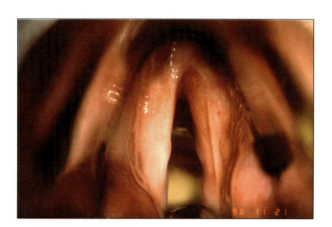

Fig 11–30. (4×) This patient presented after having her vocal folds stripped for polypoid corditis. She was extremely hoarse. Scarring of the vocal fold epithelium was noted bilaterally.

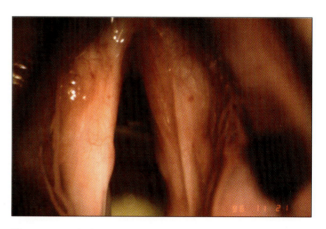

Fig 11–31. (7×) A web was noted anteriorly. The scarring was much more severe on the right and there was no epithelial vibration or flexibility.

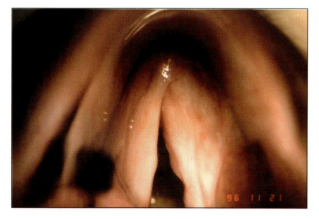

Fig 11–32. (4×) A subepithelial infusion of saline and adrenaline is done to distend the vocal fold.

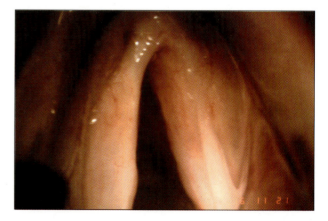

Fig 11–33. (7×) Figure 11–32 at higher magnification.

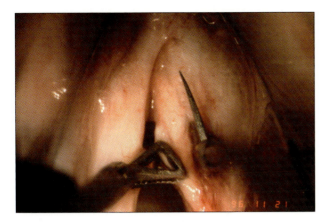

Fig 11–34. (7×) An epithelial cordotomy is performed with an upturned scissors and the microflap is retracted with an angled forceps.

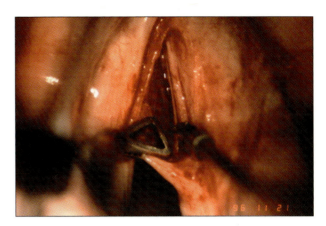

Fig 11–35. (7×) Due to the severe fibrosis, a full-length microflap is developed with a curved microscissors.

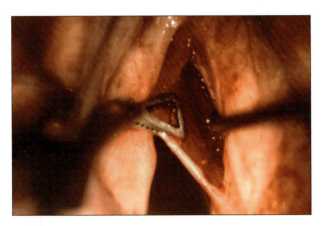

Fig 11–36. (7×) At the subcordal aspect of the vocal fold, there was less scarring and a curved dissector could be used to create a cavity.

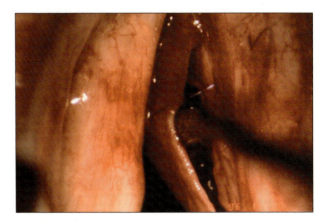

Fig 11–37. (10×) A suture has been placed in each side of the epithelium. A curved dissector is situated in the cavity to better delineate it.

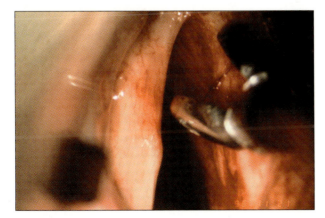

Fig 11–38. (7×) The knot is tightened by abducting the specialized forceps.

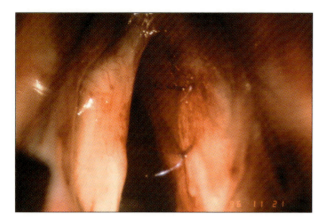

Fig 11–39. (7×) A second suture is placed more posteriorly.

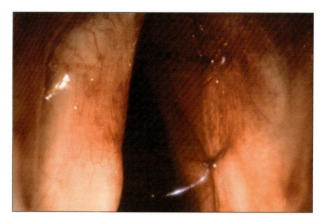

Fig 11–40. (10×) Figure 11–39 at higher magnification.

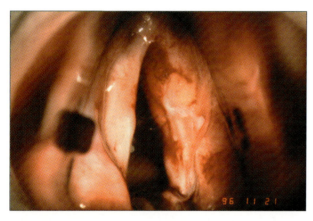

Fig 11–41. (4×) Fat has been retrieved from the right axilla and sectioned into small pieces. It is then placed under the microflap with a curved dissector.

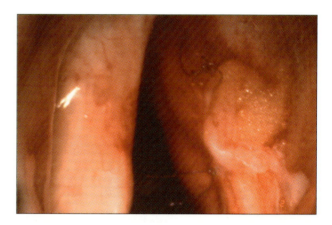

Fig 11–42. (10×) Figure 11–41 at higher magnification.

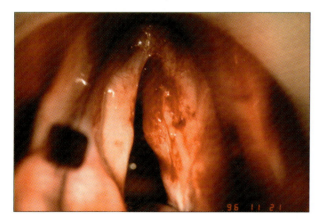

Fig 11–43. (4×) The scarred neocord on the right has now undergone augmentation of the lost SLP with axillary fat.

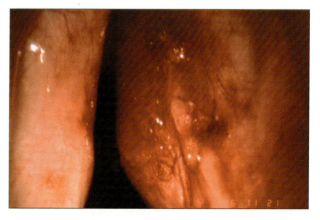

Fig 11–44. (10×) As the cavity of the subepithelial space is filled with fat, there is more inherent tension on the suture line, which maintains the fat within the cavity.

Case 11F

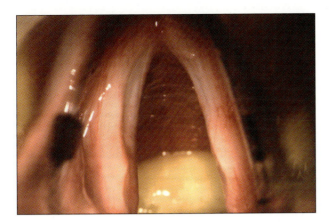

Fig 11–45. (4×) This patient presented with severe hoarseness. He has never had laryngeal trauma or vocal fold microsurgery. Bilateral medial-surface sulcus deformities are easily visible.

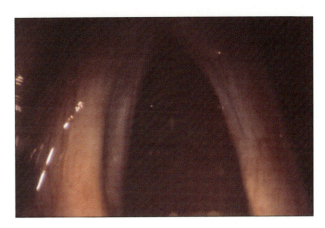

Fig 11–46. (7×) Figure 11–45 at higher magnification.

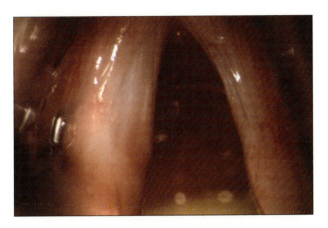

Fig 11–47. (7×) A subepithelial infusion has been performed on the left.

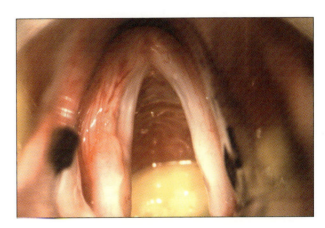

Fig 11–48. (4×) An epithelial cordotomy has been performed on the superior surface of the left vocal fold.

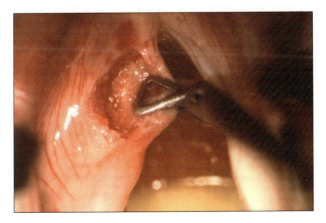

Fig 11–49. (7×) An epithelial microflap is dissected and severe scarring and fibrosis is noted.

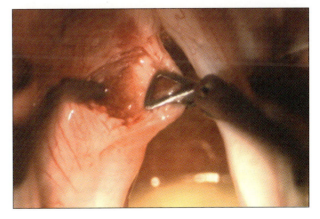

Fig 11–50. (7×) A dissector is utilized to enhance visualization of the cavity that is being developed.

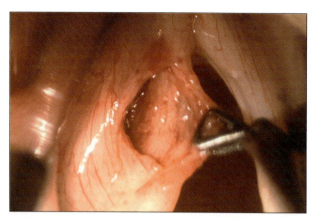

Fig 11–51. (7×) A fairly deep cavity for fat placement is now developed.

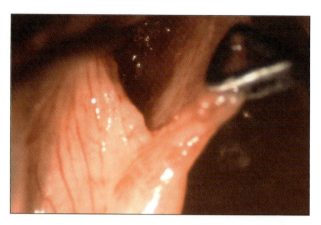

Fig 11–52. (10×) A similar image at higher magnification.

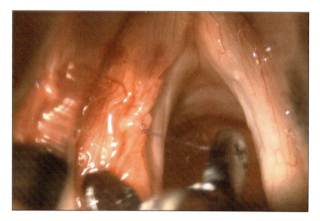

Fig 11–53. (7×) The knot from a suture in the midregion of the flap is being tightened. The phalanges of the endoscopic knot tier are opened widely to create tension on the knot.

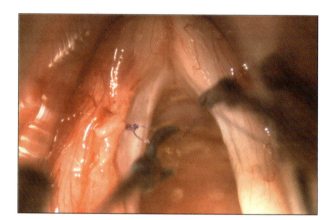

Fig 11–54. (7×) The suture is retracted with an alligator forceps and a microscissors is used to cut it.

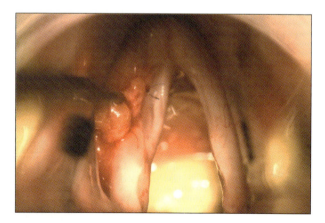

Fig 11–55. (4×) Axillary fat is being placed under the flap with a curved microdissector.

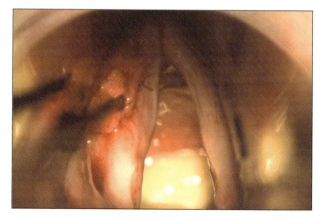

Fig 11–56. (4×) The fat has been sectioned into small lobules and the dissector is used to advance it toward the depth of the cavity.

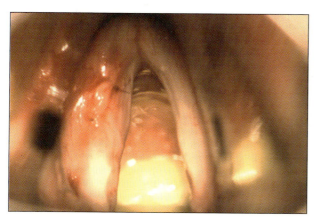

Fig 11–57. (4×) The cavity has been distended with fat. A small amount is seen at the edge of the epithelial cordotomy.

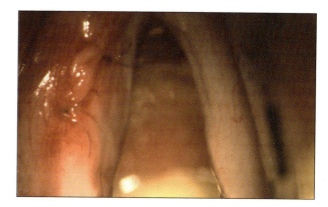

Fig 11–58. (7×) Figure 11–57 at higher magnification.

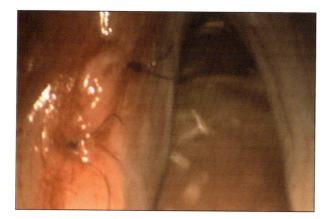

Fig 11–59. (10×) Figure 11–57 at even higher magnification.

Case 11G

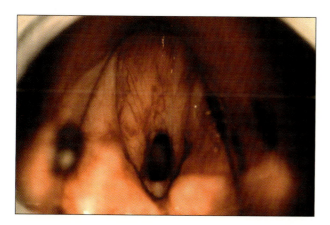

Fig 11–60. (4×) This patient has relapsing polychondritis and had undergone multiple prior microlaryngoscopic procedures for glottic stenosis. An extremely small aperture is noted posteriorly. She had nearly complete arytenoid fixation bilaterally.

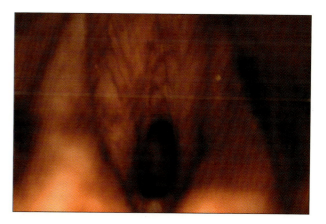

Fig 11–61. (7×) Figure 11–60 at higher magnification.

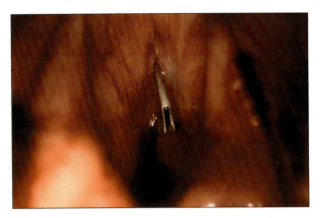

Fig 11–62. (7×) An upturned microscissors is utilized to incise the extensive web.

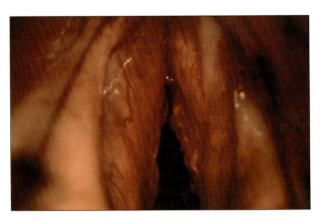

Fig 11–63. (7×) The area was extremely avascular and the segment was very long at its base near the anterior thyroid lamina.

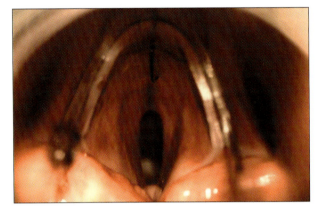

Fig 11–64. (4×) A thin sheet of Silastic was contoured for placement within the glottal introitus and sutured in place endoscopically. The patient, who had a tracheotomy, was ultimately decannulated a number of months later.

Case 11H

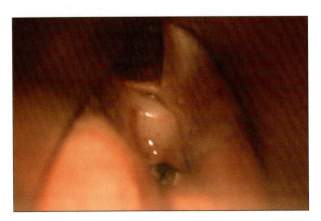

Fig 11–65. (7×) A 24-year-old female presented with more than a 20-year history of dyspnea on exertion. She underwent cardiac surgery as a child for a congenital anomaly. An interarytenoid synechia causing glottic stenosis was noted. (Courtesy of Endocraft LLC.)

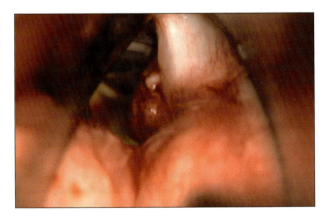

Fig 11–66. (7×) After incising the synechia with a microscissors the arytenoids separated and she has had no further airway difficulties. (Courtesy of Endocraft LLC.)

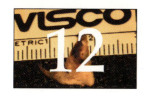

Arytenoidectomy and Posterior Cordectomy/Cordotomy

These procedures are used primarily to treat bilateral impaired mobility of the vocal folds. Patients with bilateral vocal fold paralysis can usually be distinguished from those with fixation because the former group will usually have a poor or unstable voice due to denervation. Laryngeal electromyography can be of great assistance if the diagnosis is unclear. However, great care should be taken when placing a needle in the glottal tissue if the airway is narrow and if the patient does not have a tracheotomy.

Patients should be carefully counseled that, because of the bilateral immobility, they are making a choice regarding voice quality and the airway and that the procedures permanently disturb the normal anatomy. Many of these patients developed the problem subsequent to a severe illness and a prolonged intubation. Therefore, the decision to proceed with an irreversible procedure should be approached in a deliberate fashion, especially if the patient has a fresh tracheotomy or if return of function is possible.

There are a variety of arytenoidectomy procedures in which varying amounts of cartilage and/or posterior musculomembranous vocal fold tissue are removed. The arytenoid can be excised or ablated with a laser or resected with cold instruments. It is often advantageous to leave the body of the arytenoid on the cricoid facet and to simply excise the portion of the arytenoid that is inside the airway. The operations are significantly more successful in patients who have bilateral vocal fold paralysis. The underlying soft tissue, cartilage, and joint are usually normal and heal without significant scarring and stenosis. This is not the case with posterior glottic stenosis and/or cricoarytenoid joint ankylosis. In the latter scenario, suture lateralization may be necessary to maintain a glottal aperture adequate for respiration.

Case 12A

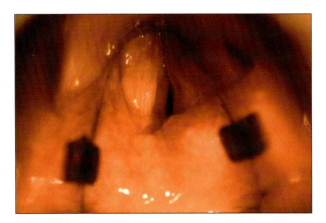

Fig 12–1. (4×) This patient had bilateral arytenoid fixation with no significant glottal aperture.

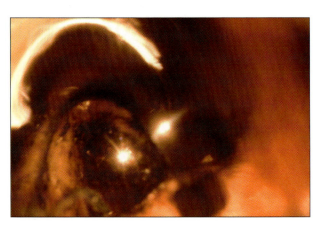

Fig 12–2. (4×) An arytenoidectomy is being performed with the microspot CO_2 laser. The image was taken during impact to display the characteristic flare that occurs with the combustion of the cartilage.

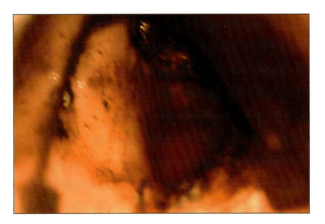

Fig 12–3. (7×) The arytenoid has been excised as well as a portion of the posterior musculo-membranous vocal fold.

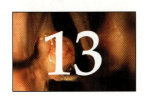

13

Benign Neoplasms

These cases represent a wide spectrum of vocal fold pathology that may relate to a systemic disorder. The management of these cases requires careful preoperative assessment and a thoughtful surgical approach that provides for flexible decision-making as the intraoperative findings dictate the ideal course of intervention.

Case 13A

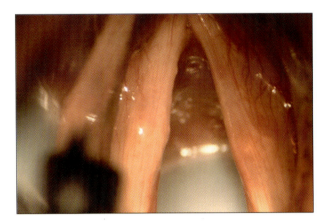

Fig 13–1. (7×) This 20-year-old female had severe dyspho-nia. Stroboscopic assessment was suggestive for bilateral subepithelial masses. The patient has a history of lupus. A light reflex is seen over a spheroid mass that was approxi-mately 3.5 mm in the mid vocal fold on the left. There is also a white area underneath the epithelium on the superior sur-face of the right vocal fold several millimeters in front of the vocal process.

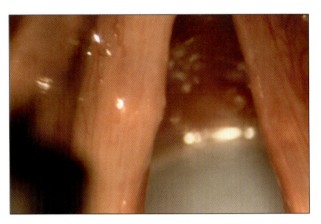

Fig 13–2. (10×) Figure 13–1 at higher magnification. The dark area in the bottom left corner is a light carrier for the laryngoscope.

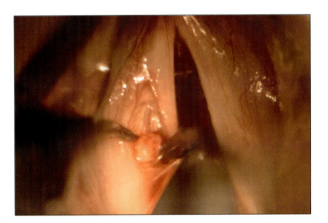

Fig 13–3. (7×) An epithelial cordotomy is performed and a subepithelial rheumatoid nodule is noted.

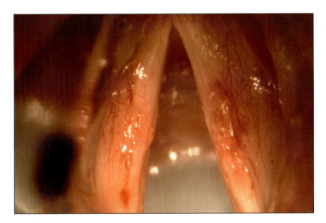

Fig 13–4. (7×) A similar lesion is noted underneath the epithelium on the right. Both lesions were resected with maximum preservation of normal epithelium and normal SLP.

Case 13B

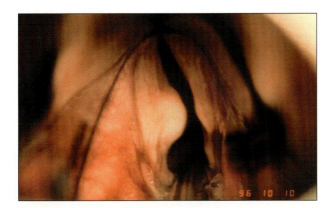

Fig 13–5. (4×) This patient is an attorney with progressive hoarseness. Note the spheroid mass was suggestive of a subepithelial cyst emanating from the left vocal fold.

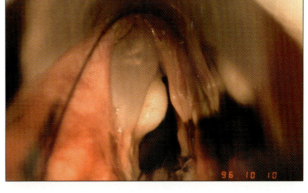

Fig 13–6. (4×) A subepithelial infusion was performed to enhance the resection. The mass was clearly adherent to the overlying epithelium.

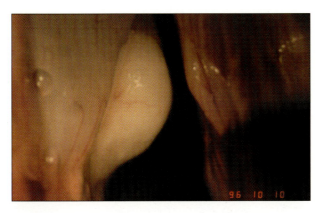

Fig 13–7. (10×) Figure 13–6 at higher magnification.

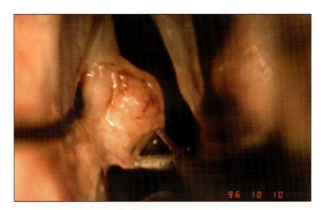

Fig 13–8. (7×) An epithelial cordotomy has been performed and the lesion was clearly noted to be solid in nature. It could not be dissected from the overlying epithelium, so this area was in turn amputated. There was maximal preservation of the underlying normal SLP.

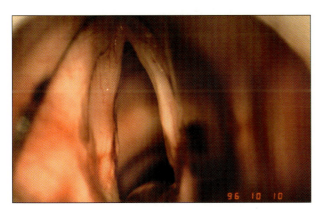

Fig 13–9. (4×) The contour of the vocal edge is significantly improved. The resultant pathology revealed a granular cell tumor. It has not recurred.

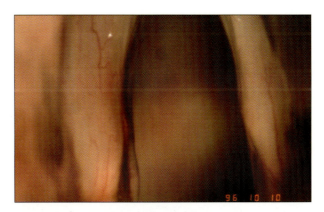

Fig 13–10. (10×) Figure 13–9 at higher magnification. The lesion could not be dissected from the overlying epithelium due to the pseudo-epitheliomatous hyperplasia. The patient's postoperative course was uneventful and his voice was dramatically improved.

Case 13C

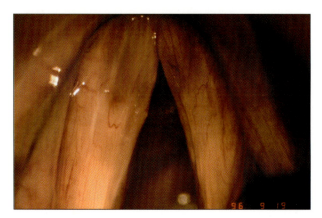

Fig 13–11. (7×) Asymmetric edema greater on the left than on the right. At the center of the superior surface of the left vocal fold there is a subepithelial white mass with an unusual vascular pattern at its perimeter. This patient had a history of arthritis and dysphonia, but did not have ankylosis of his cricoarytenoid joints.

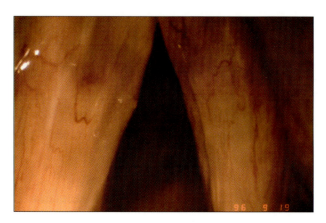

Fig 13–12. (10×) Figure 13–11 at higher magnification.

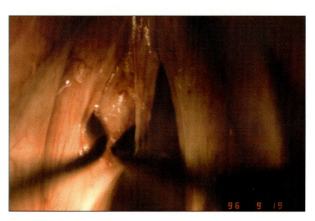

Fig 13–13. (7×) After a subepithelial infusion, an epithelial cordotomy is performed and the mass is dissected from the overlying epithelium.

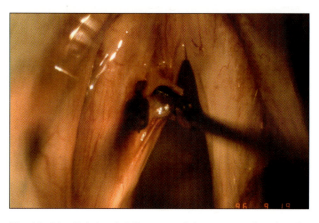

Fig 13–14. (7×) A solid fibrous nodule was noted and withdrawn from the SLP with an angled microcup forceps. A curved microscissors is utilized to complete the resection.

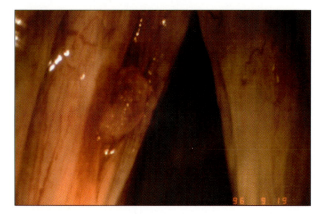

Fig 13–15. (10×) The mass is seen prior to delivery from the left vocal fold.

Case 13D

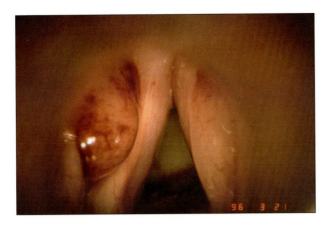

Fig 13–16. (7×) A saccular cyst is seen through a circular narrow glottiscope. This smaller laryngoscope was necessary because of difficulty in exposure and the unavailability of one of the triangular scopes in this small size. Microlaryngoscopic excision had been attempted by another surgeon, and the initial team could not intubate her due to severe retrognathia and an unusually cephalad-positioned larynx.

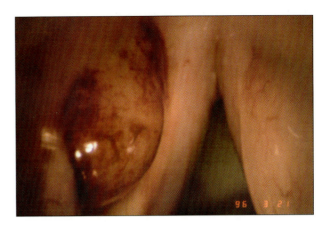

Fig 13–17. (10×) The mass is seen at higher magnification.

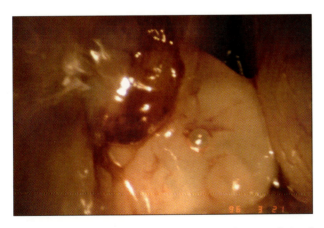

Fig 13–18. (7×) During marsupialization, the cyst drained its mucoid fluid.

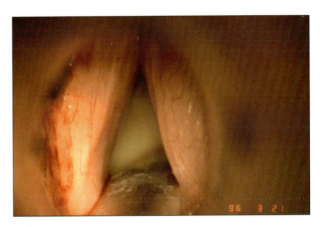

Fig 13–19. (7×) The normal vocal folds are seen subsequent to marsupialization of the cyst.

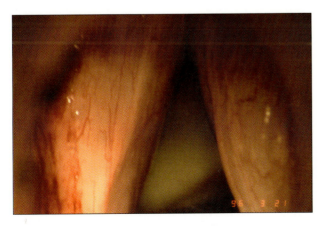

Fig 13–20. (10×) Figure 13–19 at higher magnification.

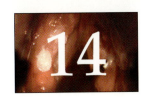

Multiple Lesions

It is not uncommon to observe multiple lesions during the clinic stroboscopic examination and it is even more likely other pathology will be discovered during microlaryngoscopy. The surgeon must perform a careful endoscopic survey of the larynx and pharynx as well as a complete microlaryngoscopic assessment of the entire glottis prior to surgical manipulation of the obvious pathology. Intraoperatively, both magnification and tissue retraction enhance the assessment of the larynx. Furthermore, patients who develop vocal fold pathology that is not initially vocally induced (ie, neoplasms, Teflon granuloma) often develop further subsequent lesions as a result of vocal overuse and abuse. Patients should give consent for surgery of both vocal folds despite a clinic examination that suggests unilateral pathology.

Case 14A

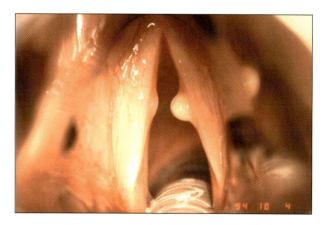

Fig 14–1. (4×) A cyst is noted on the right vocal fold and a fibrovascular nodule is noted on the left.

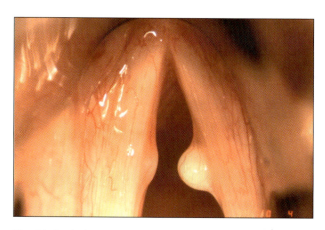

Fig 14–2. (7×) Figure 14–1 at higher magnification.

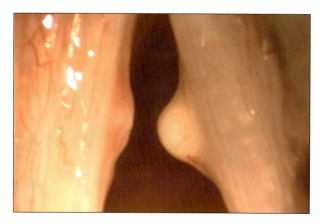

Fig 14–3. (10×) Figure 14–1 at even higher magnification.

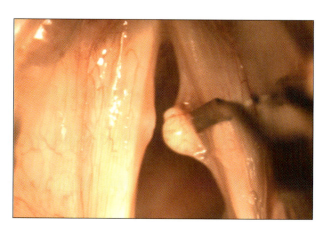

Fig 14–4. (7×) After an epithelial cordotomy is done on the right, a curved dissector is used to separate the cyst from the underlying normal SLP.

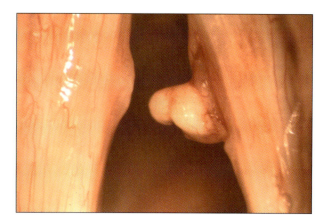

Fig 14–5. (10×) The epithelial cordotomy is well seen. The cyst was subsequently resected with preservation of an inferior microflap.

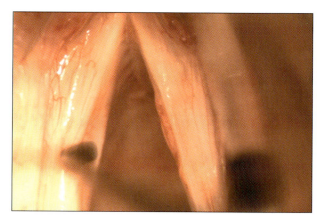

Fig 14–6. (7×) The left-sided nodule has been resected. A curved dissector is used to retract the vocal fold, displaying the excellent apposition of the epithelium. The cyst has been resected from the right.

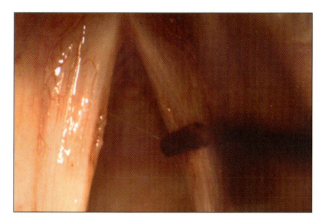

Fig 14–7. (7×) A curved dissector is now retracting the right vocal fold to show the excellent coaptation on that side.

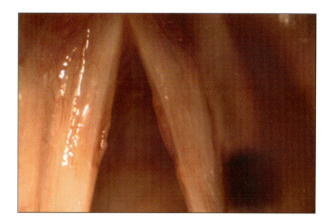

Fig 14–8. (7×) Figure 14–7 without dissectors retracting the vocal folds.

Case 14B

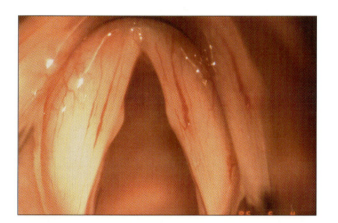

Fig 14–9. (7×) This pop singer is noted to have bilateral vocal fold nodules as well as prominent varices on the superior surface of the vocal folds.

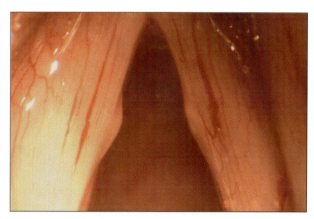

Fig 14–10. (10×) Figure 14–9 at higher magnification.

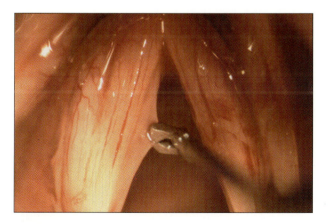

Fig 14–11. (7×) The left nodule is grasped with a microcup forceps.

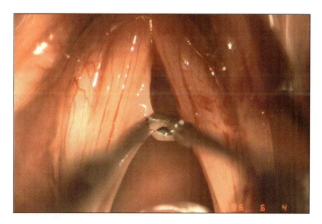

Fig 14–12. (7×) The nodule is amputated.

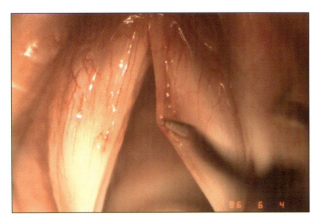

Fig 14–13. (7×) Subsequently, all of the varices are resected with cold instruments by means of multiple epithelial cordotomies. A sharp pick is seen dissecting the most prominent varix, which was situated on the right vocal fold.

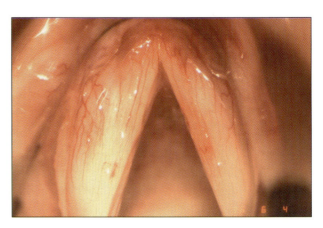

Fig 14–14. (7×) The glottal appearance is significantly improved. There has been maximal preservation of normal epithelium and normal SLP.

Case 14C

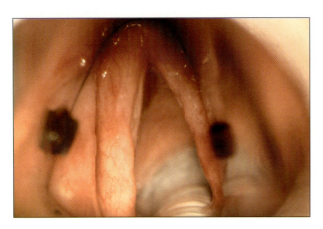

Fig 14–15. (4×) This heavy smoker was noted to have progressive hoarseness. There were keratotic areas of both vocal folds noted in bilateral sulcus deformities. The aberrant epithelium appeared worse on the right than the left.

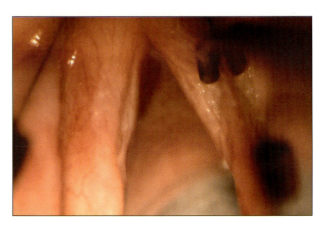

Fig 14–16. (7×) A curved dissector is used to retract the vocal fold to better visualize the keratotic area over the sulcus.

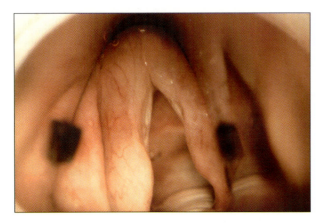

Fig 14–17. (4×) Subepithelial infusions are performed bilaterally, which demarcates the edge of the sulcus deformities.

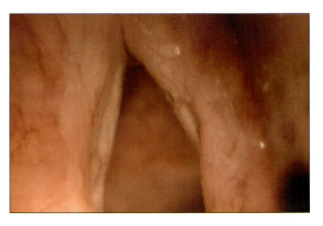

Fig 14–18. (10×) Figure 14–17 at higher magnification.

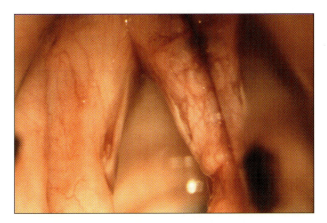

Fig 14–19. (7×) An epithelial microflap has been outlined on the right.

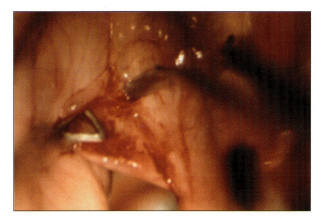

Fig 14–20. (10×) The epithelial microflap is being separated from the fibrotic underlying vocal ligament. During this dissection, it appeared that there was invasive cancer growing into the ligament.

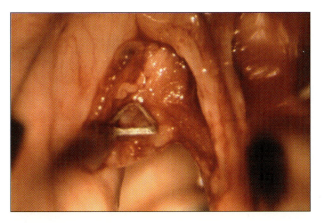

Fig 14–21. (7×) Because of the previous finding, an incision was made through the vocal ligament, which was then kept in continuity with the overlying epithelium. The vocalis muscle is well seen and the dissection now continues between the vocal ligament and the vocal muscle.

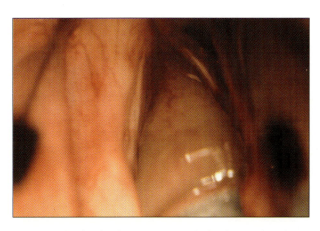

Fig 14–22. (10×) The resection of the lesion has been completed.

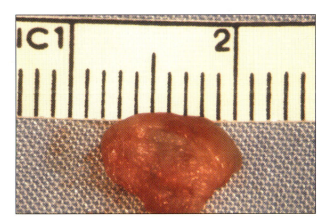

Fig 14–23. The keratotic surface of the specimen is seen, which ultimately contained microinvasive carcinoma.

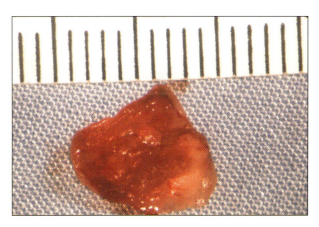

Fig 14–24. The undersurface of the specimen shows no invasion through the vocal ligament.

Case 14D

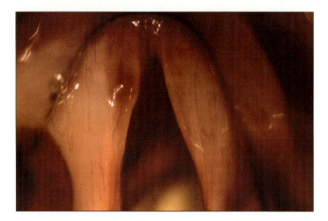

Fig 14–25. (7×) Bilateral traumatic lesions. The left-sided lesion has a more hemorrhagic appearance.

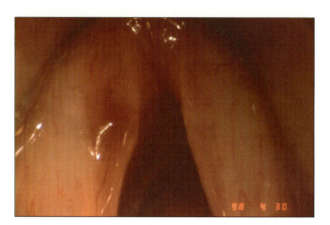

Fig 14–26. (10×) Figure 14–25 at higher magnification.

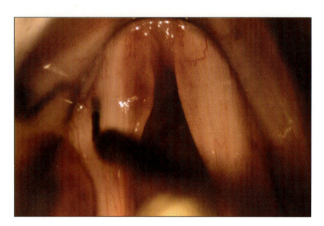

Fig 14–27. (7×) A subepithelial infusion is done. The needle is in place and can be seen through the translucent epithelium.

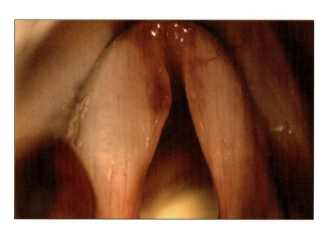

Fig 14–28. (7×) The infusion has been completed.

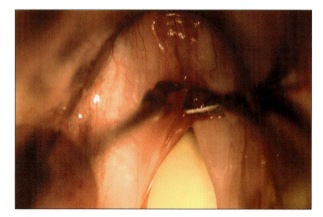

Fig 14–29. (7×) The hemorrhagic lesion is retracted with an angled forceps and an epithelial cordotomy is performed with a curved microscissors.

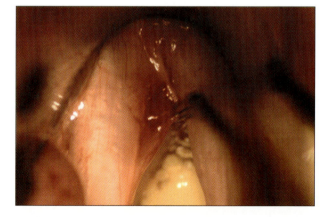

Fig 14–30. (7×) The edge of the microflap is retracted with an alligator forceps to expose the hemorrhagic fibrovascular mass.

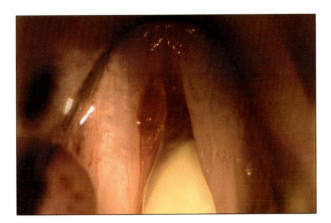

Fig 14–31. (7×) The fibrovascular mass is seen coming through the epithelial cordotomy.

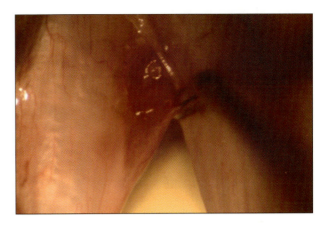

Fig 14–32. (10×) The epithelial microflap is retracted and the mass has been further mobilized.

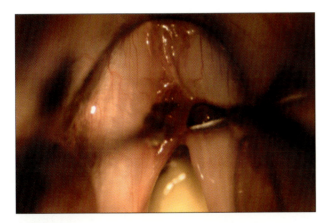

Fig 14–33. (7×) The fibrovascular mass has been grasped with an angled forceps and its base is severed from the underlying normal SLP.

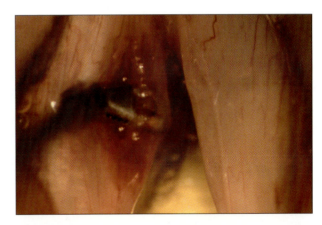

Fig 14–34. (10×) The angled triangular forceps is placed underneath the epithelium to remove any residual fibrovascular tissue from the basement membrane of the microflap.

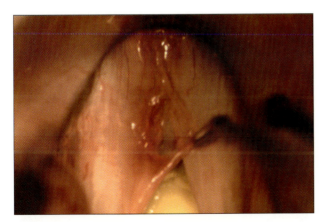

Fig 14–35. (7×) The cavity from the resected fibrovascular mass can be seen as a microalligator forceps retracts the microflap.

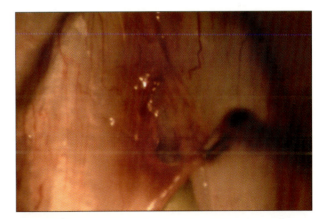

Fig 14–36. (10×) Figure 14–35 at higher magnification.

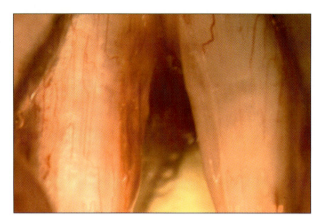

Fig 14–37. (10×) The epithelial microflap has been redraped and there is excellent coaptation of the epithelial edges.

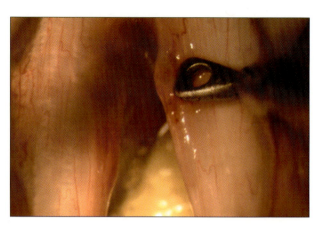

Fig 14–38. (10×) A fibrovascular nodule is noted on the medial surface of the right vocal fold which is defined by the edge of the angled forceps.

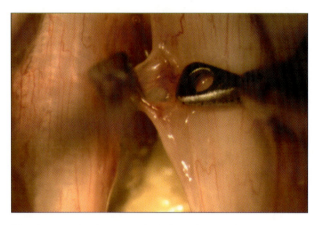

Fig 14–39. (10×) An epithelial cordotomy has been performed and the contents of the fibrovascular nodule are being removed with the angled forceps.

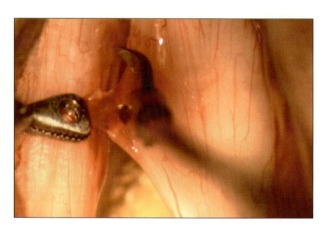

Fig 14–40. (10×) The final subepithelial resection of the fibrovascular mass is completed with the microscissors.

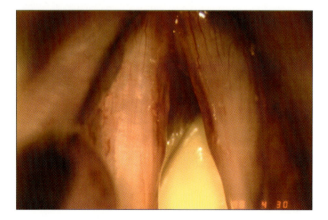

Fig 14–41. (7×) The epithelial microflaps are redraped. The vocal fold edges are well contoured and are smooth and straight.

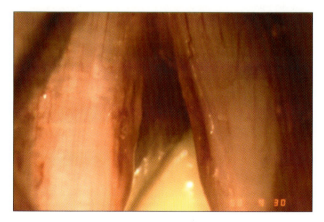

Fig 14–42. (10×) Figure 14–41 at higher magnification.

Case 14E

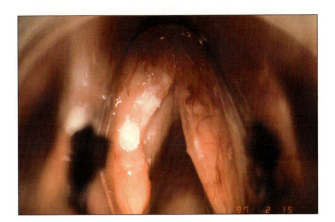

Fig 14–43. (4×) This 40-year-old pop performer had a history of heavy smoking and severe progressive hoarseness. The left vocal fold revealed a severe sulcus deformity. The overlying epithelium in both the region of the sulcus vergeture as well as the superior surface contained thick keratosis. The contralateral fold revealed severe microvascular injection and a pocket sulcus deformity.

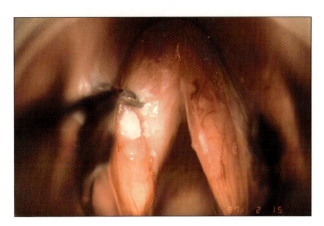

Fig 14–44. (4×) The left vocal fold is retracted to better reveal the magnitude of the keratosis on the medial surface sulcus deformity.

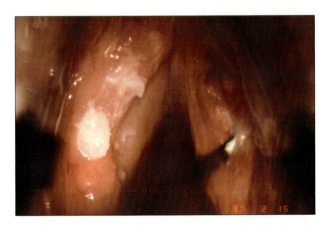

Fig 14–45. (7×) A blunt probe is placed within the pocket sulcus deformity on the right. Keratin was noted in the depth of the sulcus.

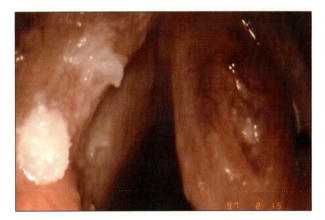

Fig 14–46. (10×) The right vocal fold is retracted laterally to better reveal the pocket sulcus deformity and the keratosis in the depth of its base.

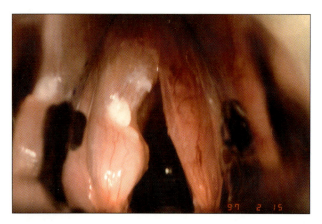

Fig 14–47. (4×) A subepithelial infusion has been performed on the left, which clearly delineates the edge of the sulcus and adherence of the epithelium to the vocal ligament. There was a significant concern for premalignant epithelium and/or microinvasive carcinoma.

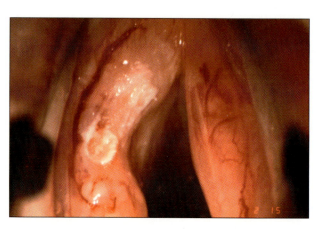

Fig 14–48. (7×) An epithelial microflap is outlined with a microscissors on the superior surface to help delineate the nature of the epithelial pathology before committing to an aggressive procedure.

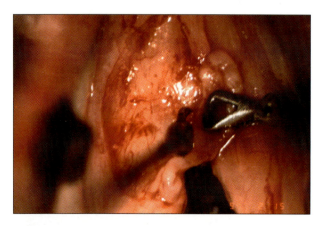

Fig 14–49. (7×) The epithelial microflap was retracted with an angled triangular forceps and a mini-microscissors was used to dissect the epithelium from the underlying residual normal superficial lamina propria.

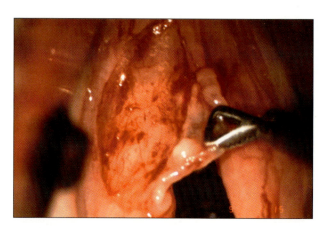

Fig 14–50. (7×) There was no obvious invasion through the undersurface of the lesion into the vocal ligament.

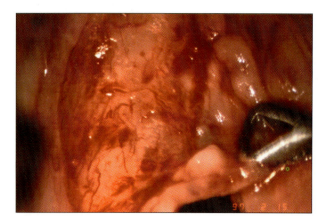

Fig 14–51. (10×) The superficial lamina propria on the superior surface of the left vocal fold does not show any neoplastic changes.

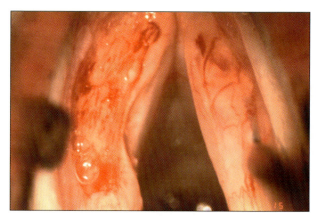

Fig 14–52. (7×) The epithelial resection is confined to the superior surface to minimize the effect on the voice prior to obtaining definitive information about the pathology.

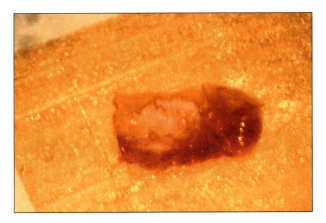

Fig 14–53. (7×) The lesion is mounted on a carrier for whole mount section analysis.

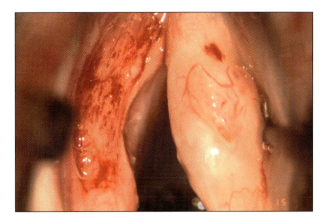

Fig 14–54. (7×) A subepithelial infusion is performed on the right. The vasoconstriction is clearly seen. A discrete varix is seen coursing around the perimeter of the sulcus deformity.

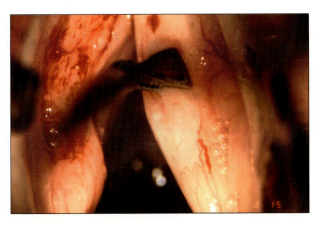

Fig 14–55. (7×) The edge of the sulcus is grasped with an angled forceps to allow for an epithelial incision at the margin of the sulcus.

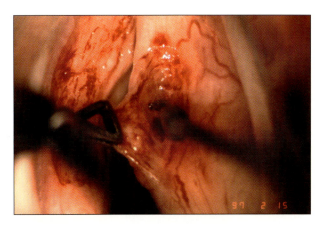

Fig 14–56. (7×) A curved microscissors is utilized to dissect the sulcus from any underlying normal SLP.

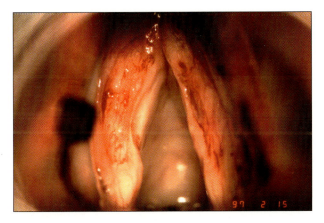

Fig 14–57. (4×) The sulcus has been completely excised from the right and a representative sample of epithelium from the left has been resected.

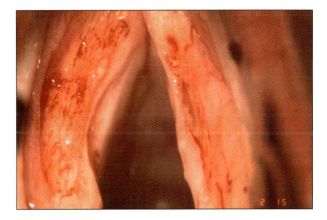

Fig 14–58. (7×) Figure 14–57 at higher magnification.

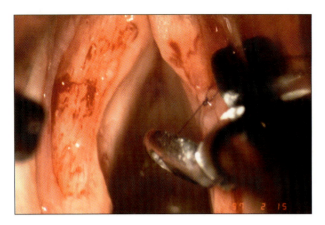

Fig 14–59. (7×) A suture is being tied to achieve primary closure of the epithelium and any normal residual SLP from the subcordal and superior surfaces for enhanced healing.

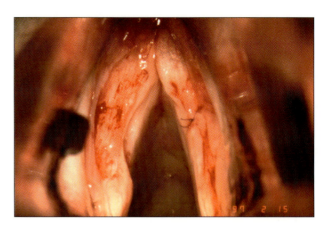

Fig 14–60. (4×) The final surgical result with the suture in place.

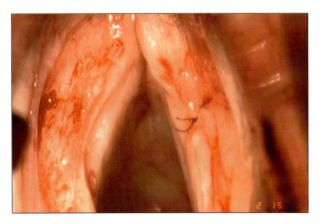

Fig 14–61. (7×) Figure 14–60 at higher magnification. The suture has brought some normal superficial lamina propria from the subcordal region to the medial valving surface of the vocal fold.

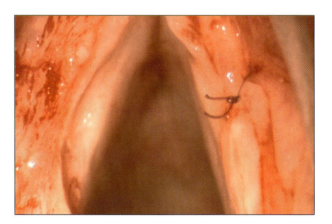

Fig 14–62. (10×) Figure 14–60 at even higher magnification further exhibiting the repositioning of the right vocal fold epithelium. Subsequent to this procedure, the patient had a dramatically improved voice. The resultant pathology could not be determined on frozen section (verrucous vulgaris versus verrucous carcinoma.) The final pathology was verrucous vulgaris. This patient was then determined to be HIV positive.

Case 14F

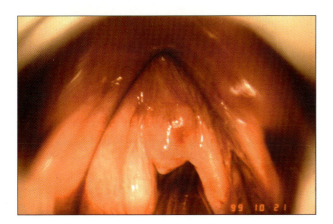

Fig 14–63. (4×) Large hemorrhagic polyp arising from the medial surface of the right musculo-membranous vocal fold.

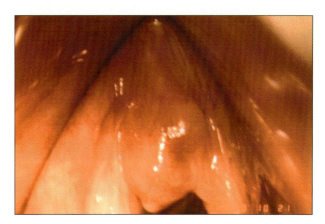

Fig 14–64. (7×) Figure 14–63 at higher magnification.

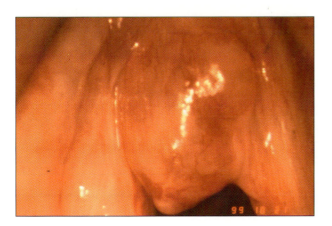

Fig 14–65. (10×) Figure 14–63 at the highest magnification

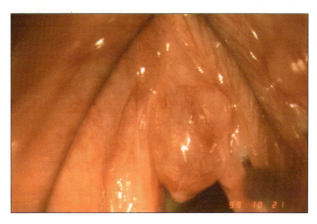

Fig 14–66. (7×) The infusion needle has been placed at the epithelium lateral to the lesion.

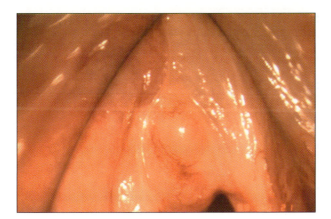

Fig 14–67. (7×) A subepithelial infusion has been done with saline and 1/10,000 adrenaline, which has placed the epithelium on tension.

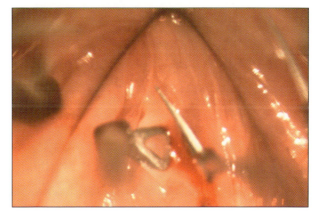

Fig 14–68. (7×) An upturned scissors is used to make an epithelial cordotomy.

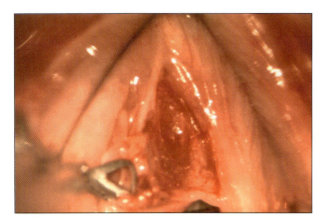

Fig 14–69. (7×) Blunt dissection is done to separate the base of the dense fibrovascular tissue from the loose SLP.

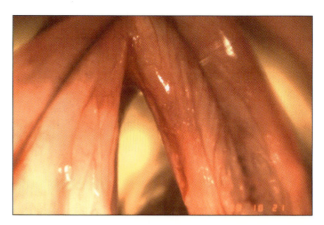

Fig 14–70. (7×) The polyp has been resected and an inferiorly based microflap has been preserved to provide coaptation of the epithelial edges.

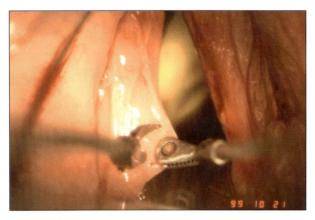

Fig 14–71. (7×) Left-sided polypoid corditis changes are resected by means of an epithelial cordotomy. It is limited in the left mid-fold region by the collision trauma from the right fold.

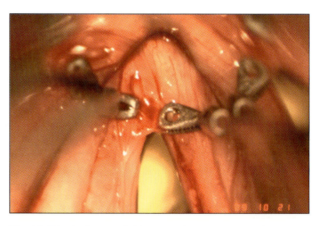

Fig 14–72. (7×) A small fibrovascular mass is noted on anterior aspect of the left fold. A subepithelial resection is done by retracting the microflap and removing the mass with a mini-microcup forceps.

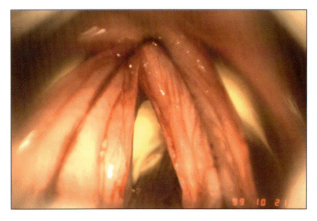

Fig 14–73. (4×) The three lesions have been resected with maximal preservation of the vocal folds' epithelium and laminae propria.

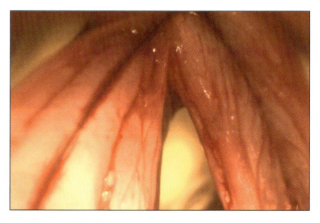

Fig 14–74. (7×) The postresection image at higher magnification

Case 14G

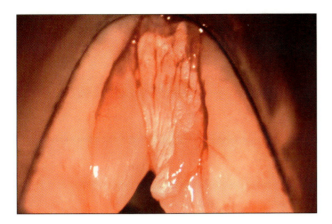

Fig 14–75. (7×) Bilateral polypoid corditis (Reinke's edema) in a male with extensive right-sided keratosis.

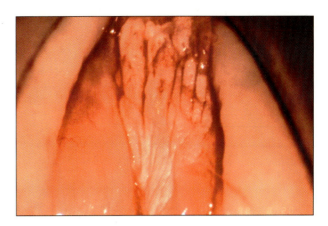

Fig 14–76. (10×) Figure 14–75 at higher magnification.

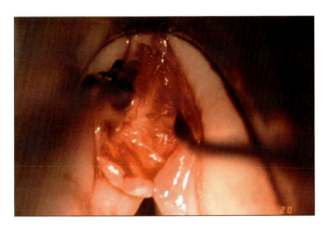

Fig 14–77. (7×) After an epithelial cordotomy is done, the keratotic epithelium is resected as a microflap.

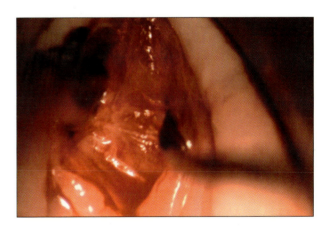

Fig 14–78. (10×) Figure 14–77 at higher magnification.

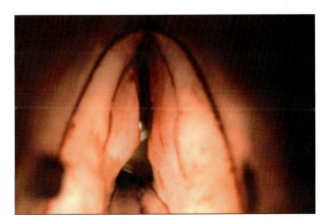

Fig 14–79. (4×) The postresection image of the vocal folds. The left fold was not dissected and the patient's vocal quality improved considerably.

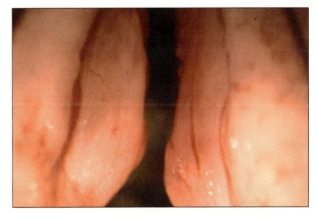

Fig 14–80. (10×) Figure 14–79 at higher magnification.

Case 14H

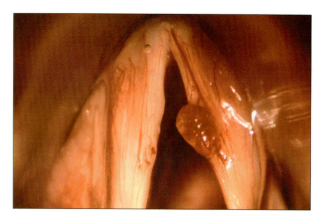

Fig 14–81. (7×) The patient was a 25-year-old female rock singer with progressive dysphonia. Multiple traumatic vascular lesions are noted including varices, ectasias, and a polyp.

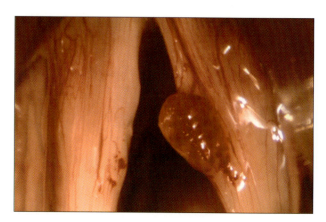

Fig 14–82. (10×) Figure 14–81 at higher magnification.

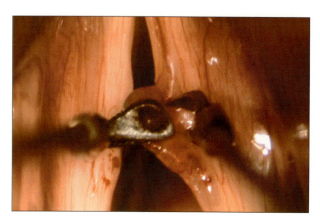

Fig 14–83. (10×) The polyp is retracted and a epithelial cordotomy is made adjacent to the edge of the lesion.

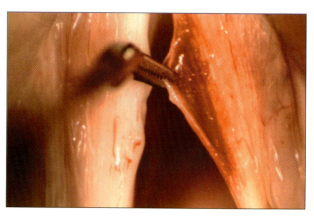

Fig 14–84. (10×) The edge of the microflap is retracted with an alligator forceps demonstrating the subepithelial resection of the polyp.

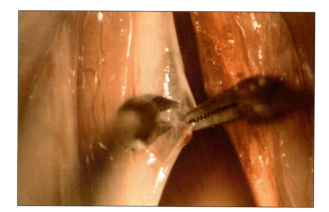

Fig 14–85. (10×) There is a sessile fibrovascular nodule on the left, which is also excised by means of an epithelial cordotomy and subepithelial resection. The microscissors is used to dissect the fibrovascular tissue, while retracting the translucent normal epithelium with an alligator forceps.

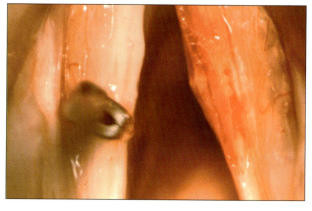

Fig 14–86. (10×) The fibrovascular tissue is removed without the epithelium by means of a microcup forceps.

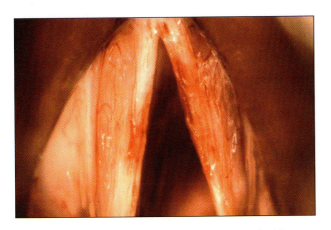

Fig 14–87. (7×) All the lesions have been excised with maximal preservation of the epithelium and SLP.

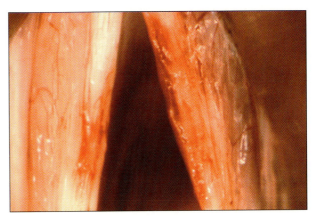

Fig 14–88. (10×) Figure 14–87 at higher magnification.

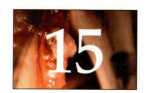

Vocal Fold Atypia/Dysplasia and Carcinoma

DISEASE PRESENTATION

Premalignant vocal fold epithelium and early glottic cancer are primarily smoking-induced diseases. Lesions frequently are confined geographically to the superior ventricular surface of the vocal fold.[65] This allows for complete preservation of layered microstructure on the medial valving surface of the glottis. Keratotic[168] lesions of the vocal fold comprise most of the dysplastic lesions of the glottis. Unfortunately, the magnitude and appearance of the surface keratosis does not belie the severity of the underlying cellular atypia or the presence of microinvasive carcinoma.[65] Erythroplasia (red lesions) is an infrequent finding and typically contains carcinoma in situ. Isolated ulceration of the musculo-membranous vocal fold in an immunocompetent smoking host, who does not have an infectious process, typically reflects carcinoma.

PHILOSOPHY OF MANAGEMENT

Since any adequate treatment for T1 glottic cancer (endoscopic excision, transcervical excision, radiation therapy) results in a cure rate of 85–90%,[169] a primary parameter by which the clinician should judge the success of the treatment is the resulting quality of the voice. Recently, laryngologists have incorporated physiological principles of laryngeal sound production into the design of the oncological procedures. The surgeon; however, must not lose sight of the fact that a variety of circumstances might dictate a particular treatment approach.

A primary goal of the endoscopic management of T1 glottic cancer is to narrow the cancer-free margin to minimize patient morbidity, while not altering the cure rate. Phonomicrosurgical procedures can precisely accommodate the narrow deep resection margin of T1 vocal fold cancer to the depth of invasion (invisible third dimension) (Figures 15–1 and 15–2). A small amount of extra tissue that is excised with the deep margin can have a profound effect on the vocal outcome, while not necessarily improving the cure rate. This is especially so for lesions that are confined to the epithelium or that minimally invade the superficial lamina propria.

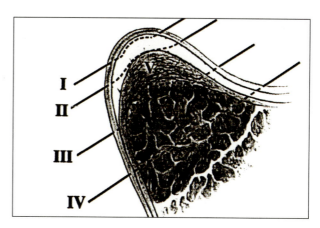

Fig 15–2. The coronal section of the vocal fold delineates the depth of potential resection margins for vocal fold atypia and cancer. (From Hartig G, Zeitels SM: *Operat Tech Otolaryngol Head Neck Surg.* 1998;9:214–223 with permission.)

   I. The dissection is performed just underneath the basement membrane with preservation of most of the underlying superficial lamina propria.

  II. The dissection is performed well within the superficial lamina propria, but does not include the vocal ligament.

 III. The dissection is performed between the vocal ligament and vocalis muscle.

 IV. The dissection is performed deep within the vocalis muscle.

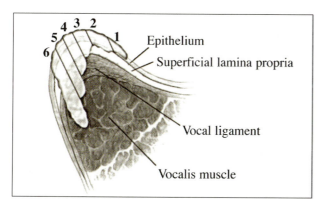

Fig 15–1. Diagram displays how a surface vocal fold lesion may harbor a variety of invasion patterns. (From Hartig G, Zeitels SM: *Operat Tech Otolaryngol Head Neck Surg.* 1998; 9: 214–223 with permission.)

Reinke's space infusion (Chapter 2) has helped to precisely determine the depth of invasion of T1 cancers before committing to the depth of the excision.[65,104] In a number of patients with T1 cancers, the infusion has allowed for preservation of all of the vocal ligament and vocalis muscle as well as part of the deep portion of the superficial lamina propria.[65,156] We have had one microinvasive local failure in approximately 30 patients in whom this graded microsurgical approach was used[151] and that patient has been controlled by means of a subsequent superficial endoscopic resection. The majority now have more than 3 years of follow-up.

Endoscopic excision is associated with a very low complication rate, which consists mainly of minor postoperative bleeding[170–173] and granuloma formation.[171–174] An en bloc excisional biopsy provides an accurate diagnosis as well as an effective treatment,[170,175] and does so with minimal morbidity. Whole-mount-section histological examination of resected specimens prevents overtreatment or undertreatment of small glottic lesions.

All treatment options, including further transoral resections, are preserved after endoscopic excision. Unlike radio-

therapy (Figure 15–3), endoscopic resection treats only the lesion without ablating the remaining normal glottal tissue. Postradiotherapy videostroboscopic exams suggest that both normal and cancerous tissues reflect fibrotic changes and impaired mucosal oscillation.[176] The use of radiotherapy for early cancers precludes its further use for tumor recurrence or for new primaries, and may even induce carcinogenesis in atypical epithelium.[177,178] The cost of endoscopic excision is significantly less than open laryngeal surgery or radiation since either of these latter procedures are typically preceded by a staging endoscopy.[179] Also, the patient sustains the increased burden of time and travel commitments required by radiotherapy.

DISEASE IN THE ANTERIOR COMMISSURE

The anterior commissure tendon, or Broyle's ligament, is a confluence of the vocal ligament, the thyroepiglottic ligament, the conus elasticus, and the internal perichondrium of the thyroid alae (Figure 15–4). There is a misconception that T1 cancers at the anterior commissure have a great predilection for understaging and that many of these lesions have occult invasion of the thyroid cartilage (T4 stage).[180,181] This is based on the misunderstanding that the anatomy of the dense anterior-commissure ligament is a less resilient tumor barrier than the adjacent thin thyroid perichondrium. Kirchner[180,181] has made it clear that T1a and T1b carcinomas rarely transgress Broyle's ligament to invade thyroid cartilage. Anterior commissure tumors that have thyroid cartilage invasion typically display cephalad surface-invasion of the infrapetiole region of the supraglottis or caudal surface invasion of the subglottis (both T2 by surface staging criteria) (Figures 15–5 and 15–6)

There has been divergent opinion as to whether cancer can be endoscopically eradicated from the anterior commissure. The proscriptions imposed by some are based primarily on the difficulty in obtaining adequate surgical exposure in this area.[182] The rate-limiting factors for resection of early cancer in the anterior commissure are the true extent of the disease (is it invading cartilage?) and the endoscopic exposure required to encompass the lesion. Davis[175] and the Boston University group and later Koufman et al[171] demonstrated that cancer could be removed from the anterior commissure; however, it required great skill to excise the lesion without vaporizing the specimen. Vaporizing cancer without clear en bloc resection margins is inadequate surgical oncological technique. This factor, as well as underestimating the extent of disease, probably led to the reported failures by a number of investigators.[182–185]

Because of the treatment failures mentioned above, poor outcome of the cancer was mistakenly attributed to the biological behavior of the disease rather than the inadequate exposure and the compromised resection. Therefore, a procedure was designed to facilitate the diagnostic staging and treatment of early glottic cancer at the anterior commissure.[186,187] It is composed of resecting the supraglottal tissue (infrapetiole region and anterior vestibular folds) cephalad to the anterior commissure tendon to determine whether limited anterior glottic cancer had invaded the thyroid cartilage. A CO_2 laser resection of the uninvolved supraglottis is done

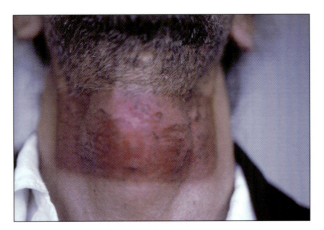

Fig 15–3. The appearance of the neck of an individual at the conclusion of radiation for a T1 glottic carcinoma.

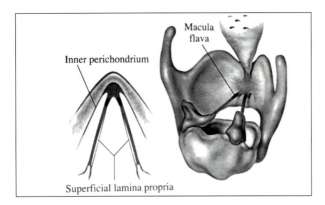

Fig 15–4. Diagrammatic representation of the anterior commissure tendon. (From Hartig G, Zeitels SM: *Operat Tech Otolaryngol Head Neck Surg.* 1998;9:214–223 with permission.)

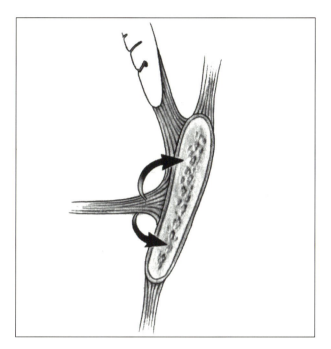

Fig 15–5. Diagrammatic representation of how cancer spreads around the anterior commissure tendon to invade the thyroid cartilage. (From Hartig G, Zeitels SM: *Operat Tech Otolaryngol Head Neck Surg.* 1998;9:214–223 with permission.)

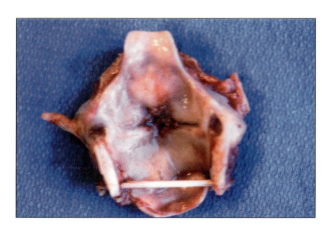

Fig 15–6. Old laryngectomy specimen. The patient failed radiotherapy and had severe pulmonary compromise. Diffuse soft-tissue invasion cephalad and caudal to the anterior commissure tendon correctly portended thyroid cartilage invasion.

in any case where the perimeter of the lesion cannot be visualized in its entirety. This allows for positioning of the triangular glottiscope adjacent to the inner thyroid lamina above the AGC, which facilitates clear resection of part or all of the anterior commissure tendon. There have been no resection failures in a limited number of cases thus far.[122] If the cancer is confined to the anterior commissure tendon and if resection of the tendon is not in the patient's best interest (ie, post-op voice quality), radiation can commence promptly knowing there is true T1 disease.

If one accepts Kirchner's histopathological data regarding the invasion pattern of T1 glottic cancer, there is no reason to believe that an adequate soft-tissue resection of small-volume soft-tissue disease is not adequate treatment. This premise is further substantiated by a number of reports that did not find a correlation between anterior commissure involvement with T1 glottic cancer and failure of radiotherapy as a curative modality.[188,189]

The extensive European experience reported by Steiner,[190] Eckel and Thumfart,[172] and Rudert[191] substantiates that glottal cancer in the anterior commissure can be removed transorally. The problem with any surgical approach to the anterior commissure (for true T1a, T1b, and T2 lesions) is that when these procedures disturb the structural integrity of both sides of the anterior commissure tendon vocal quality is significantly impaired. Lesions that are invading cartilage are T4 by stage, require open partial laryngectomy and are not suitable for endoscopic excision. An endoscopic exploration of the infrapetiole region of the supraglottis allows for definitive determination about whether a presumed T1 lesion has cartilage invasion (T4).[186] This procedure facilitates precise staging (without disarticulating Broyle's ligament), commensurate management, and optimal post-treatment voice quality.

ENDOSCOPIC TECHNIQUE

The goal of endoscopic treatment of an isolated T1 lesion of the musculo-membranous vocal fold is eradication of the disease with maximal preservation of the normal layered microstructure. This approach results in the optimal postoperative voice without compromising oncological cure. There are 4 basic procedures based on the depth of excision (see Figure 15–2).[151]

1. Dissection just deep the epithelial basement membrane in the superficial aspect of the superficial lamina propria for atypical epithelium and microinvasive cancer,
2. Dissection within the deeper aspect of the superficial lamina propria microinvasive cancer that is not attached to the vocal ligament,
3. Dissection between the deep lamina propria (vocal ligament) and the vocalis muscle for lesions that are attached to the ligament but not through it, and
4. Dissection within the thyroarytenoid muscle for lesions penetrating the vocal ligament and invading the vocalis muscle.

This approach can be fine-tuned further by performing partial resections of any of the layered microstructure. The specimen is always oriented for whole-mount histological analysis and frozen-section margin assessment is employed selectively to verify a complete excision.[65,151]

If dissection is performed within the SLP, cold instruments facilitate precise tangential dissection around the curving vocal fold. This allows for maximal preservation of the superficial lamina propria and for pliability of the regenerating epithelium.[65,77] Dissection between the vocal ligament and the vocalis muscle can be performed equally well with cold instruments alone or with assistance of the CO_2 laser. Dissection within the muscle is performed most precisely with the CO_2 laser, which allows for improved visualization because of its hemostatic cutting properties.

In addition to improving pre-excisional assessment of lesion depth, the subepithelial saline-epinephrine infusion into Reinke's space assists with the surgeon's technical execution of the surgery in a number of ways:

1. The infusion facilitates mucosal incisions by improving visualization of the lateral border of the lesion and by distending the SLP so that the overlying epithelium is under tension;
2. The infusion also increases the depth of the superficial lamina propria, which facilitates less traumatic dissection in this layer and leads to regenerated epithelium that is more flexible;
3. The epinephrine and hydrostatic pressure of the infusion vasoconstrict microvasculature in the SLP and this improves visualization and precise dissection; and
4. If the laser is used, the saline acts as a heat sink, which decreases thermal trauma to the normal vocal fold tissue.

VOCAL OUTCOME AFTER ENDOSCOPIC RESECTION OF THE MUSCULO-MEMBRANOUS REGION

The laryngologist can precisely accommodate a micro-controlled excision to the 3-dimensional characteristics of the vocal-cord cancer. Unlike radiation,[176] this approach avoids trauma to uninvolved tissue, such as the contralateral fold, during treatment of a unilateral lesion. As to be expected, increasing the magnitude of the resection, especially its depth, leads to deteriorating vocal function.[65,192,193] Therefore, the graded resection approach that was suggested by Hirano[192] and Koufman[171] was developed further.[65,151]

The mucosal microflap technique that is useful for resection of epithelial atypia and microinvasive cancer can sometimes be confined to the superior surface of the vocal fold. After reepithelialization, typically, the patient can comfortably increase subglottal driving pressures to achieve perceptually and objectively measured (acoustical analysis) normal voice at conversational levels. Maximal-range tasks reveal some mild limitation of frequency variation (dynamic range) and loudness capability. These vocal findings show mild progression in a similar pattern with extension of the resection to the medial vocalizing surface of the vocal fold.[65] When the surgical dissection is confined to the SLP in one vocal fold, the perceptual assessment of the resulting voice is usually normal. Stroboscopy reveals mild impairment of mucosal-wave propagation with regard both to amplitude and magnitude wherever there has been dissection in the SLP.

As the deep resection margin extends to include the vocal muscle, there is further acoustic, aerodynamic, and stroboscopic, impairment. When the SLP is excised as a component of the cancer resection, the regenerated epithelial surface is adherent to the underlying body of the vocal cord.[65,156] This results in unavoidable stiffness in the vibratory characteristics of the regenerated epithelium. We have not seen evidence that the pliable SLP regenerates after removal in the way that epithelium does. However, after a resection of the vocal fold epithelium and its underlying laminae propria, the healed neocord is usually smooth and straight and glottal closure is usually normal. Vocal limitations may still not be perceptible at conversational levels in some patients if glottal closure is complete. Aerodynamic valvular incompetence that leads to obvious hoarseness is usually observed when complete glottal closure does not occur because of tissue loss and a resulting vocal-edge excavation.[65,156]

Case 15A

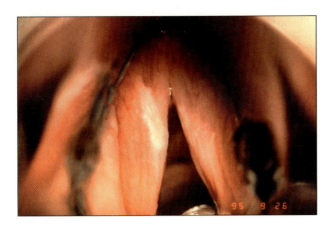

Fig 15–7. (4×) There is distinct geographic focus of keratosis with atypia on the left vocal fold. There is less poorly defined thin keratosis on the right vocal fold.

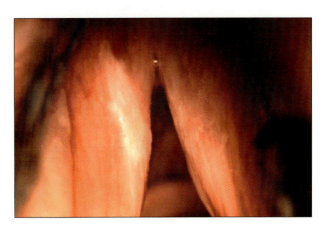

Fig 15–8. (7×) Figure 15–7 at higher magnification.

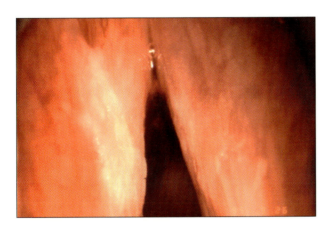

Fig 15–9. (10×) Figure 15–7 at even higher magnification.

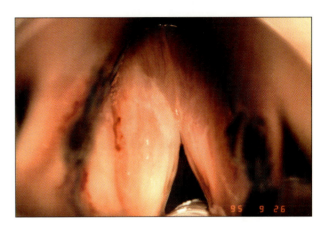

Fig 15–10. (4×) A subepithelial infusion of saline and adrenaline has been placed on the left. Note the convex contour of the left vocal fold, as well as the vasoconstriction of the vasculature. The puncture site was at the lateral aspect of the vocal folds where the blood is now seen.

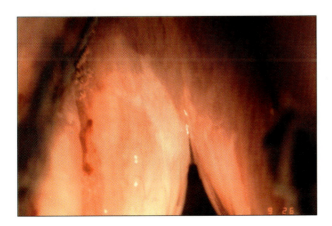

Fig 15–11. (7×) Figure 15–10 at higher magnification.

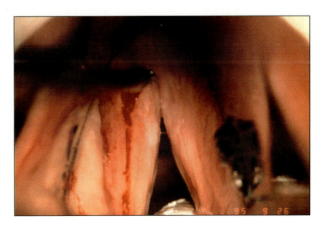

Fig 15–12. (4×) A perimeter incision is made with a curved microscissors.

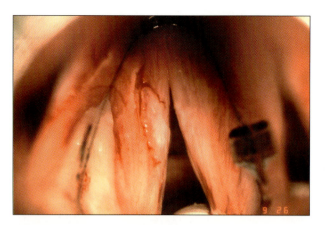

Fig 15–13. (4×) The posterior lateral and anterior perimeter incision has been made around the lesion.

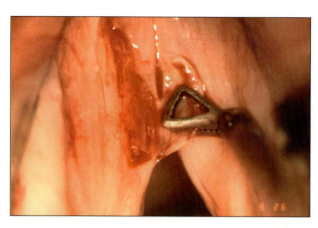

Fig 15–14. (7×) An angle forceps is used to retract the microflap, which has been mostly dissected from the underlying normal SLP.

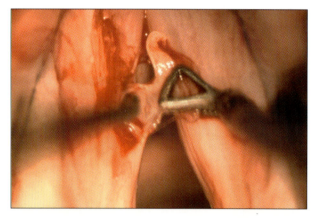

Fig 15–15. (7×) A curved dissector is used to complete the dissection of the basement membrane of the epithelium from the underlying normal superficial lamina propria.

Case 15B

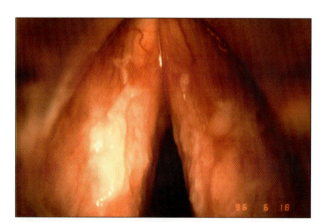

Fig 15–16. (7×) There is diffuse keratosis with atypia of both musculo-membranous vocal folds as seen. Due to chronic vocal trauma, there are associated fibrous changes of the SLP bilaterally.

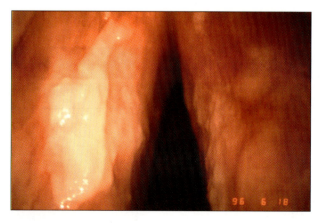

Fig 15–17. (10×) Figure 15–16 at higher magnification.

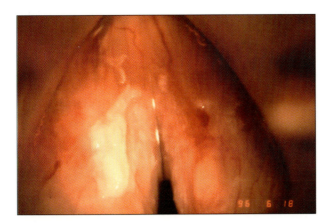

Fig 15–18. (7×) A subepithelial infusion of saline and adrenaline has been performed on the left.

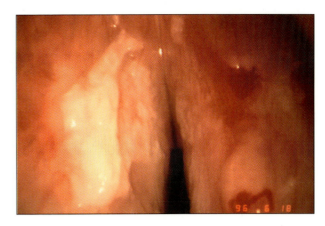

Fig 15–19. (10×) Figure 15–18 at higher magnification.

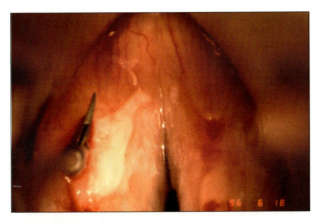

Fig 15–20. (7×) A perimeter incision is made around the lesion with a microscissors.

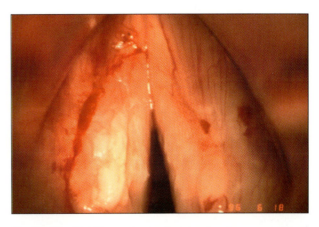

Fig 15–21. (7×) The perimeter incision has been completed.

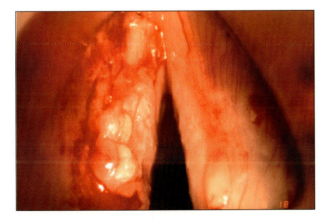

Fig 15–22. (7×) Most of the superior surface of the right vocal fold has been mobilized due to the need for a margin.

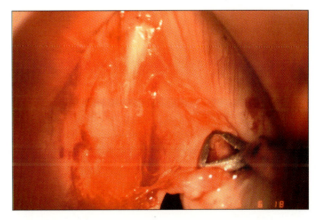

Fig 15–23. (7×) The microflap containing the keratosis with atypia is retracted. The residual normal superficial lamina propria and its associated microvasculature are seen on the left.

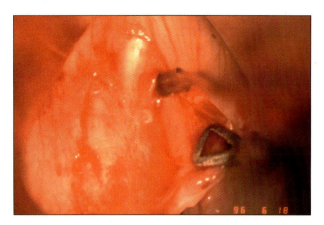

Fig 15–24. (7×) A curved dissector is utilized to enhance the preservation of the superficial lamina propria on the medial and subcordal surface, as it is dissected from the basement membrane of the lesion.

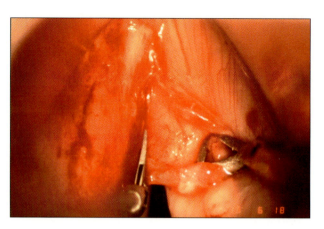

Fig 15–25. (7×) Once the caudal edge of the keratosis has been dissected from the underlying normal superficial lamina propria, an upturned scissors is used to complete the excision.

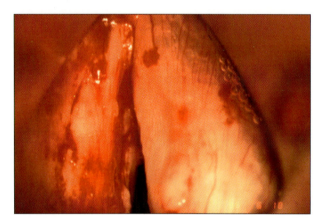

Fig 15–26. (7×) The lesion on the left has been resected in its entirety. The residual mild bleeding and microvasculature are an indication of the preservation of the superficial lamina propria. Due to the dissection into the anterior commissure, the right-sided lesion must be resected in a second stage after left-sided healing.

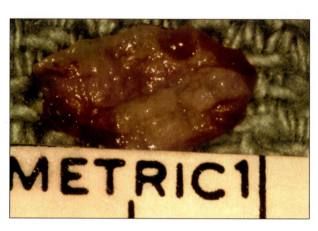

Fig 15–27. The surface of the specimen is visualized.

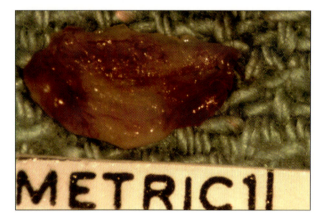

Fig 15–28. The undersurface or basement membrane side of the lesion is visualized.

Case 15C

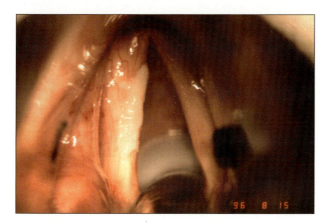

Fig 15–29. (4×) There is a distinct area of keratosis on the superior and medial surface of the left vocal fold.

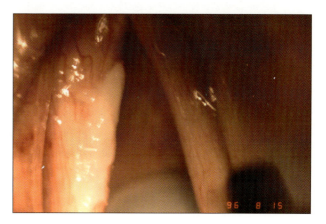

Fig 15–30. (7×) Figure 15–29 at higher magnification.

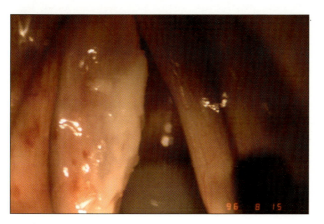

Fig 15–31. (7×) A subepithelial infusion of saline and adrenaline has been performed revealing that the lesion is not adherent to the vocal ligament.

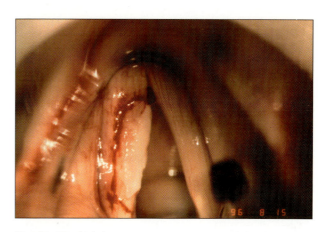

Fig 15–32. (4×) A perimeter incision around the lesion has been performed.

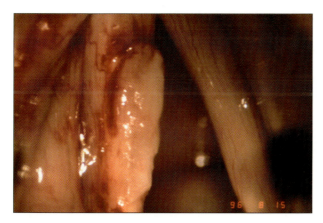

Fig 15–33. (7×) Figure 15–32 at higher magnification.

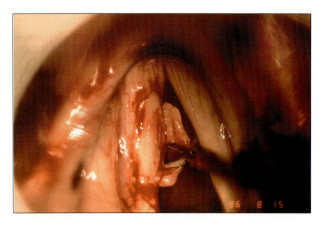

Fig 15–34. (4×) The epithelial lesion is retracted as a microflap.

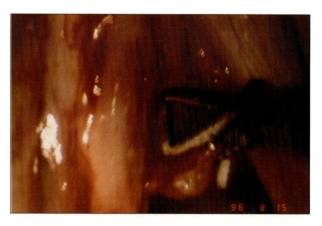

Fig 15–35. (10×) Figure 15–34 at higher magnification.

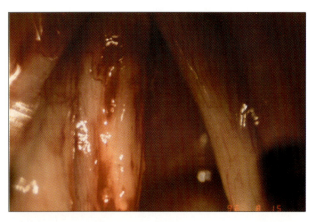

Fig 15–36. (7×) The lesion has been resected in its entirety.

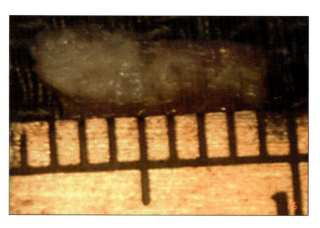

Fig 15–37. The keratotic surface of the lesion is well visualized.

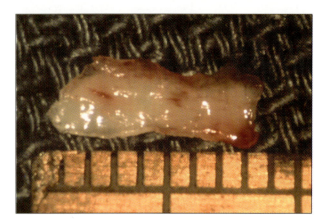

Fig 15–38. The basement membrane surface of the lesion is well visualized. One can appreciate the translucent normal epithelium at the margin of the lesion and the lack of significant microvascularity, which is part of the normal SLP which was preserved. The keratosis is seen through the undersurface of the translucent epithelium.

Case 15D

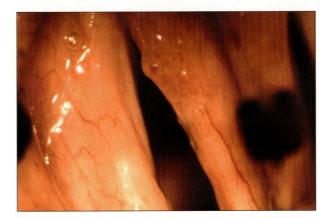

Fig 15–39. (7×) Erythroplasia of the right anterior vocal fold on the superior and medial surface. The erythroplasia typically has the irregular bubbled appearance and invariably reveals carcinoma in situ. The thickness of this lesion is well delineated posteriorly, as the prominent varix, which is seen on the right through the translucent epithelium, is obscured at the edge of the lesion. There is a small focus of mild thin keratosis just anterior to the vocal process on the left. A sulcus deformity was noted on the medial surface of the left vocal fold caused by vocal hyperfunction and collision forces from the lesion on the right.

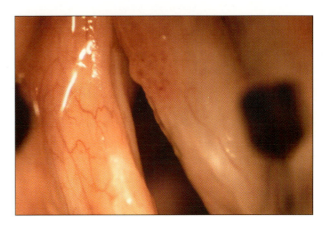

Fig 15–40. (7×) A subepithelial infusion of saline and adrenaline has been performed.

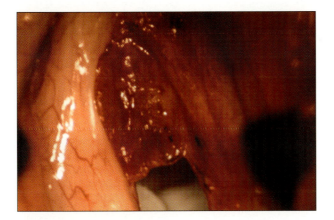

Fig 15–41. (7×) The entire lesion on the right is resected by means of an epithelial microflap. The CO_2 laser was used to enhance the excision where there were a few prominent vessels. The majority of the dissection and resection was performed with cold instrumentation.

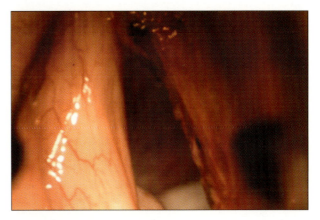

Fig 15–42. (7×) The right-sided lesion has been resected in its entirety and the resultant pathology revealed carcinoma in situ. The left-sided lesion was then resected and this revealed simply hyperplasia.

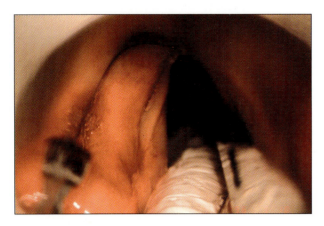

Fig 15–43. (4×) Without external counterpressure, the anterior glottal lesions are not seen.

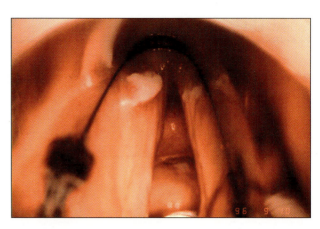

Fig 15–44. (4×) Subsequent to external counterpressure with a laryngeal cushion and 1-inch silk tape, bilateral keratotic lesions are seen of the anterior musculo-membranous vocal folds. The lesion on the left is more prominent than the one on the right.

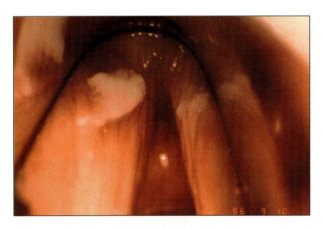

Fig 15–45. (7×) The prior lesion is seen at higher magnification encroaching on the anterior glottal commissure.

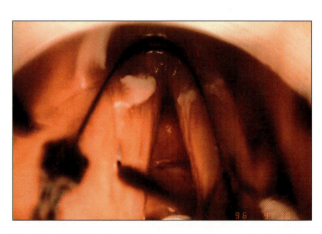

Fig 15–46. (4×) A subepithelial infusion needle has been placed and can be seen through the translucent epithelium.

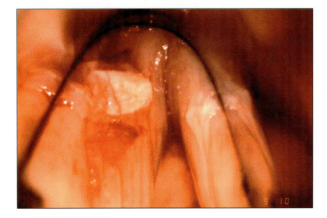

Fig 15–47. (7×) The lesion on the left has been mobilized as a microflap.

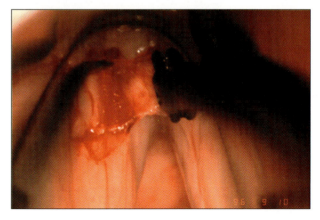

Fig 15–48. (7×) The lesion is being retracted and the underlying normal SLP is dissected from the basement membrane with a sharp pick.

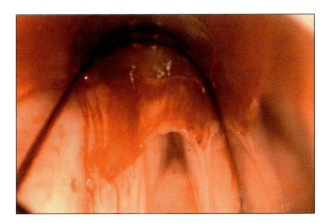

Fig 15–49. (7×) The microflap is seen in preparation for excision.

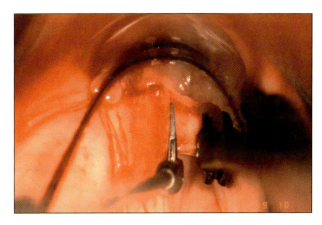

Fig 15–50. (7×) The microflap is retracted and an upturned scissors is used to complete the resection.

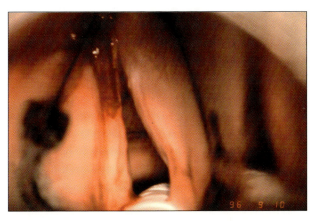

Fig 15–51. (4×) The left-sided lesion has been resected. A subepithelial infusion has been performed on the right to prepare that lesion for resection.

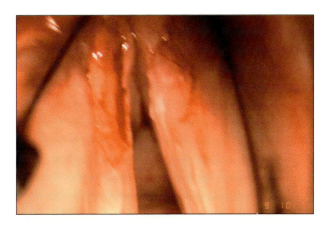

Fig 15–52. (7×) A perimeter incision has been made around the right-sided lesion.

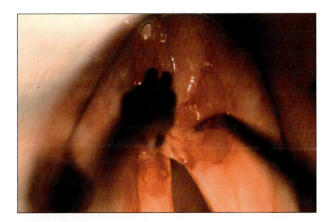

Fig 15–53. (7×) The right-sided lesion is retracted and a sharp pick is used to mobilize the normal SLP from the basement membrane.

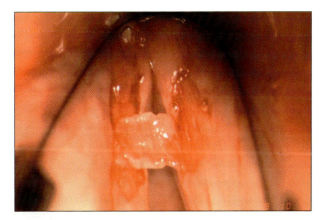

Fig 15–54. (7×) The microflap containing the epithelial atypia is visualized from the basement membrane surface.

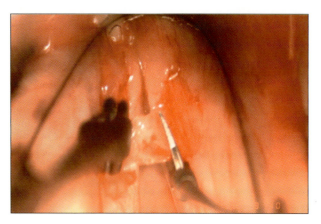

Fig 15–55. (7×) The microflap is retracted by means of a straight triangular forceps and an upturned scissors is used to complete the caudal margin.

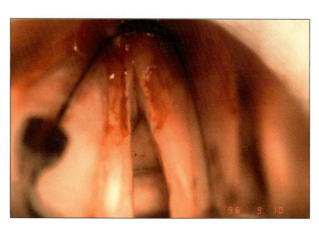

Fig 15–56. (4×) Both anterior lesions had been resected in their entirety.

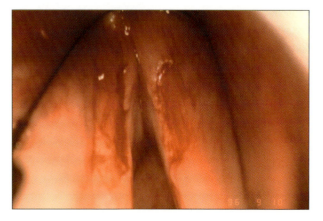

Fig 15–57. (7×) Figure 15–56 at higher magnification. There has been maximum preservation of normal epithelium and normal superficial lamina propria.

Case 15E

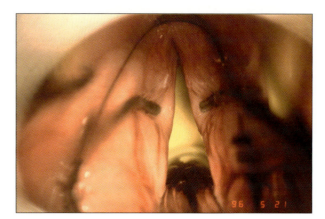

Fig 15–58. (4×) Bilateral keratosis with atypia on the medial surface of the musculo-membranous vocal folds.

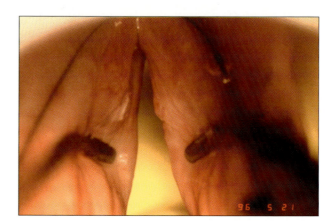

Fig 15–59. (7×) Figure 15–58 at higher magnification. There is chronic edema of the SLP of both vocal folds and retraction allows for better visualization of these lesions.

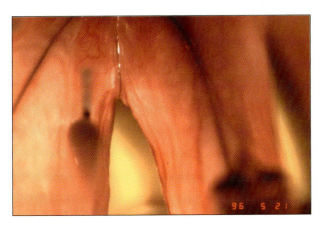

Fig 15–60. (7×) A subepithelial infusion of saline and adrenaline will be performed by means of a special needle. The needle can be seen through the translucent epithelium.

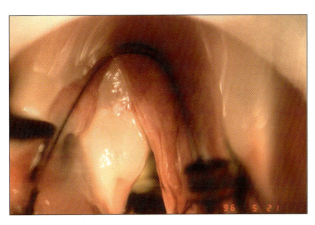

Fig 15–61. (4×) A subepithelial infusion has been performed on the left. The obvious vasoconstriction is well seen, as well as the narrowing of the glottal aperture. The infusion is quite dramatic because of chronic underlying edema that is already present. The keratotic area is now more clearly seen on the superior surface of that vocal fold anteriorly.

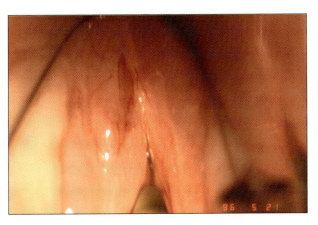

Fig 15–62. (7×) An anterior epithelial cordotomy incision is made.

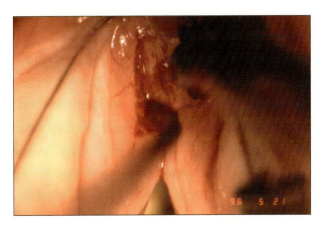

Fig 15–63. (7×) The microflap encompassing the lesion is retracted with a straight triangular forceps and the normal SLP is preserved by means of a curved dissector.

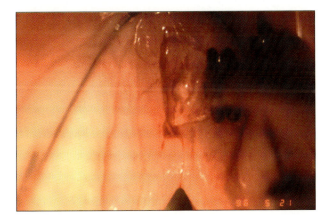

Fig 15–64. (7×) The microflap is retracted with the triangular forceps and the keratotic lesion can be seen through the undersurface of the microflap.

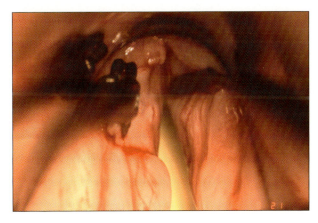

Fig 15–65. (7×) The microflap encompassing the keratotic lesion is retracted so that the caudal margin can be delineated. The right vocal fold is retracted with the dissector to allow for better visualization.

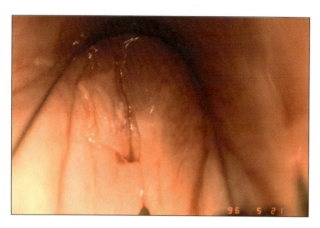

Fig 15–66. (7×) The redundant epithelium with the micro-flap is seen with the lesion at its center.

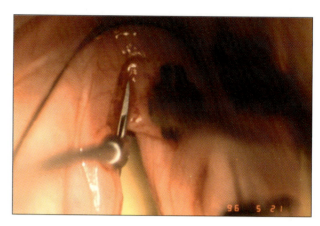

Fig 15–67. (7×) The lesion is retracted and an upturned scissors is used to complete the resection.

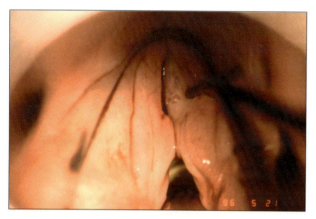

Fig 15–68. (4×) The lesion on the right is delineated by means of retraction with a curved dissector.

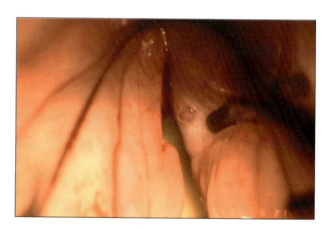

Fig 15–69. (7×) Figure 15–68 at higher magnification.

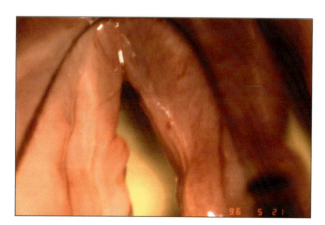

Fig 15–70. (7×) The right-sided lesion has been resected.

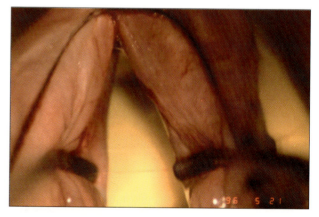

Fig 15–71. (7×) Bilateral curved dissectors are utilized to enhance visualization of the medial surface of the vocal folds. Due to the chronic edema of the SLP and the infusion, there is maximal preservation of normal epithelium and SLP and there is excellent coaptation of the epithelial edges.

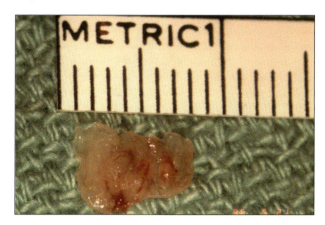

Fig 15–72. The epithelial lesion from the left can be visualized through the basement membrane surface of the resected microflap.

Case 15F

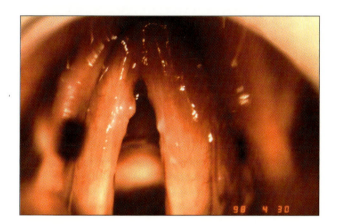

Fig 15–73. (4×) There are bilateral irregular lesions of the superior and medial surface of the vocal folds. There is a T1, N0, M0 squamous cell carcinoma on the left and keratosis with atypia on the right.

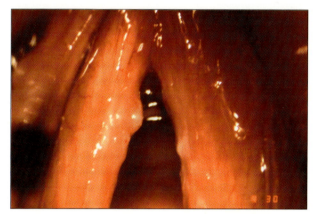

Fig 15–74. (7×) Figure 15–73 at higher magnification.

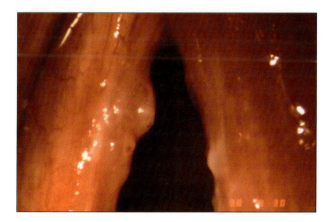

Fig 15–75. (10×) Figure 15–73 at even higher magnification.

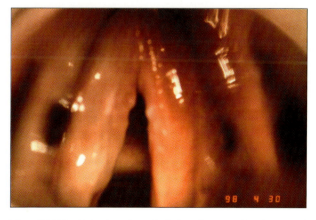

Fig 15–76. (4×) A subepithelial infusion of saline and adrenaline has been placed on the left.

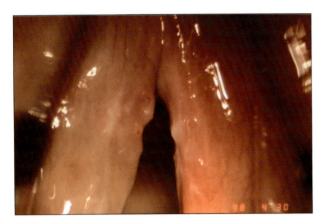

Fig 15–77. (7×) Figure 15–76 at higher magnification.

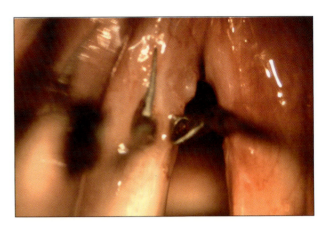

Fig 15–78. (7×) A perimeter incision is made lateral to the left-sided lesion.

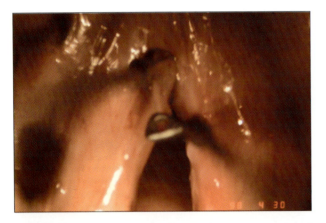

Fig 15–79. (7×) The epithelial microflap is retracted and a microscissors is used to complete the anterior limiting incision.

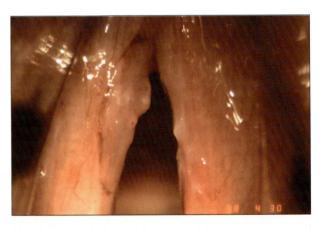

Fig 15–80. (7×) The incision around the perimeter around the left T1 cancer is delineated.

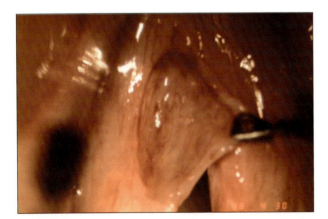

Fig 15–81. (7×) The dissection within the normal superficial lamina propria is performed to encompass the entire right lesion. The dissection on the medial and subcordal surface has not begun yet.

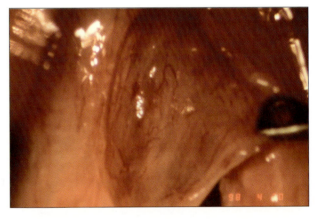

Fig 15–82. (10×) Figure 15–81 at higher magnification.

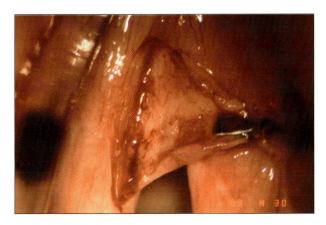

Fig 15–83. (7×) There has been further dissection toward the subcordal surface of the left vocal fold and the epithelial microflap is retracted.

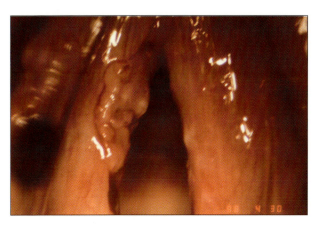

Fig 15–84. (7×) The mobilized epithelial lesion is redraped.

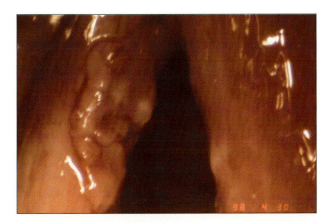

Fig 15–85. (10×) Figure 15–84 at higher magnification.

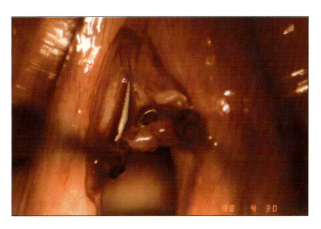

Fig 15–86. (7×) The microinvasive carcinoma is excised at its caudal margin with an upturned scissors.

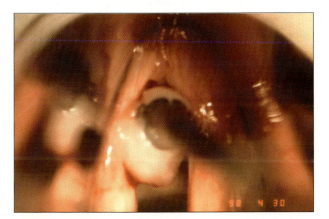

Fig 15–87. (4×) A loose cottonoid with 1/10,000 saline and adrenaline is applied.

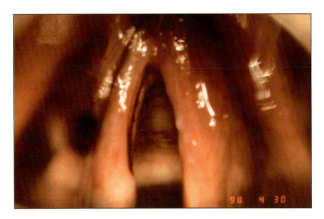

Fig 15–88. (4×) The left-sided lesion has been completely resected. Due to the extension to the anterior glottal commissure, the right-sided lesion will require resection at a second stage.

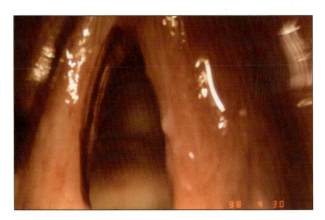

Fig 15–89. (7×) Figure 15–88 at higher magnification.

Case 15G

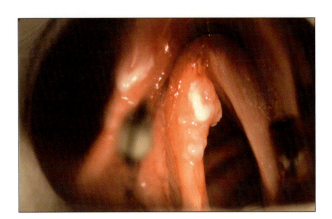

Fig 15–90. (4×) There is a T1, N0, M0 squamous cell carcinoma of the superior and medial surface of the left vocal fold. It caused severe hoarseness and dysphonia because of its bulky nature near the anterior glottal commissure.

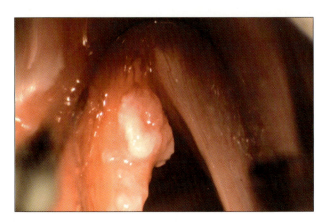

Fig 15–91. (7×) Figure 15–90 at higher magnification.

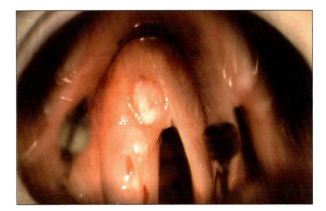

Fig 15–92. (7×) A subepithelial infusion has been performed. Despite the fact that the infusion revealed no adherence of the undersurface of the lesion to the vocal ligament, there was no substantive mucosal wave vibration through this area.

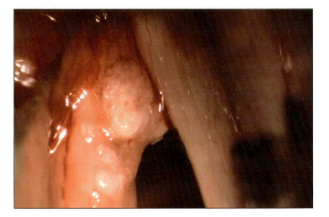

Fig 15–93. (7×) A perimeter 1-mm incision is made for a resection margin by means of an upturned scissors.

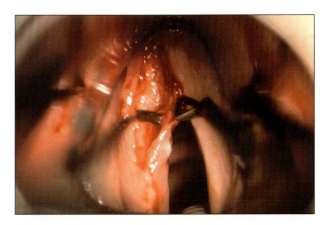

Fig 15–94. (4×) The lesion and the epithelial microflap are retracted with the forceps and the underlying normal superficial lamina propria is dissected from the undersurface of the neoplasm. Invasion to the vocal ligament (if present) can be easily appreciated by means of palpation and inspection and was not noted.

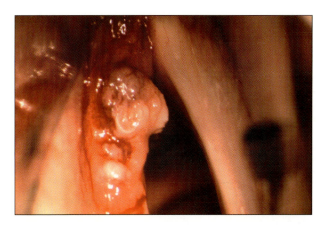

Fig 15–95. (7×) The lesion has been completely mobilized except for its attachment on the subcordal surface.

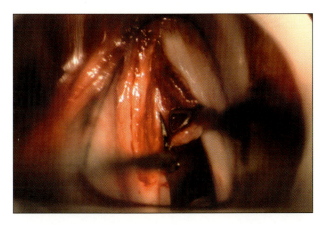

Fig 15–96. (4×) The lesion is retracted and an upturned scissors is used to complete the resection.

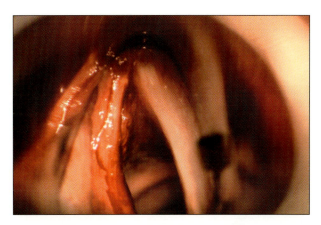

Fig 15–97. (4×) The T1 cancer has been resected with maximal preservation of normal epithelium and normal superficial lamina propria. This patient is 6 years postop without recurrence.

Case 15H

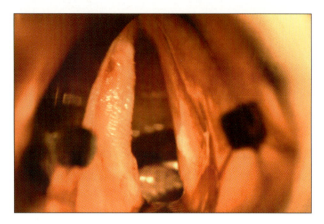

Fig 15–98. (4×) The patient is status post phonomicrosurgical resection of a right-sided keratotic lesion, which revealed severe atypia. There is mild residual keratosis at the right vocal process. The procedures were staged due to the extension on both sides to the anterior glottal commissure. The diffuse keratotic changes are seen encompassing the superior and medial surface of the left vocal fold.

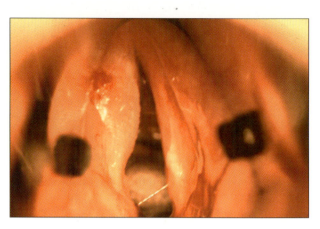

Fig 15–99. (4×) A subepithelial infusion of saline and adrenaline has been performed.

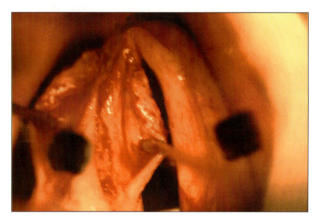

Fig 15–100. (4×) The epithelial microflap has been developed to encompass the entire lesion on the left. It is being retracted with a dissector.

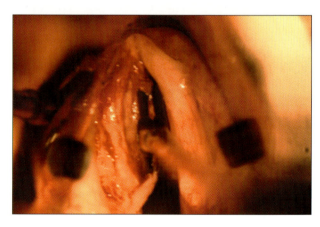

Fig 15–101. (4×) The epithelial microflap is further retracted with a straight triangular forceps.

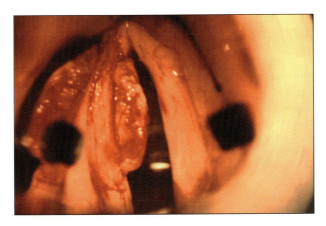

Fig 15–102. (4×) The epithelial microflap is seen attached by its caudal margin.

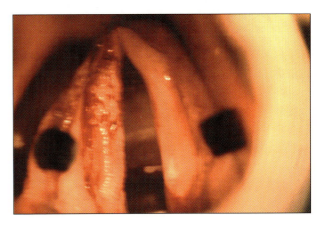

Fig 15–103. (4×) The microflap is redraped to determine the inferior extent of the disease.

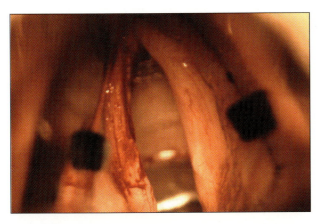

Fig 15–104. (4×) The lesion has been resected in its entirety.

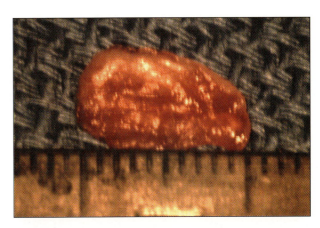

Fig 15–105. The lesion is seen through the undersurface of the basement membrane and a whole mount section was performed. This revealed microinvasive carcinoma.

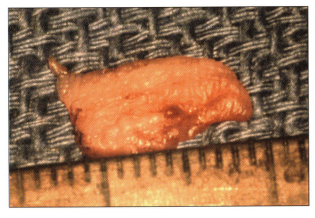

Fig 15–106. The keratotic irregular lesion is seen from the surface; histopathology revealed microinvasive carcinoma.

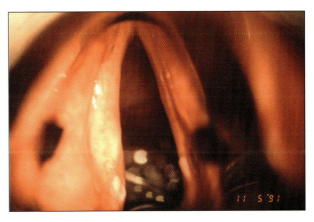

Fig 15–107. (4×) The patient continued to have keratotic areas overlying the medial surface of the arytenoids bilaterally. There was also a small left vestibular fold abnormality.

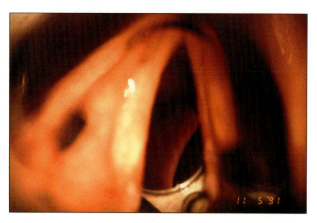

Fig 15–108. (4×) A mirror has been placed below the level of the glottal aperture to demonstrate the excellent healing that occurred from the prior phonomicrosurgical resections.

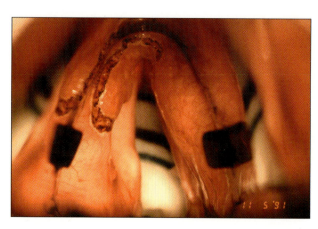

Fig 15–109. (4×) The laryngoscope has been withdrawn slightly to a level above the vestibular folds, so that the microspot CO_2 laser can be used to excise the left vestibular fold lesion. This revealed carcinoma in situ.

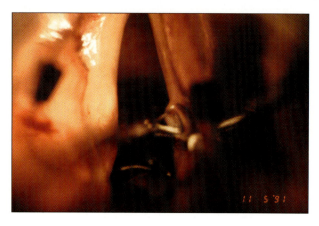

Fig 15–110. (4×) The right-sided keratotic lesion was excised in its entirety.

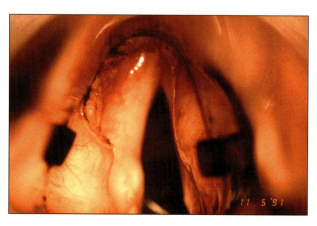

Fig 15–111. (4×) One can see the vestibular fold resection as well as the right-sided arytenoid epithelial lesion. Ultimately, the left-sided arytenoid lesion was removed as well. The patient has had no further surgery and no recurrence since 1991.

Case 15I

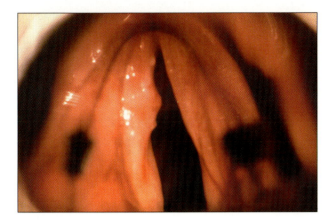

Fig 15–112. (4×) This patient had previously undergone microlaryngoscopic removal of carcinoma in situ from the left vocal fold approximately 10 years prior to this presentation. Stroboscopic assessment revealed diffuse stiffness of the left vocal fold epithelium, even in areas where the lesion was not present.

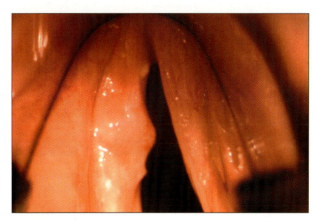

Fig 15–113. (7×) The lesion, which was a T1 cancer, is seen at higher magnification.

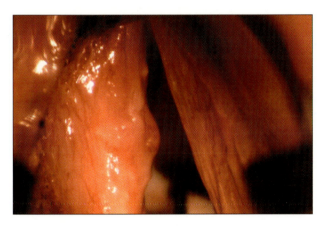

Fig 15–114. (7×) A CO_2 laser resection of the left vestibular fold has been performed to improve exposure of the lesion, especially in its lateral aspect. A subsequent subepithelial infusion had revealed diffuse adherence of both the epithelium, both in the region of the lesion as well as outside the perimeter of the lesion. This was presumably present as a result of the prior microlaryngoscopic procedure.

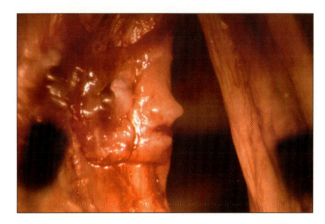

Fig 15–115. (7×) The entire lesion was dissected as an epithelial microflap. The retraction of the tissue to be excised is clearly seen and is typical.

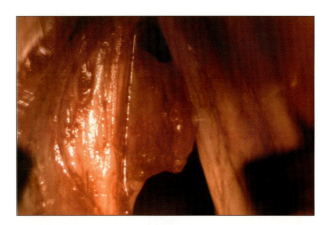

Fig 15–116. (7×) One can see there is no gross tumor invasion through the fibrosis that occurred as a result of the prior procedure. There was no normal SLP that could be preserved. The fibers of the preserved vocal ligament can be seen on the left.

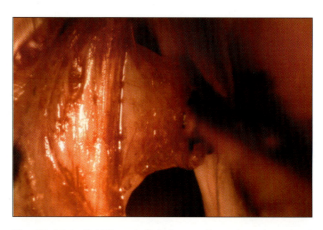

Fig 15–117. (7×) The epithelial microflap is being retracted to allow for a clean excision at the caudal margin of the lesion.

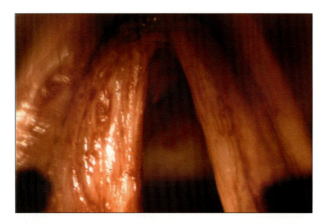

Fig 15–118. (7×) The entire superior and medial surface of the left vocal fold epithelial lesion has been resected. The patient had an uneventful postoperative course, and recovered his voice to normal conversational levels. This was documented by means of acoustic and aerodynamic measures. His cancer has not recurred, nor has he required subsequent surgery since this procedure in 1992.

Case 15J

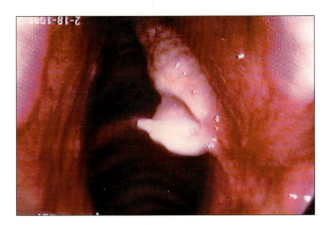

Fig 15–119. Clinic exam of a verrucous carcinoma.

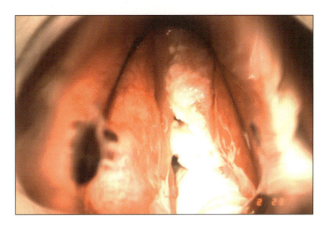

Fig 15–120. (4×) There is an exophytic verrucous carcinoma of the right vocal fold. Because of subglottic extension, it was staged as a T2, N0, M0 lesion. There was no substantive mucosal wave through that lesion.

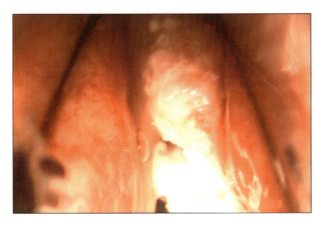

Fig 15–121. (7×) The prior lesion at higher magnification.

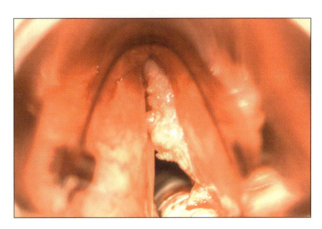

Fig 15–122. (4×) The laryngoscope has been withdrawn slightly to perform a vestibular fold resection to enhance visualization of the lateral margin of the lesion.

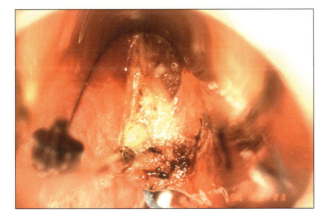

Fig 15–123. (4×) The Helium-neon aiming beam for the microspot CO_2 laser can be seen as the vestibular fold is being resected through the paraglottic fat.

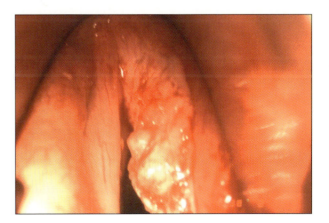

Fig 15–124. (7×) The vestibular fold has been resected, which facilitates visualization of the anterior and lateral margin of the lesion.

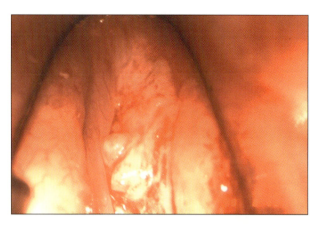

Fig 15–125. (7×) A subepithelial infusion is done on the right, which enhances visualization of the margins. There is no evidence of adherence of the lesion to the underlying vocal ligament based upon the subepithelial infusion.

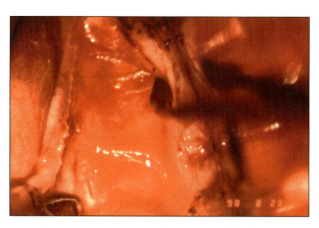

Fig 15–126. (7×) After beginning the procedure by performing an epithelial cordotomy with the microspot CO_2 laser, cold instruments are utilized to dissect the normal superficial lamina propria from the overlying neoplastic lesion.

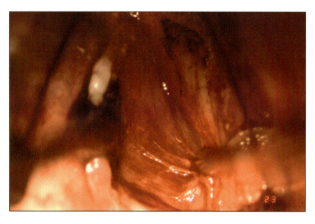

Fig 15–127. (7×) The undersurface of the lesion and the normal superficial lamina propria is well seen. A dissector is used to enhance the caudal margin of the resection. Anteriorly one can see the carbonization from the initial incision with the CO_2 laser.

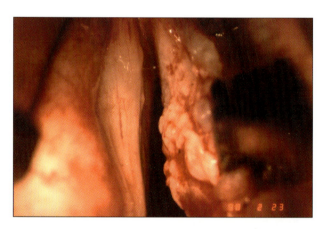

Fig 15–128. (7×) A large straight triangular forceps is used to withdraw and mobilize the flap to check for the extent of the caudal margin.

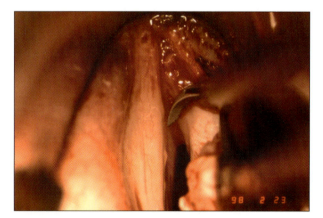

Fig 15–129. (7×) A left microscissors was used to complete the excision which extends through the epithelium in the anterior glottal commissure.

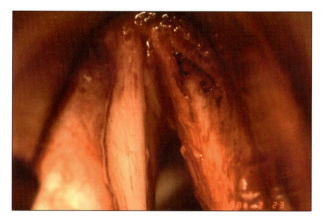

Fig 15–130. (7×) The lesion has been resected to its inferior extent at the beginning of the subglottis. There has been maximal preservation of normal superficial lamina propria and normal epithelium.

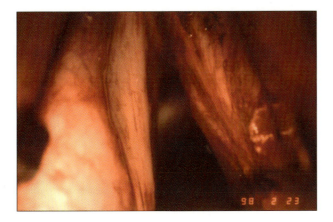

Fig 15–131. (7×) A dissector is in place on the posterior medial aspect of the fold demonstrating the caudal extent of the resection.

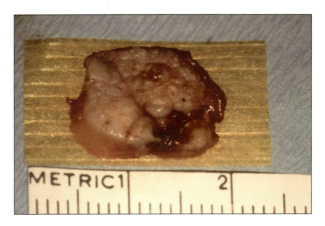

Fig 15–132. The extensive keratotic lesion is placed on a carrier for whole mount sectioning.

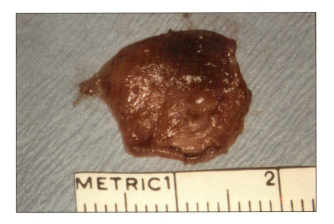

Fig 15–133. The undersurface of the neoplasm is visualized from the basement membrane side of the lesion.

Case 15K

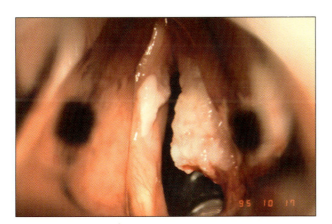

Fig 15–134. (4×) There are bilateral keratotic lesions. The lesion on the right revealed a microinvasive squamous cell carcinoma. Although the left-sided lesion was not resected during this procedure, it ultimately revealed keratosis with severe atypia.

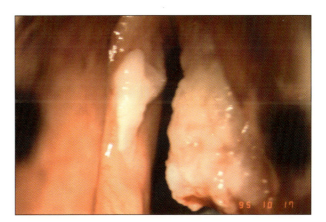

Fig 15–135. (7×) The prior lesion at higher magnification.

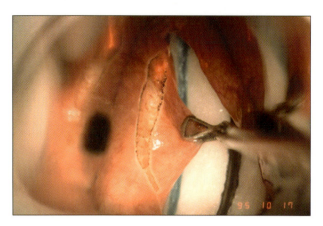

Fig 15–136. (4×) The left vestibular fold resection is performed with the microspot CO_2 laser to enhance visualization of the glottis. A cottonoid is placed in the ventricle to avoid trauma to the true vocal folds.

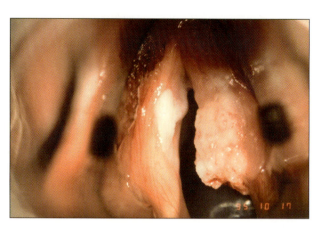

Fig 15–137. (4×) Both vestibular folds had been resected. There is improved visualization of the glottis.

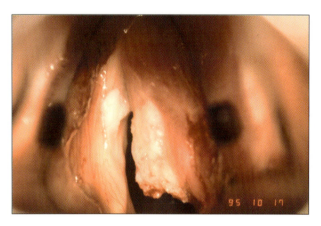

Fig 15–138. (4×) A subepithelial infusion has been performed on the right which demonstrated that the lesion was not invading the vocal ligament. The lateral margin of the lesion is now well seen and there is increased normal mucosa laterally to create a safe margin.

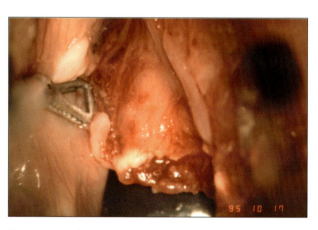

Fig 15–139. (7×) An epithelial cordotomy is performed with an upturned scissors and the microflap within the SLP, which encompasses the entire lesion, was developed with cold instruments.

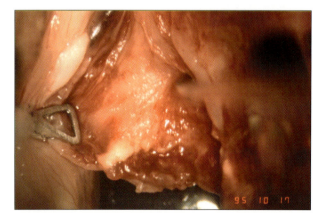

Fig 15–140. (7×) The lesion is retracted and a curved dissector is used to continue the caudal dissection of the flap.

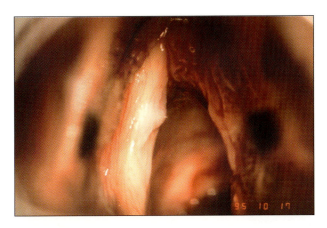

Fig 15–141. (4×) After the caudal dissection of the tumor was completed, the tumor was excised en bloc.

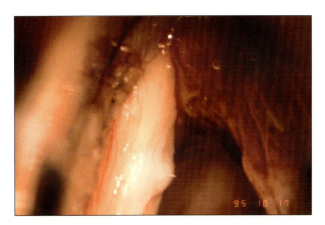

Fig 15–142. (7×) Figure 15–141 at higher magnification. Because of the anterior dissection and the extent of the disease on the medial surface anteriorly on the left, the left vocal fold lesion was resected later.

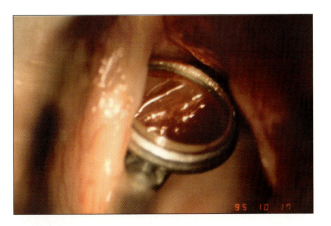

Fig 15–143. (7×) A mirror is employed to demonstrate the normal mucosa at the caudal margin.

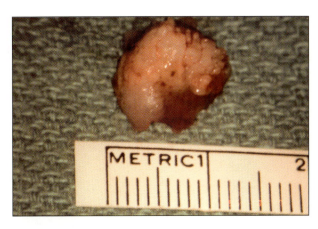

Fig 15–144. The keratotic surface of the lesion is well seen.

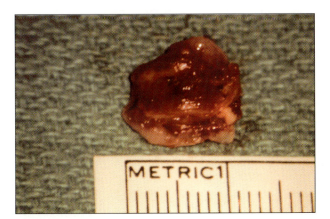

Fig 15–145. The lesion is visualized through the undersurface with no deep invasion. This patient had no substantive mucosal wave through this keratotic epithelium despite the fact there was no invasion to the vocal ligament.

Case 15L

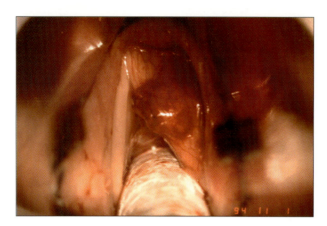

Fig 15–146. (4×) There is an exophytic T1, N0, M0 squamous cell carcinoma of the right vocal fold.

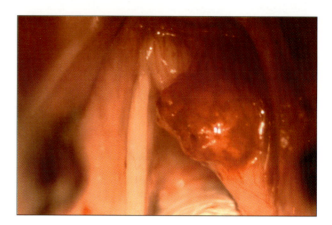

Fig 15–147. (7×) The prior lesion seen at higher magnification.

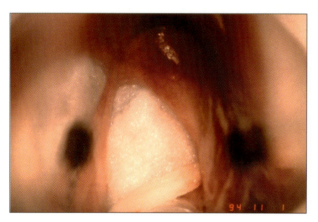

Fig 15–148. (4×) The laryngoscope is withdrawn to perform a vestibular fold resection to enhance visualization and exposure of the cancer. A cottonoid is placed in the ventricle to protect the vocal fold.

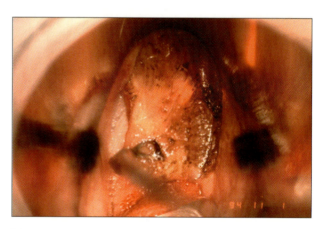

Fig 15–149. (4×) The microspot CO_2 laser is utilized to resect the vestibular fold.

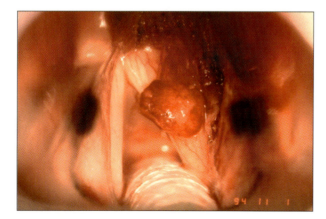

Fig 15–150. (4×) The vestibular fold has been resected, which provides excellent exposure of the right vocal fold cancer.

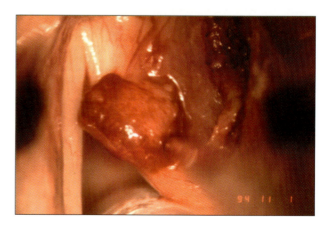

Fig 15–151. (7×) The prior lesion is seen at higher magnification.

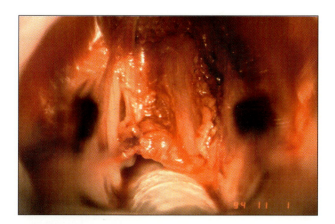

Fig 15–152. (4×) The lesion was attached to the vocal ligament; therefore, the resection proceeds between the vocal ligament and the vocalis muscle. The lesion is retracted medially and caudally through the glottal aperture.

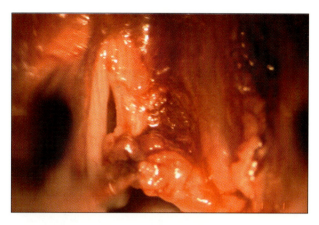

Fig 15–153. (7×) The dissection is performed so that very little of the vocal muscle is disturbed and the vocal ligament is used as a margin.

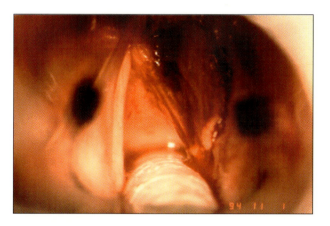

Fig 15–154. (4×) The right vocal fold cancer has been resected en bloc with the vocal ligament as a margin. The right neocord is remarkably well contoured considering the extent of the resection.

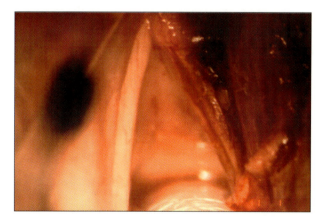

Fig 15–155. (7×) Figure 15–154 at higher magnification.

Case 15M

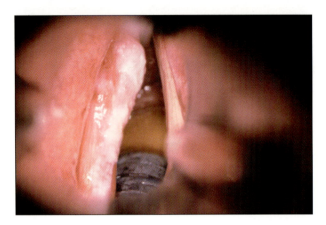

Fig 15–156. (4×) T1, N0, M0 squamous cell carcinoma of the left vocal fold exposed by means of Dedo laryngoscope. Note the limitations and exposure with this instrumentation. Also note that, due to the circular shape of this instrument distally, the edge of the laryngoscope could not distract the vestibular folds well.

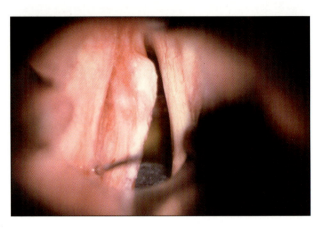

Fig 15–157. (4×) A subepithelial infusion is performed, which reveals that the lesion is attached to the vocal ligament.

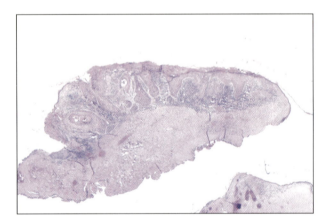

Fig 15–158. The resected specimen showing invasion to the vocal ligament.

Case 15N

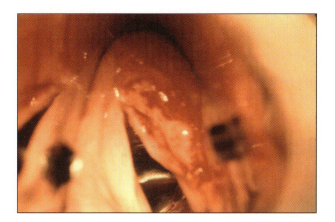

Fig 15–159. (4×) A large ulcerating T1, N0, M0 squamous cell carcinoma of the right vocal fold and initial anterior incision was made with cold instruments, which produced a significant amount of bleeding. This obscured visualization initially of the anterior glottis.

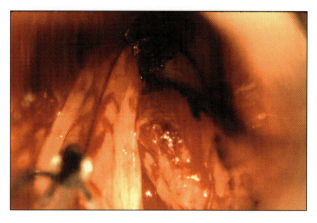

Fig 15–160. (4×) The CO_2 laser was utilized to control the bleeding anteriorly. Then a modified Rosen knife was utilized to hand dissect the lesion from the anterior thyroid lamina which is seen just lateral to the carbonized perichondrium anteriorly.

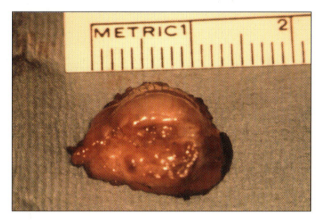

Fig 15–161. (4×) The entire vocal fold including the underlying muscle was resected en bloc.

Case 15O

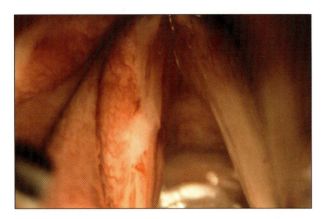

Fig 15–162. (7×) This patient presented with a previous biopsy. The resultant pathology revealed a spindle cell carcinoma or a carcino-sarcoma. There was no substantive mucosal wave through any of the left vocal folds. The full length of that vocal fold was unusually rigid by palpation during the laryngoscopy.

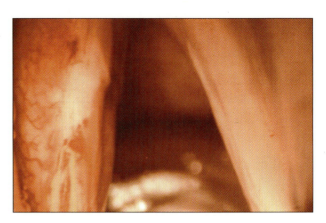

Fig 15–163. (10×) Figure 15–162 at higher magnification.

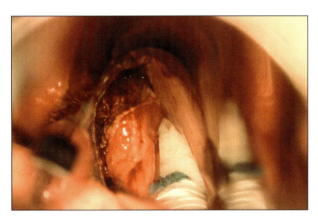

Fig 15–164. (4×) A perimeter incision around the thyroarytenoid muscle and its overlying mucosa is made with the microspot CO_2 laser.

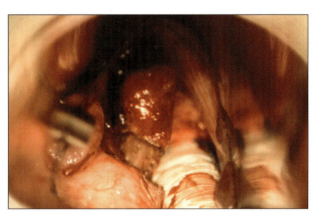

Fig 15–165. (4×) A transmural excision of the lesion is performed.

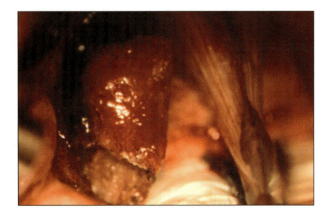

Fig 15–166. (7×) Figure 15–165 at higher magnification.

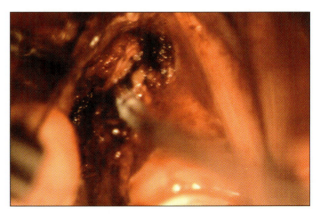

Fig 15–167. (7×) The thyroid cartilage is seen at the edge of the carbonization on the left. A biopsy is done to ensure for clear deep margins.

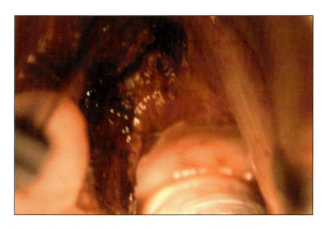

Fig 15–168. (7×) The resultant postsurgical defect.

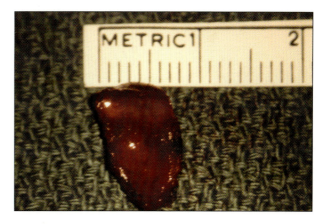

Fig 15–169. The resected specimen had submucosal disease.

Case 15P

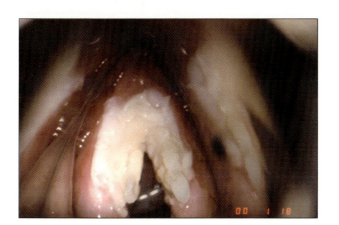

Fig 15-170. (4×) Verrucous keratosis of both vocal folds.

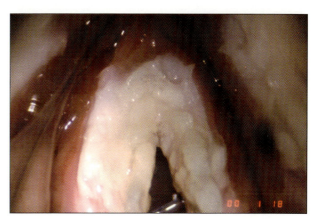

Fig 15–171. (7×) Figure 15–170 at higher magnification.

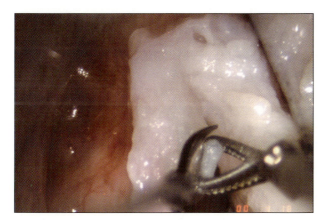

Fig 15–172. (10×) The necrotic keratin is partially removed prior to use of a pulsed-dye laser.

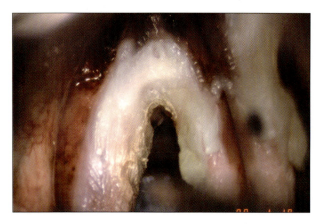

Fig 15–173. (7×) A pulsed-dye laser is used to photocoagulate the subepithelial microvasculature. The fiber is directed at the left fold.

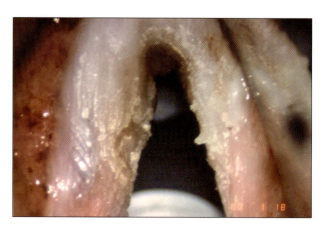

Fig 15–174. (10×) Figure 15–173 at higher magnification.

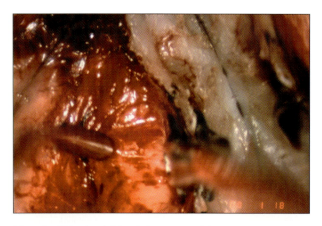

Fig 15–175. (10×) The left verrucoid lesion is resected by means of a microflap with a dissector. Despite prior resections and resultant epithelial scarring, the laser facilitated the resection by enhancing hemostasis and by creating a dissection plane between the lesion and the underlying SLP.

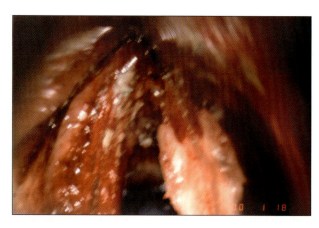

Fig 15–176. (7×) The left-sided lesion has been resected; the right will be done subsequent to epithelialization at the anterior commissure.

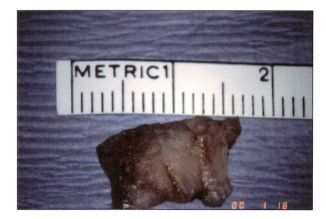

Fig 15–177. The specimen from the left-sided resection including the anterior commissure.

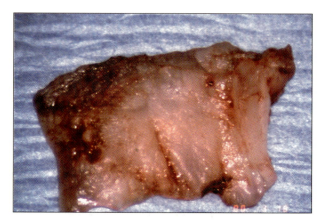

Fig 15–178. Figure 15–177 at higher magnification.

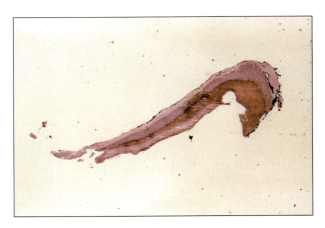

Fig 15–179. H&E of the resected specimen displaying the contours of the anterior commissure; the histopathology only revealed hyperplasia.

Case 15Q

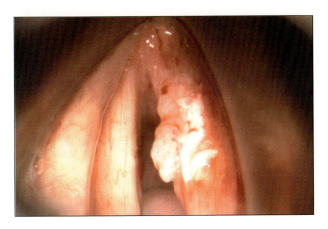

Fig 15–180. (4×) A T1, N0, M0 squamous cell carcinoma is seen on the right vocal fold in a Shakespearean actor. (Courtesy of Endocraft LLC.)

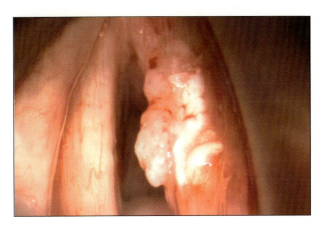

Fig 15–181. (7×) Figure 15–180 seen at higher magnification. (Courtesy of Endocraft LLC.)

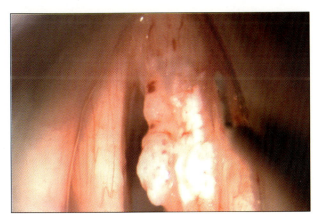

Fig 15–182. (7×) An infusion needle is seen lateral to the cancer margin. The lesion did not invade the vocal fold. (Courtesy of Endocraft LLC.)

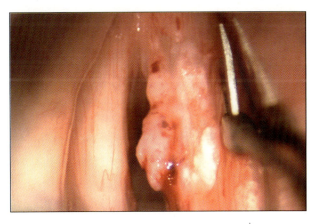

Fig 15–183. (7×) An upturned scissors is used to perform a perimeter incision lateral to the lesion. (Courtesy of Endocraft LLC.)

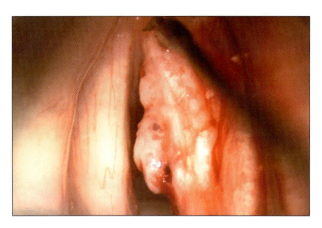

Fig 15–184. (7×) The incision is completed. (Courtesy of Endocraft LLC.)

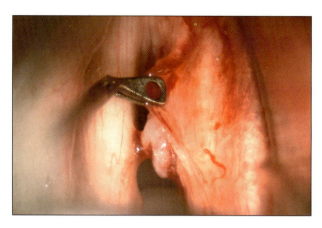

Fig 15–185. (7×) The lesion is retracted medially as a micro-flap. Cancer is not seen invading through the SLP to the vocal ligament. (Courtesy of Endocraft LLC.)

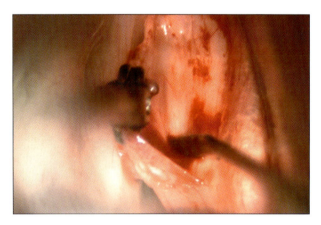

Fig 15–186. (7×) A curved dissector is used to continue the caudal deep dissection. (Courtesy of Endocraft LLC.)

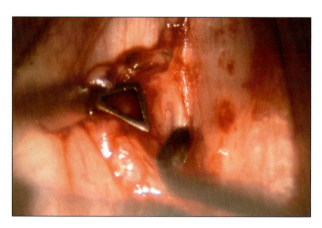

Fig 15–187. (7×) The curved dissector is utilized to continue the caudal deep dissection. (Courtesy of Endocraft LLC.)

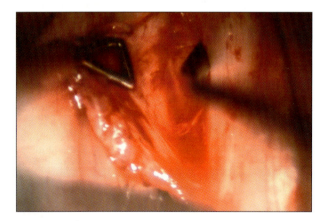

Fig 15–188. (7×) The lesion is retracted. Note the normal deep SLP. (Courtesy of Endocraft LLC.)

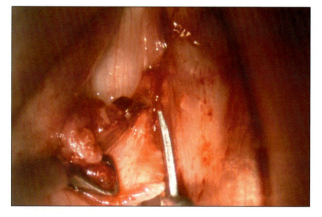

Fig 15–189. (7×) An upturned scissors is used to complete the caudal resection of the cancer. (Courtesy of Endocraft LLC.)

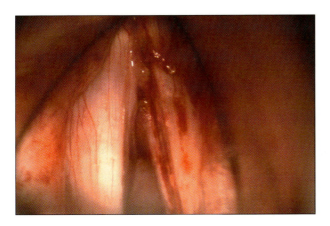

Fig 15–190. (4×) The completed cancer resection. Note that there is residual microvasculature in the deep SLP. (Courtesy of Endocraft LLC.)

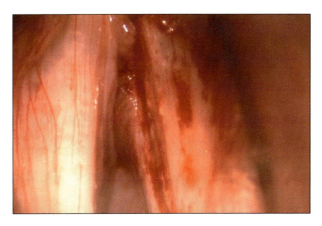

Fig 15–191. (7×) Figure 15–190 at higher magnification. (Courtesy of Endocraft LLC.)

Case 15R

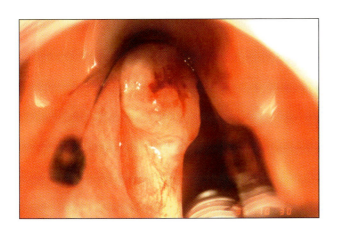

Fig 15–192. (4×) A cancer is seen at the anterior commissure, arising from the left vocal fold. The anterior limit of the lesion cannot be determined.

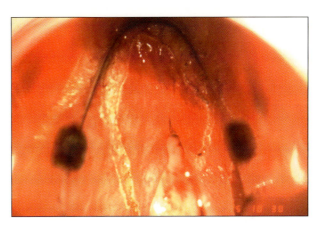

Fig 15–193. (4×) The scope has been withdrawn and the CO_2 laser is used to excise the lower anterior supraglottis.

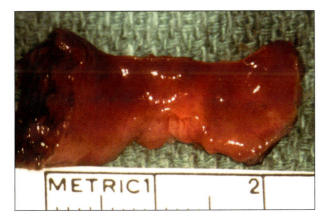

Fig 15–194. Both anterior vestibular folds and the infrapetiole region have been resected.

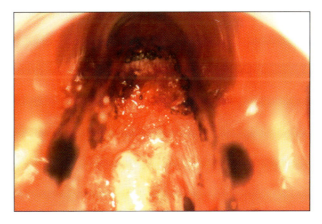

Fig 15–195. (4×) It can now be seen that the cancer is not grossly invading the thyroid cartilage.

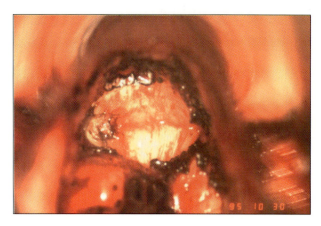

Fig 15–196. (4×) The anterior commissure tendon can be retracted from the underlying cartilage to ensure that there is no occult cancer invasion.

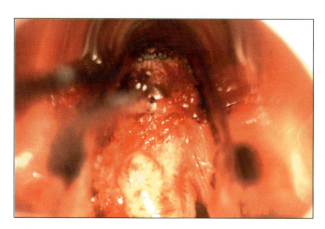

Fig 15–197. (4×) A biopsy and frozen section confirmed that this was a T1 lesion.

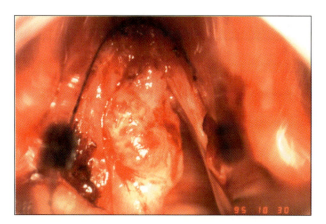

Fig 15–198. (4×) The resection could have been done but potentially would have required resection of the right side of the anterior commissure tendon. Preoperatively, the patient had elected to undergo radiation therapy if this scenario was encountered. Note that the tendon naturally repositions if it is not completely disassociated from the cartilage.

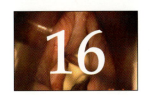

Glottic Reconstruction and Voice Rehabilitation

When a significant amount of vocalis muscle is removed as part of the deep margin, the healed neocord is usually concave. The excavated neocord results in incomplete glottal closure during phonation. This leads to a stiff, leaking glottal-valve and a hoarse disordered voice. As the depth of an excision leads to valvular incompetence of the glottis, there is increased: subglottal pressures and flows, acoustical instability (jitter and shimmer), and supraglottal muscle strain patterns. Stroboscopy reveals no substantive mucosal-wave oscillation but rather a mass vibration of the stiff neocord body.[65]

Once the neocord is healed, phonosurgical reconstruction may ensue if the vocal edge is excavated. Initially, this may consist of microlaryngoscopic fat injection. It may take one or two injections based on how much tissue was initially resected and how much of the fat implant is resorbed. As necessary a medialization laryngoplasty can be performed once there is adequate glottal tissue medial to the thyroid lamina. Goretex has been ideal in this setting because it can be molded in vivo to conform to the abnormal postresection contours.[194] The advantage of the medialization is that it is done under local anesthesia with intravenous sedation, which allows for phonatory feedback during the procedure. The vocal outcome is often dependent on the flexibility of the normal layered microstructure of the uninvolved vocal fold.

Case 16A

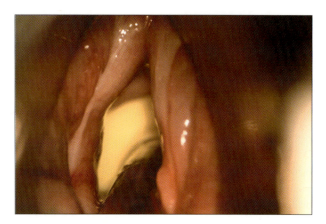

Fig 16–1. (4×) The patient has undergone phonomicrosurgical resection of a left T1a carcinoma and now has an excavated vocal fold in the musculo-membranous region.

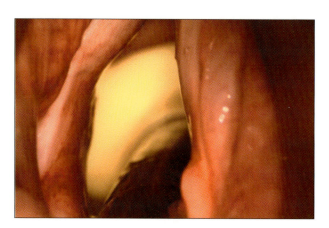

Fig 16–2. (7×) Figure 16–1 at higher magnification.

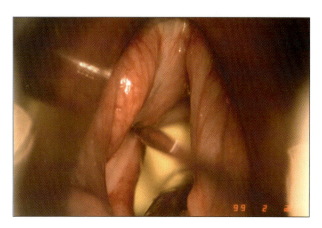

Fig 16–3. (4×) A Brünings injection needle is placed lateral to the concavity in the paraglottic space.

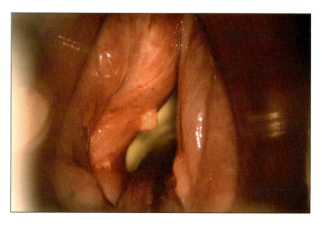

Fig 16–4. (4×) The vocal fold has been augmented with fat. A small amount of the graft is extruding from the puncture site and should be removed with cold instruments to avoid a granuloma. Note the new convexity of the vocal fold.

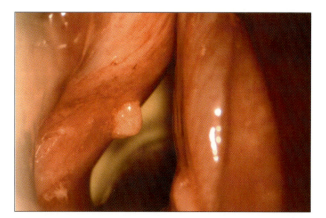

Fig 16–5. (7×) Figure 16–4 at higher magnification.

Case 16B

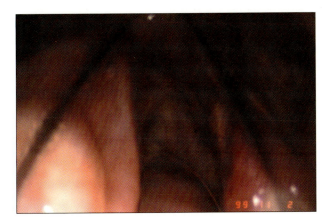

Fig 16–6. (7×) A T1 carcinoma, which extended to the anterior commissure tendon, was previously resected from the right vocal fold. Note the large defect anteriorly, which resulted in severe aerodynamic leakage as noted on stroboscopy. The healed mucosa was adjacent to the thyroid cartilage without underlying paraglottic muscle or fat.

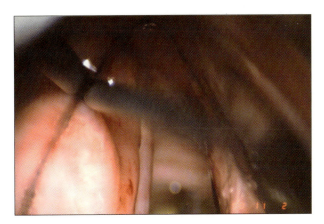

Fig 16–7. (7×) Initially fat is injected into the anterior paraglottic region of the healthy left fold.

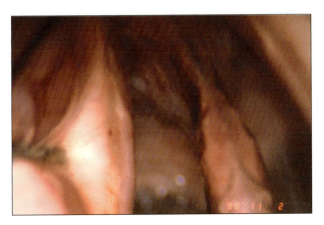

Fig 16–8. (7×) The left vocal fold is now convex in contour.

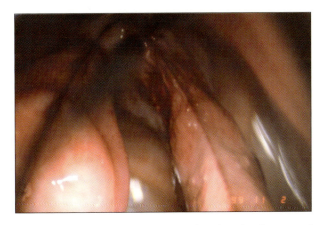

Fig 16–9. (7×) The needle is then placed under the scarred mucosa in the right anterior commissure in an attempt to close the persistent anterior keyhole aperture. Very little fat could be placed. Although improved from this procedure, the patient ultimately required an open laryngoplasty under local-regional anesthesia to close the anterior commissure gap.

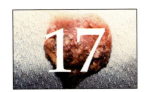

Supraglottic Cancer

THE PHILOSOPHY OF SUPRAGLOTTAL SURGERY

Endoscopic supraglottal surgery is done far less frequently than glottal surgery.[77] The surgical field is typically much larger and therefore requires different laryngoscopes and hand instrumentation (Figure 17–1). A bivalved adjustable supraglottiscope (Figure 17–2) was designed[121] to facilitate endoscopic supraglottal surgery. This instrument was a modification of Steiner's[195] laryngoscope. A number of bivalved instruments suitable for supraglottal surgery are available from the major manufacturers. The surgeon should compare the distal distension strength prior to purchasing one. In principle, bivalved laryngoscopes better accommodate the large supraglottal surgical field and the larger lesions that require increased hand-instrument angulation for tissue retraction. Larger and more sturdy supraglottic hand instruments are now available. The premicroscope era instruments can still be purchased as well or they can often be obtained from the mediastinoscopy set.

If the airway is stable, there are different primary functional concerns between endoscopic surgery of the glottis and supraglottis. In glottal surgery, the most common functional concern is preservation of the voice; in supraglottal surgery, it is swallowing. In turn, the microspot CO_2 laser is a very effective instrument for supraglottal surgery. Thermal-induced fibrosis of residual supraglottal tissues results in beneficial cicatricial scarring and re-establishment of a competent supraglottic swallowing valve.[196]

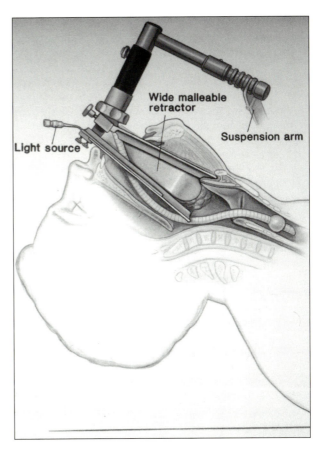

Fig 17–2. Diagrammatic representation of the Adjustable Supraglottiscope in place with the patient and Jackson position. The upper blade is situated in the vallecula glosso-epiglottica. The lower blade distracts the endotracheal tube. (From Shapiro J, Zeitels SM, Fried MF. *Operat Tech Otolaryngol Head Neck Surg.* 1992;3:84–92 with permission.)

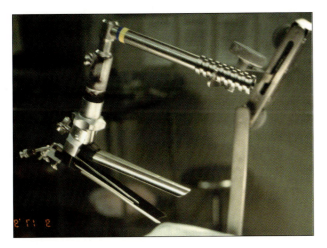

Fig 17–1. Zeitels adjustable supraglottiscope.

BACKGROUND OF ENDOSCOPIC MANAGEMENT

Direct laryngoscopic resection of supraglottic cancer dates back to the early 20th century. Jackson[197–199] described the use of a tubular laryngoscope and a punch biopsy forceps for resecting suprahyoid epiglottic cancer. The lesion was resected by cutting around the lesion with the punch, and if the tissue specimens within the punch were without cancer, the resection was considered curative. In 1941, New et al[133] performed transoral ablation (by means of surgical diathermy) of several supraglottic carcinomas by employing a Lynch suspension laryngoscope,[126,127] which was a modification of Killian's system.[48,49] Vaughan[76] first described microscopically controlled CO_2 laser resection of supraglottic cancer in 1978. Subsequently, other Boston University trainees including Davis et al[200,201] and Zeitels et al[196,202,203] reported several series of CO_2 laser supraglottic cancer resections. Steiner,[195,204] Eckel and Thumfart,[172] and Rudert[191] have also been strong advocates of endoscopic management of supraglottic cancer.

These investigators in the United States and Germany incorporated technological advancements in microlaryngeal surgery to expand Jackson's concepts. However, for a number of reasons, most surgeons in North America have not adopted the endoscopic excision approach despite its value and merit. First, most surgeons are not familiar with the details of the technique and the endoscopic approach represents a paradigm shift. Second, larger lesions are technically difficult to resect if one is not familiar with the details of the method. Furthermore, teaching the technique is not effectively done in continuing education courses. Finally, surgical resection of laryngeal cancer is declining at many centers at which there has been a proliferation of chemotherapy-radiation protocols.

CURATIVE ENDOSCOPIC RESECTION

Endoscopic resection of supraglottic cancer can be performed as a single modality treatment. Small lesions are excised during the staging endoscopy and the resection is both diagnostic and therapeutic.[203] Therefore, any further treatment such as open surgery or radiation becomes superfluous and cost-ineffective. With this endoscopic approach, there has not been significant loss of laryngeal function. Most patients return to a normal diet within several days and no patient has required artificial airway intervention.

Transoral excision of supraglottic cancer as a single modality is successful when lesions are selected for small size and endoscopic accessibility. Small volume lesions that arise on the suprahyoid epiglottis, aryepiglottic fold, and vestibular fold are amenable to en bloc endoscopic resection because they are more perpendicular to the distal lumen of the laryngoscope.

Specimen margins are ideally established through multiple section analysis of the en bloc resected specimen rather than by means of frozen sections from the patient. Decisions about postoperative radiotherapy and treatment of "the necks" should be based on the pathological assessment of the lesion. Controlling neck metastasis is critical for curing patients of supraglottic cancer.[205–207] Consideration should be given to the volume of the cancer, the depth and location of its penetration, and the pattern of its invasion. Even small

lesions of the aryepiglottic fold and vestibular fold will demonstrate early invasion of the paraglottic space. This places the neck at risk for occult metastasis. In contrast, early suprahyoid epiglottic carcinomas rarely invade the pre-epiglottic space and rarely metastasize to the neck if there is no occult tongue-base invasion.[208]

It is not clear whether radiation to the larynx is necessary if an adequate endoscopic resection has been performed. Currently, the first multi-institutional study is being conducted to assess the reliability of endoscopic resection (without radiation) of any accessible supraglottic cancer. The initial data should be available in 2001. There are many T2 and T3 lesions in this series. The participants are Davis, DeSanto, Gluckman, Haughey, Hoffman, Pearson, Strome, and Zeitels.

ENDOSCOPIC RESECTION FOLLOWED BY RADIATION THERAPY

Transoral resection of larger supraglottic cancers followed by full-course radiotherapy to the primary site and both necks offers a more aggressive treatment approach for individuals who otherwise would have undergone radiotherapy as a sole treatment. The endoscoscopic resection is a neoadjuvant therapy with a histopathologically controlled result. This approach stresses laryngeal *function preservation* (airway, swallowing and voice) rather than *organ preservation*.[209]

These endoscopic supraglottic resections are considered excisional biopsies since margins are frequently close and the deep compartments (pre-epiglottic and paraglottic spaces) are not excised completely. However, the patients have no clinical evidence of cancer when they commence radiotherapy. The success of obtaining clear margins on these excisional biopsies is based on the typical pattern of invasion, which is broad and pushing with a pseudocapsule.[180,181,208] This pseudocapsule probably arises from the epiglottic perichondrium and the quadrangular membrane.[196,208]

SURGICAL TECHNIQUE

Lesions that are larger and those arising on the infrahyoid epiglottis and upper false vocal fold are more difficult to resect transorally because they are visualized tangentially.[196,210] The surgeon must decide whether the neoplasm will be excised en bloc or in a piecemeal fashion. The philosophy of endoscopic en bloc excision maintains a more standard surgical oncological approach. However, larger lesions gradually fill the laryngoscope lumen as they are mobilized. This makes en bloc excision technically difficult. Some groups in Germany[190,211] section the specimen and resect the tumor in a piecemeal fashion. There is little question that this makes the procedure technically easier. These investigators also maintain that transecting the lesion facilitates a precise assessment of the depth of invasion. They have not noted increased rates of local, regional, or distant failure.

LARYNGEAL FUNCTION AFTER ENDOSCOPIC EXCISION

The airway and voice are not typically impaired by an endoscopic supraglottic resection. Often however, the airway is improved when an exophytic lesion is excised. On occasion, a patient may require a late tracheotomy secondary to late stenosis from severe gastroesophageal reflux.[203]

Laryngeal protective function may be impaired temporarily depending on the extent of the supraglottic tissues excised. There has not been permanent swallowing impairment in patients who have otherwise normal swallowing mechanisms. Previous impairment, such as that sustained from a stroke or previous head and neck surgery, is a relative contraindication to any partial laryngeal resection.

Limited resections of the suprahyoid epiglottis, aryepiglottic fold or vestibular fold did not impair swallowing function because most of the sphincteric function of the supraglottis is unaffected. The epiglottis is a vestigial organ in man and often contains olfactory epithelium in mammals.[212] More extensive resections may predispose to aspiration that may last from several days to 6 weeks depending on the magnitude of the resection. Although patients may require nasogastric feeding during this time, none has sustained an aspiration pneumonia during swallowing rehabilitation or from salivary soilage.

The favorable swallowing rehabilitation after extensive transoral supraglottic resections occurs for several reasons.[203,213] Most importantly, the superior laryngeal nerves are not disturbed proximal to the larynx. Therefore, the neo-supraglottic region becomes fully sensate. Secondly, laryngeal elevation is not impaired either by disturbance of the suprahyoid musculature or by performing a tracheotomy. Finally, since the supraglottic defect heals completely by secondary fibrosis and epithelialization, there is favorable cicatrization that results in a new supraglottic valve. Hospitalization from this procedure is usually 1 to 3 days.

Case 17A

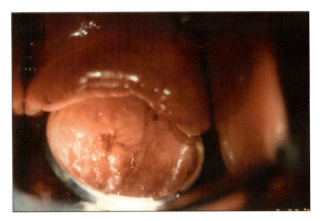

Fig 17–3. (4×) There is an ulcerated cancer on the laryngeal surface of the suprahyoid epiglottis. It is not well appreciated due to the tangential image, and therefore, a mirror is utilized to display the carcinoma.

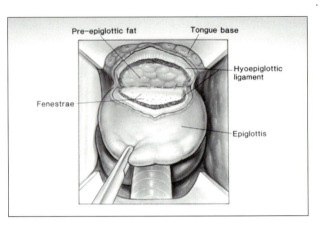

Fig 17–4. Diagrammatic representation of the initial incision in the vallecula through the hyoepiglottic ligament. (From Shapiro J, Zeitels SM, Fried MF. *Operat Tech Otolaryngol Head Neck Surg.* 1992;3:84–92 with permission.)

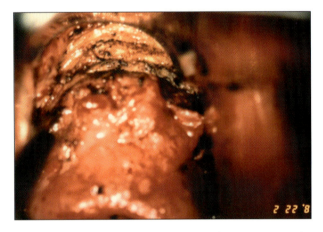

Fig 17–5. (4×) The dissection proceeds anterior to the epiglottis through the pre-epiglottic fat.

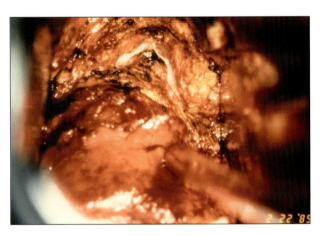

Fig 17–6. (4×) Continued dissection is performed until the petiole of the epiglottis is resected.

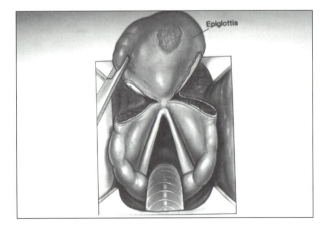

Fig 17–7. Diagrammatic representation of the previous resection. (From Shapiro J, Zeitels SM, Fried MF. *Operat Tech Otolaryngol Head Neck Surg.* 1992;3:84–92 with permission.)

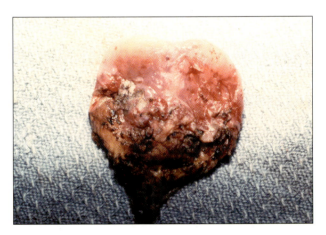

Fig 17–8. The epiglottis has been resected en bloc. The image is from the lingual surface.

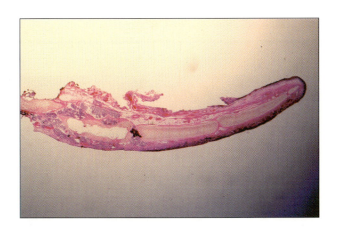

Fig 17–9. A whole mount section is performed on the specimen and confirms the carcinoma in the suprahyoid region. The final staging was that of a T1, N0, M0 SCCA of the suprahyoid epiglottis.

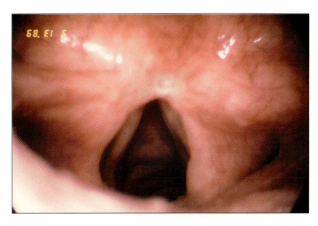

Fig 17–10. Telescopic visualization of the healed neolarynx. The defect healed secondarily with overlying smooth mucosa and a fusion of the vestibular folds to create a neosupraglottic valve.

Case 17B

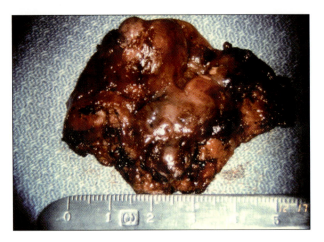

Fig 17–11. A T2, N0, M0 squamous cell carcinoma is situated on the lingual surface of the suprahyoid epiglottis. The disease extended just onto the aryepiglottic fold, as well as the laryngeal surface of the epiglottis. It has been resected en bloc by means of the microspot CO_2 laser.

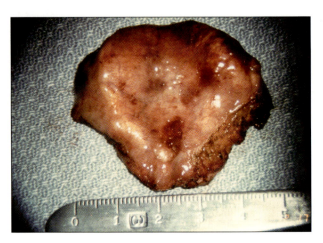

Fig 17–12. The prior lesion is seen from the laryngeal surface. As previously noted, there was less significant disease in the introitus of the larynx.

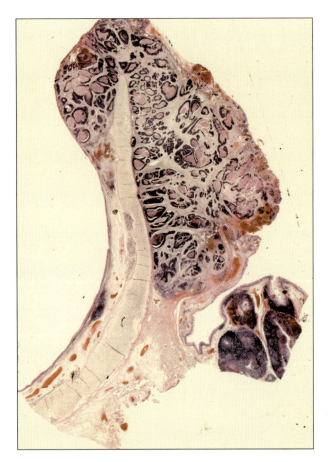

Fig 17–13. This is a whole mount section of the specimen that established wide clear margins on this lesion. There is a basophilic conglomeration of cells anteriorly and inferiorly, which represents lymphocytes from the lingual tonsils.

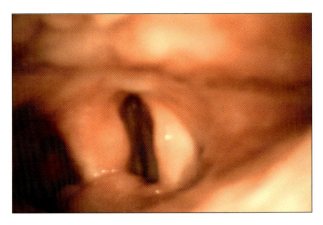

Fig 17–14. This patient has not had a recurrence and the clinic examination shows the neosupraglottic valve.

Case 17C

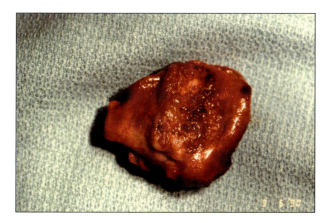

Fig 17–15. The specimen from an endoscopic resection of a T3, N0, M0 carcinoma that extended submucosally at the left aryepiglottic fold. Clear mucosal margins on the laryngeal surface of the epiglottis are well seen. This patient is a professional comedian.

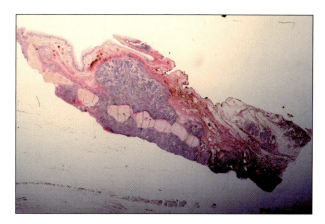

Fig 17–16. The whole mount section of the lesion displays clear margins on the tumor. The typical pattern of invasion is seen with progression of disease through the preformed fenestra of the epiglottis into the pre-epiglottic space. There is a pseudocapsule that forms around the lesion, which is also typical. The lesion is limited superiorly by the hyoepiglottic ligament.

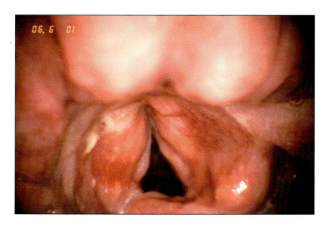

Fig 17–17. Clinic examination 1 month subsequent to the resection, which revealed almost complete epithelialization (respiratory phase).

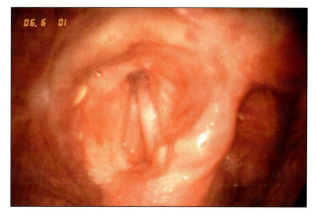

Fig 17–18. The prior patient is seen during phonation with excellent glottal closure. The patient was taking a full per oral diet within 10 days. Anteriorly, the superior edge of the thyroid lamina can be seen as the white rim. The patient did receive radiotherapy since no neck dissection was performed. He has been without recurrence for 10 years.

Case 17D

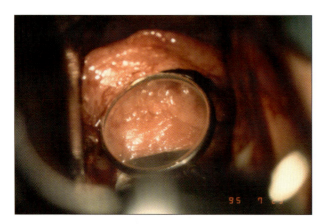

Fig 17–19. (4×) There is a large ulcerating and exophytic lesion covering the entire laryngeal surface of the epiglottis. A mirror is utilized to enhance the tangential visualization.

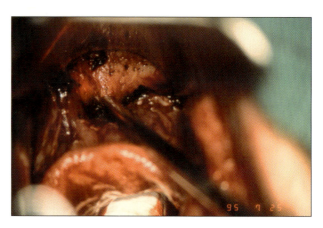

Fig 17–20. (4×) An incision is made through the mucosa of the vallecular epiglottica. A suction is used to retract the mucosa to expose the hyoepiglottic ligament.

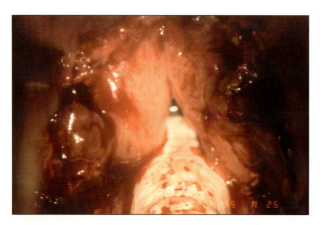

Fig 17–21. (4×) The resection has been completed and the vocal folds are shown to be free of disease despite the edema that has ensued. The patient was extubated at the end of the case.

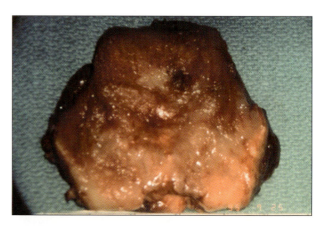

Fig 17–22. The completed en bloc resection of the neoplasm is seen with grossly normal mucosal margins. Frozen section analysis confirmed the clear margins initially and this was further established by permanent histopathological analysis.

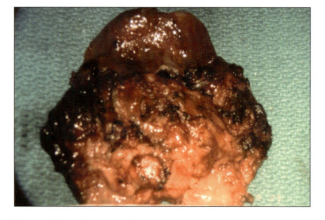

Fig 17–23. The resected specimen including the pre-epiglottic fat is well seen.

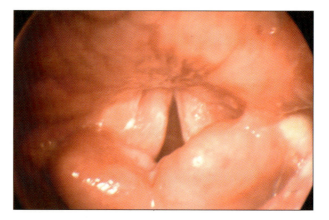

Fig 17–24. Clinic exam of a healed neosupraglottis of a patient who underwent an identical resection.

Case 17E

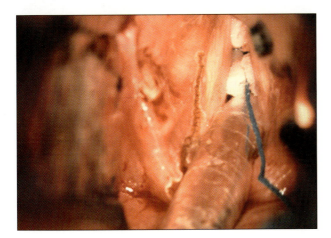

Fig 17–25. (4×) A left aryepiglottic fold ulceration is noted. An incision is made with the CO_2 laser along the anterior face of the arytenoid, as well as along the vestibular fold for resection of the aryepiglottic fold lesion. The upper blade of the supraglottiscope is underneath the laryngeal surface of the epiglottis.

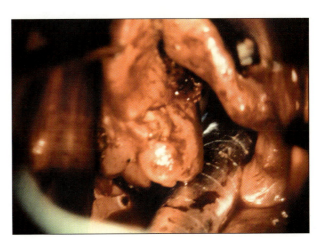

Fig 17–26. (4×) The supraglottiscope is then readjusted so that the upper blade is in the vallecula. Subsequently, the epiglottis is sagitally split to allow for resection of the left hemisupraglottis.

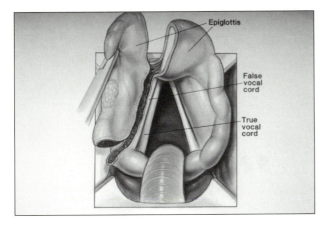

Fig 17–27. Diagrammatic representation of the prior image. (From Shapiro J, Zeitels SM, Fried MF. *Operat Tech Otolaryngol Head Neck Surg.* 1992;3:84–92 with permission.)

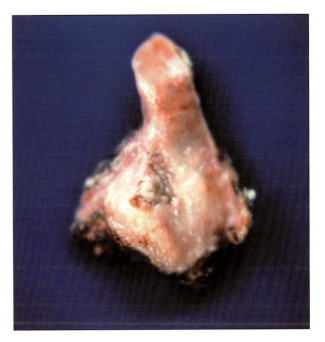

Fig 17–28. The specimen revealed an invasive carcinoma of the left aryepiglottic fold.

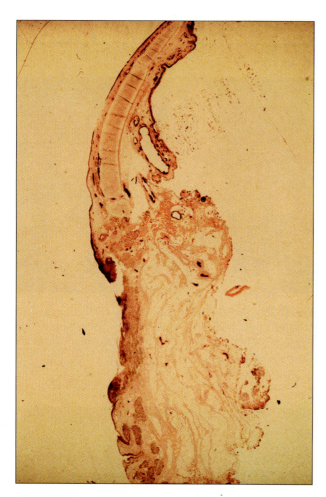

Fig 17–29. Whole mount section of the cancer reveals wide clear margins.

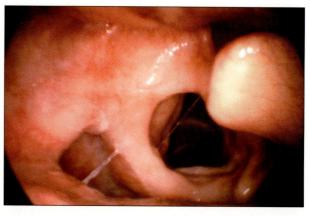

Fig 17–30. The clinic examination of the patient during respiration after healing.

Case 17F

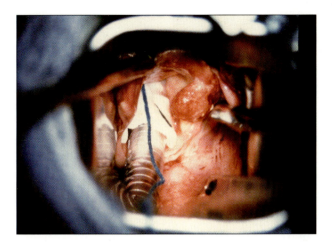

Fig 17–31. (2.5×) There is a right-sided exophytic lesion of the right aryepiglottic fold. The epiglottis is retracted to reveal the aryepiglottic fold lesion, which is exophytic and superficial.

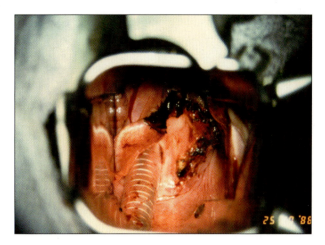

Fig 17–32. (2.5×) The epiglottis is being sagittally split and the lesion has been resected. The laser has left carbonized debris at the resection site.

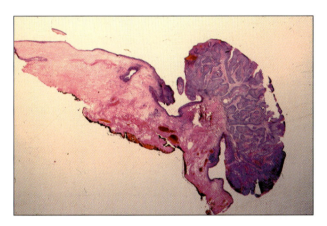

Fig 17–33. Whole mount section of the resected neoplasm shows the exophytic lesion, which was resected with clear margins.

Case 17G

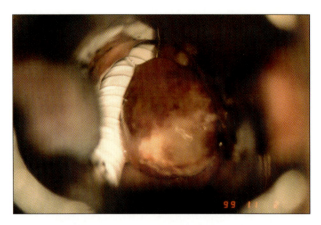

Fig 17–34. (2×) A patient presented with intermittent stridor and change in the resonance of her voice. There is a spheroid mass arising from the right aryepiglottic fold.

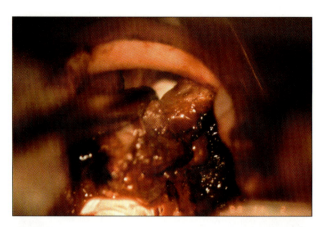

Fig 17–35. (2×) An incision is made with the CO_2 laser through the right paraglottic space through the medial wall of the pyriform sinus in the cuneiform region.

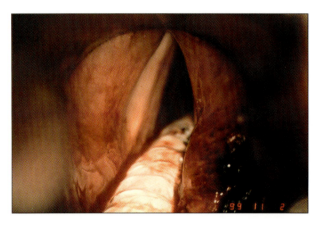

Fig 17–36. (2×) The mass is resected and the airway is normal.

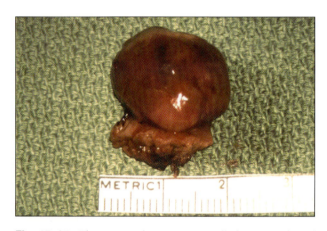

Fig 17–37. The resected mass was well-demarcated and firm; note the pedunculated narrow base.

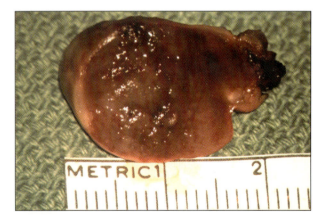

Fig 17–38. The specimen has been sectioned and histopathology revealed a neuroendocrine carcinoma.

Case 17H

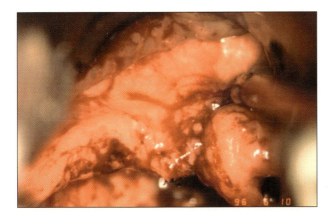

Fig 17–39. (2.5×) There is a large left aryepiglottic fold carcinoma extending along the pharyngoepiglottic fold and into the pyriform sinus. The suction is in the vallecula and the edge of the curled epiglottis is seen at the right inferior corner of the image.

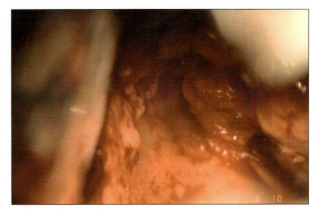

Fig 17–40. (4×) The laryngoscope is advanced into the pyriform sinus. There was increased neoplastic change on the left medial wall to pyriform which is seen on the right side of the image. The caudal extent of the lateral wall in the pyriform is seen at the center of the field.

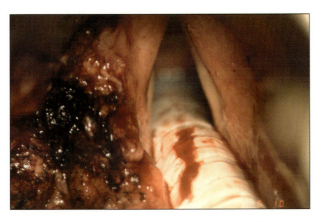

Fig 17–41. (2.5×) The lesion has been resected. This image of the laryngeal introitus shows no evidence of obstruction or impairment of the airway.

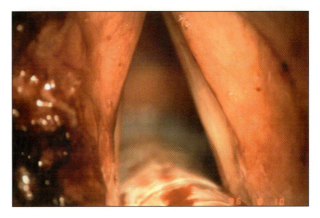

Fig 17–42. (4×) Figure 17–41 seen at higher magnification.

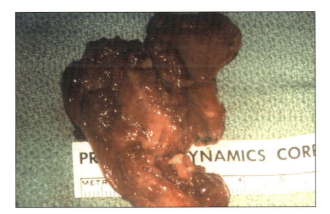

Fig 17–43. The entire left aryepiglottic fold and epiglottis have been resected en bloc with the left pyriform sinus. Frozen section analysis revealed clear margins.

Case 17I

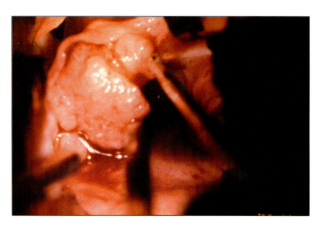

Fig 17–44. (2.5×) T1, N0, M0 exophytic squamous cell carcinoma of the right medial wall of the pyriform sinus. The thin aryepiglottic fold is seen on the left side of the lesion. The more central opaque area is the pyriform sinus.

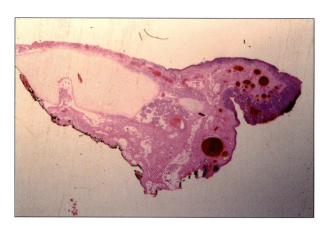

Fig 17–45. The exophytic carcinoma can be seen as well as the edge of the cartilage of the epiglottis.

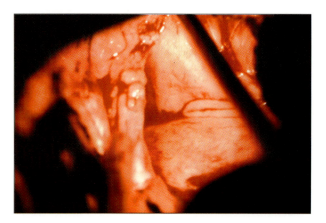

Fig 17–46. (2.5×) There is a microinvasive carcinoma of the left pharyngoepiglottic fold at the center of the field. This patient had bilateral T1 lesions.

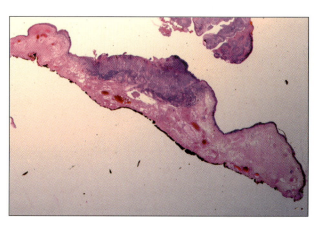

Fig 17–47. The carcinoma is at the epicenter of the specimen which shows histopathologically clear margins.

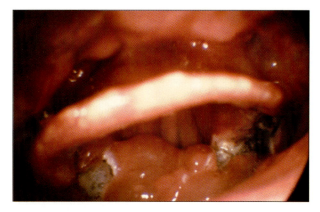

Fig 17–48. The clinic examination of the patient in the early postoperative period.

Case 17J

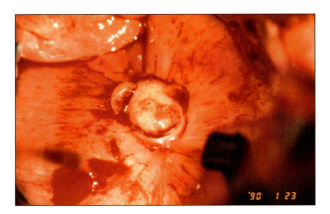

Fig 17–49. (4×) A small carcinoma is noted on the posterior pharyngeal wall. The periarytenoid region is seen in the top left.

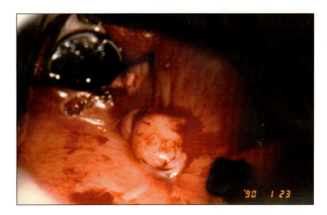

Fig 17–50. (4×) The distal margin is created by reflecting the beam of the CO_2 laser off of a mirror, since the distal incision was in an extreme tangential plain.

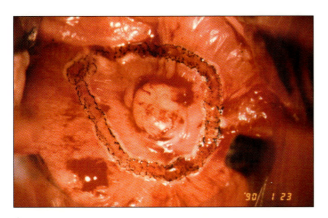

Fig 17–51. (4×) A perimeter incision is made with the CO_2 laser around the lesion.

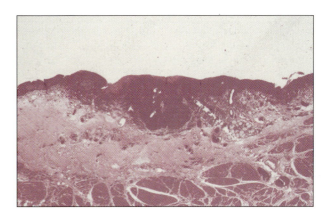

Fig 17–52. H&E staining of the specimen reveals that the necrotic exophytic area separated from the specimen. The base revealed a microinvasive carcinoma with clear margins.

Case 17K

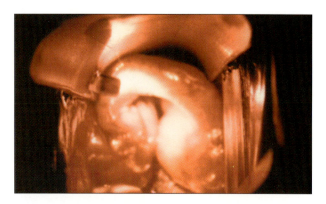

Fig 17–53. (2.5×) There is diffuse radiation-induced supraglottic edema creating airway obstruction. The majority of the edema occurred along the aryepiglottic folds and periarytenoid regions.

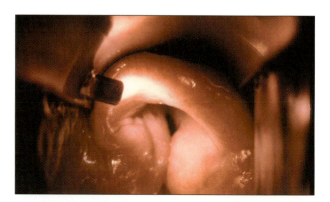

Fig 17–54. (4×) Figure 17–53 at higher magnification.

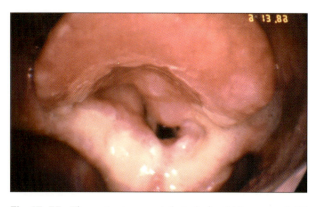

Fig 17–55. The patient was extubated after 24 hours and did not require tracheotomy. The clinic exam one week postop revealed fibrinous debris along both aryepiglottic folds with a stable airway.

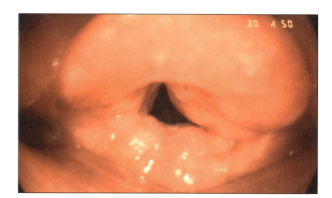

Fig 17–56. Seven months later, the clinic exam revealed that the airway remained stable and well healed.

Case 17L

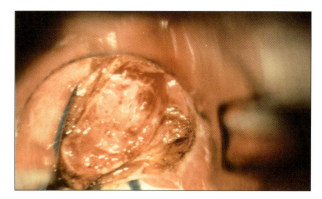

Fig 17–57. (4×) There is a neoplastic process emanating from the supraglottis obscuring the vocal folds. The lesion arose from the right false vocal fold.

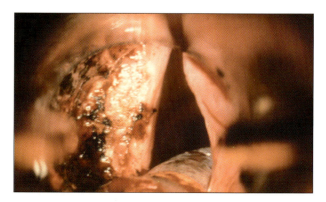

Fig 17–58. (4×) The lesion was cytoreduced for airway palliation and revealed very little disease at the level of the glottis. The patient went on to receive full course radiation therapy to the primary site in both necks.

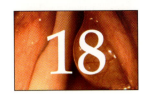

Benign Supraglottic Pathology

As stated earlier, the microspot CO_2 laser is a precise cutting and vaporizing instrument for use in the supraglottis. The most common lesion of the supraglottis is probably papillomatosis. These lesions can be managed quite well with the microspot CO_2 laser because mild thermal trauma in the supraglottis does not result in a substantive change in laryngeal function. A pulsed-dye laser may prove to be the optimal surgical approach to these lesions by ablating the subepithelial microvasculature. Carbon-dioxide laser vestibular fold resection can be performed to marsupialize saccular cysts or to improve exposure of the superior surface of the true vocal fold.[186,214] Vallecular cysts are not infrequently noted on examination and the larger ones are sometimes resected because of suspicion of neoplasia or because they cause throat discomfort when distended. Large fibroepithelial polyps that ball valve into the airway are occasionally encountered. They usually arise from a narrow stalk and are easily resected. These lesions were much more common in the pre-antibiotic era and were frequently discussed in 19th century literature. Chronic edema (ie, post radiation) that does not respond to medical management can often be vaporized to avoid a tracheotomy.[215] On rare occasions sarcoid presents as a mass in the epiglottis and can be resected with little difficulty. Vascular malformations are better managed with the neodymium-YAG laser.[216]

Case 18A

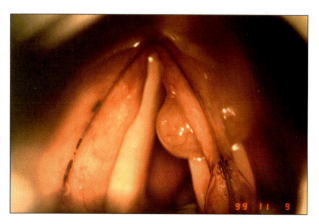

Fig 18–1. (4×) There is spheroid hypertrophy of the right vestibular fold. The mass was fairly solid to palpation. The patient had a significant smoking history. (Courtesy of Endocraft LLC.)

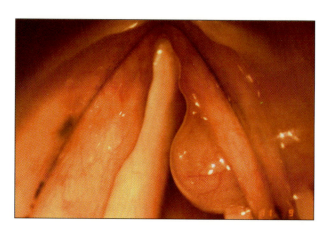

Fig 18–2. (7×) Figure 18–1 at higher magnification. (Courtesy of Endocraft LLC.)

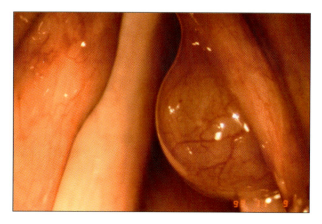

Fig 18–3. (10×) Figure 18–1 at even higher magnification. (Courtesy of Endocraft LLC.)

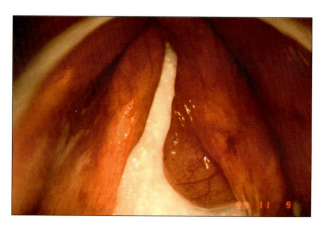

Fig 18–4. (7×) The right vestibular fold has been infused with saline and 1/10,000 epinephrine. A saline soaked cotton pad has been placed in the ventricle to protect the vocal fold from unintended laser injury. (Courtesy of Endocraft LLC.)

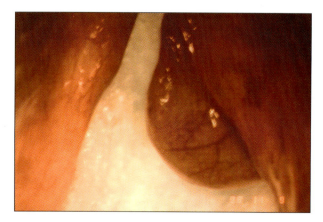

Fig 18–5. (10×) Figure 18–4 at higher magnification. (Courtesy of Endocraft LLC.)

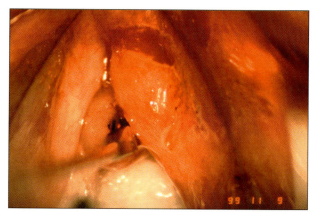

Fig 18–6. (7×) The CO_2 laser is used to make an incision in the vestibular. (Courtesy of Endocraft LLC.)

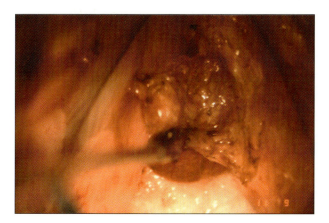

Fig 18–7. (7×) The mass is retracted placing the tissue on tension, while the mass is excised. (Courtesy of Endocraft LLC.)

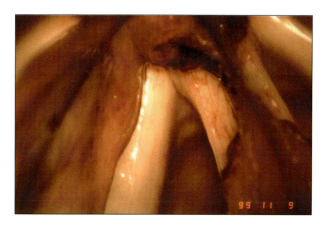

Fig 18–8. (7×) The mass has been excised with the microspot CO_2 laser. There was diffuse hypertrophy of glandular elements of the vestibular fold and there was no evidence of a cyst. (Courtesy of Endocraft LLC.)

Case 18B

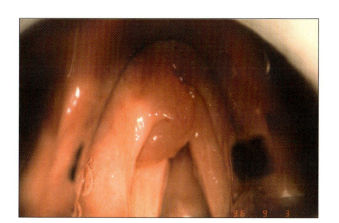

Fig 18–9. (4×) A spheroid mass is noted emanating from the left vestibular fold and left ventricle.

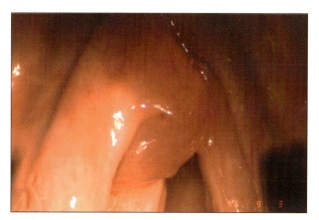

Fig 18–10. (7×) Figure 18–9 at higher magnification.

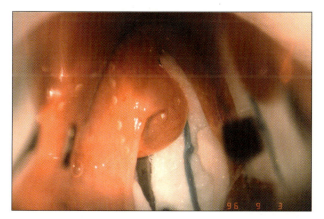

Fig 18–11. (4×) A saline soaked cotton pad is placed underneath the spheroid mass to avoid trauma to the underlying vocal folds. The microspot laser is utilized to excise the mass.

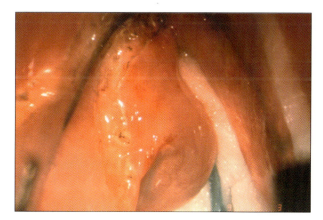

Fig 18–12. (7×) The laser is used with a repeated pulse mode, a 0.3-mm spot, and approximately 4 watts of power.

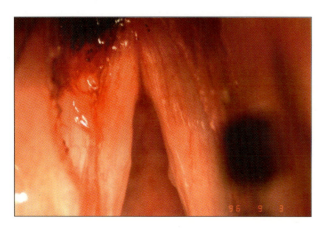

Fig 18–13. (7×) The mass has been excised en bloc. The vestibular fold is appropriately excavated and the true vocal fold has been undisturbed.

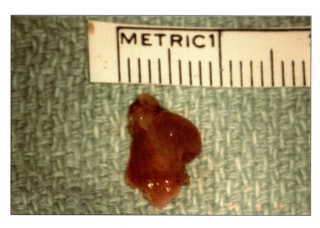

Fig 18–14. The mass was not cystic in nature, but revealed hypertrophy of glandular elements of the vestibular fold.

Case 18C

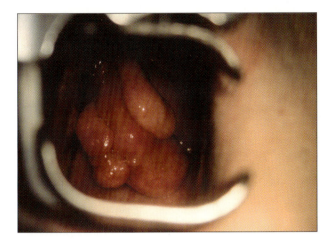

Fig 18–15. (2.5×) A multilobulated mass is noted to be rising from the medial wall of the pyriform to the edge of the left aryepiglottic fold. During inspiration, the mass would displace into the introitus of the supraglottis. It is visualized by means of the bivalve adjustable supraglottiscope.

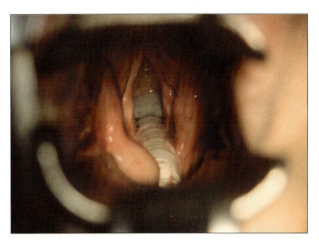

Fig 18–16. (2.5×) The mass can be displaced out of the laryngeal introitus and in fact reveals that it is not arising from the internal surface of the larynx.

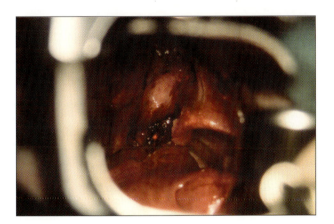

Fig 18–17. (2.5×) The CO_2 laser has been utilized to resect the lesion. The charred eschar can be seen along side the left pharyngoepiglottic fold.

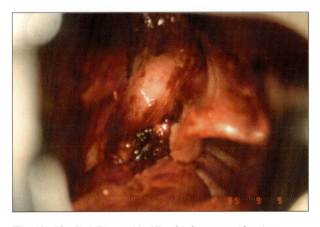

Fig 18–18. (4×) Figure 18–17 at higher magnification.

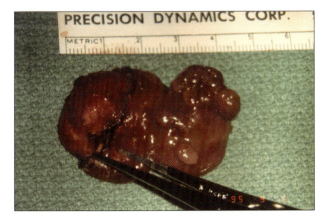

Fig 18–19. The specimen revealed a fibrovascular multilob-ulated polyp. It was remarkably noted to be 5 cm in size.

Case 18D

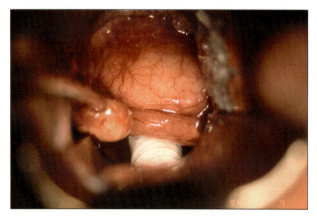

Fig 18–20. (4×) A large submucosal cyst is seen in the vallecular glossoepiglottica through the adjustable bivalve supraglottiscope.

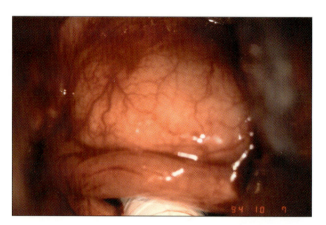

Fig 18–21. (7×) Figure 18–20 at higher magnification.

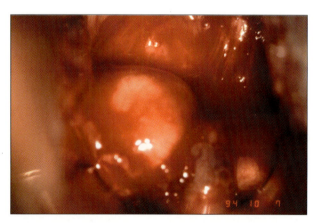

Fig 18–22. (7×) The CO_2 laser is utilized to enhance the resection of that mass. Despite the laser, there is significant bleeding. Much of the dissection is done by means of cold instruments.

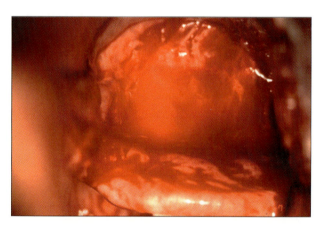

Fig 18–23. The mass has been completely excised. The epiglottis is seen horizontally at the bottom of the field.

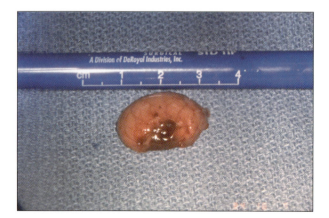

Fig 18–24. The cyst has been resected en bloc.

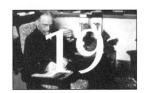

Summary and Prologue

Endoscopic surgery of the larynx is one of the earliest examples of minimally invasive surgery. It has been just over a century since Kirstein formally introduced direct laryngoscopy, which paved the way for current endoscopic surgical approaches for laryngeal disease. Every substantive innovation in endoscopic surgery of the larynx enhanced precision and in turn improved postoperative laryngeal function (airway, swallowing, and voice). Further improvements in technology (ie, laryngoscopes, mechanical tissue-handling, and lasers) will probably facilitate the expansion of endolaryngeal surgery. This work provides the reader with a comprehensive compilation of laryngeal pathology with stepwise surgical management.

The current major impetus underlying endoscopic supraglottic surgery arose from the potential expansion and growth of function-preserving management of supraglottic cancer. The text provides the reader with a foundation for understanding this approach, which is seldom taught in training programs.

The text also provides the reader with extensive detail regarding endoscopic glottal surgery for both benign and malignant disease, which has emerged as a physiologically based phonomicrosurgical approach. It has developed from the convergence of microlaryngoscopic surgical-technique theory with mucosal wave theory of laryngeal sound production. Endoscopic glottal surgery will continue to evolve as a result of the interdependent collaboration of surgeons with voice scientists, engineers, speech pathologists, and other voice professionals. Since a majority of vocal fold problems are the result of trauma (phonatory and/or instrumental), surgery will remain a mainstay of treatment for the foreseeable future. Furthermore, tissue-engineering and instrument-design initiatives should expand surgical indications, especially for rejuvenation of the vocal fold vibratory function in our active aging population.

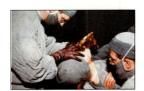

References

1. García M. Observations on the human voice. *Proc Royal Soc London.* 1855;7:397–410.

2. Bozzini P. *Der Lichtleiter oder Beschreibung einer einfachen Vorichtung, und ihrer Anwendung zur erleucht ung inherer Hohlen, und Zwischenraume des lebenden animaschen Korpers.* Weimar; 1807.

3. Cagniard de Latour C. *J l'Institut.* 1825:350. Cited by: Fournie E. *Physiologie de la. Voix et de la Parole.* Paris, France: Adrien Delahaye; 1866.

4. Senn N. *J de Progres.* 1829. Cited by: Mackenzie M. *The Use of the Laryngoscope in Diseases of the Throat With an Appendix on Rhinoscopy.* London, UK: J & A Churchill; 1865:17.

5. Babington BG. *London Med Gazette.* 1829;3:555.

6. Selligue. 1832. Cited by: Mackenzie M. *The Use of the Laryngoscope in Diseases of the Throat With an Appendix on Rhinoscopy.* London, UK: J & A Churchill; 1865:17.

7. Liston R. *Practical Surgery.* London, UK: J & A Churchill; 1837:350.

8. Baumes. *Compte Rendu des Travaux de la Societe de Medecine de Lyons.* 1836–1838;19:18.

9. Avery J. 1844. Cited by: Mackenzie M. *The Use of the Laryngoscope in Diseases of the Throat With an Appendix on Rhinoscopy.* London, UK: J & A Churchill; 1865:25.

10. Zeitels SM, Vaughan CW. "External counter-pressure" and "internal distension" for optimal laryngoscopic exposure of the anterior glottal commissure. *Ann Otol Rhinol Laryngol.* 1994;103:669–675.

11. Zeitels SM. A universal modular glottiscope system: the evolution of a century of design and technique for direct laryngoscopy. *Ann Otol Rhinol Laryngol.* 1999;108(suppl 179):1–24.

12. Trousseau A, Belloc H. *Pathisie Laryngie.* Paris, France: Chez and Bailliere; 1837.

13. Ehrmann CH. *Histoire des Polyps du Larynx.* Straasbourg, France: Imprimerie de FG Levrault; 1850.

14. Green H. *A Treatise on Diseases of the Air Passages.* New York, NY: Wiley and Putnam; 1846.

15. Green H. *Observations on the Pathology of Croup.* New York, NY: John Wiley; 1849.

16. Green H. On the subject of the priority in the medication of the larynx and trachea. *Am Med Monthly.* 1854;1:241–257.

17. Green H. Report on the use and effect of applications of nitrate silver to the throat, either in local or general disease. *Trans Am Med Assoc.* 1856;9:493–530.

18. Elsberg L. Laryngology in America [President's address]. *Trans Am Laryngol Assoc.* 1879;1:30–90.

19. Donaldson F. The laryngology of Trousseau and Horace Green. *Trans Am Laryngol Assoc.* 1890;12:10–18.

20. Clerf LH. Manuel García's contribution to laryngology. *Bull NY Acad Med.* 1956;32:603–611.

21. Green H. *Morbid Growths Within the Larynx.* New York, NY: GP Putnam; 1852.

22. Mackenzie M. *The Hygiene of the Vocal Organs.* 8th ed. New York, NY: Edgar S Werner; 1899.

23. Mackinlay MS. *García the Centenarian and His Times: Being a Memoir of Manuel García's Life and Labours for the Advancement of Music and Science.* New York, NY: D Appleton and Co; 1908.

24. Czermak JN. Ueber den Kehlkopfspiegel. *Wiener Med Wochenschrift.* 1858;8(13):196–198.

25. Turck L. On the laryngeal mirror and its mode of employment, with engravings on wood. *Zeitschrift der Gesellschaft der Aerzte zu Wein.* 1858;26:401–409.

26. Stoerk C. On the laryngoscope. *Zeitschrift der Gesellschaft der Aerzte zu Wein.* 1859;46:721–727.

27. Lewin G. *Allgemeine Medizinische Central-Zeitung.* 1861;30:654.

28. Mackenzie M. *The Use of the Laryngoscope in Diseases of the Throat With an Appendix on Rhinoscopy.* London, UK: J & A Churchill; 1865.

29. Mackenzie M. *Growths in the Larynx.* London, UK: J & A Churchill; 1871.

30. Mackenzie M. The laryngoscope and its accessory apparatus; laryngoscopy; autolaryngoscopy; infra-glottic laryngoscopy; the laryngoscope image; laryngeal instruments; dilators of the larynx. In: *Diseases of the Pharynx, Larynx, and Trachea.* New York, NY: William Wood & Co; 1880:158–195.

31. Fraenkel B. First healing of a laryngeal cancer taken out through the natural passages. *Archiv für Klinische Chirurgie.* 1886;12:283–286.

32. Elsberg L. *Laryngoscopal Medication or the Local Treatment of the Diseases of the Throat, Larynx, and Neighboring Organs, Under Sight.* New York, NY: William Wood & Co; 1864.

33. Elsberg L. *Laryngoscopal Surgery Illustrated in the Treatment of Morbid Growths Within the Larynx.* Philadelphia, Pa: Collins; 1866.

34. Zeitels SM. Jacob Da Silva Solis-Cohen: America's first head and neck surgeon. *Head Neck Surg.* 1997:342–346.

35. Solis-Cohen J. Clinical history of surgical affections of the larynx. *Med Record.* 1869;4:244–247.

36. Solis-Cohen J. Pharyngeal voice: illustrated by presentation of a patient who phonates without a larynx and without the use of the lungs. *Trans Am Laryngol Assoc.* 1893;15:114–116.

37. Solis-Cohen J. *Diseases of the Throat: A Guide to the Diagnosis and Treatment.* New York, NY: William Wood; 1872.

38. Jackson C. *Peroral Endoscopy and Laryngeal Surgery.* St. Louis, Mo: The Laryngoscope Co; 1915.

39. Elsberg, L. Laryngological instruction [President's address]. *Trans Am Laryngol Assoc.* 1880;2:4–8.

40. Sataloff RT. Education in laryngology. *Ann Otol Rhinol Laryngol.* 2000.

41. Oertel M. Ueber eine neues laryngostroboskopische Untersuchungsmethode des Kehlkopfes. *Centralblatt Medizinischen Wiss.* 1878;16:81–82.

42. Oertel M. Das laryngo-stroboskip und die Laryngo-Stroboskpische Untersuchung. *Arch Laryngol Rhinol.* 1895;3:1–16.

43. Kirstein A. Autoskopie des Larynx und der Trachea (Laryngoscopia directa, Euthyskopie, Besichtigung ohne Spiegel). *Arch Laryngol Rhinol*. 1895;3:156–164.

44. Kirstein A. *Autoscopy of the Larynx and Trachea (Direct Examination without Mirror)*. Philadelphia, Pa: FA Davis Co; 1897.

45. Boyce JW, ed. Duties of the second assistant in endoscopy per os. In: Jackson C, ed. *Tracheobronchoscopy, Esophagoscopy and Gastroscopy*. St. Louis, Mo: The Laryngoscope Co; 1907:145–147.

46. Jackson C. Position of the patient for peroral endoscopy. In: *Peroral Endoscopy and Laryngeal Surgery*. St. Louis, Mo: The Laryngoscope Co; 1915:77–88.

47. Killian G. Demonstration of an endoscopic spatula. *J Laryngol Rhinol*. 1910;25:549–550.

48. Killian G. Die Schwebelaryngoskopie. *Arch Laryngol Rhinol*. 1912;26:277–317.

49. Killian G. Suspension laryngoscopy and its practical use. *J Laryngol Otol*. 1914;24:337–360.

50. Killian G. *Die Schwebelaryngoskopie und ihre praktische Verwertung*. Wien, Germany: Urban & Schwarzenberg; 1920.

51. Israel S. The directoscope of Haslinger in diagnosis and surgery of the larynx. *Laryngoscope*. 1923;33:945–948.

52. Jackson C, Tucker G, Clerf LH. Laryngostasis and the laryngostat. *Arch Otolaryngol*. 1925;1:167–169.

53. Brünings W. Direct laryngoscopy: autoscopy by counter-pressure. In: *Direct Laryngoscopy, Bronchoscopy, and Esophagoscopy*. London, UK: Bailliere, Tindall, & Cox; 1912:110–115.

54. Lewy RE. Suspension fixation gear power laryngoscopy (with motion pictures). *Laryngoscope*. 1954;64:693–695.

55. Roberts SE, Forman FS. Direct laryngoscopy—a simplified technique. An aid to the early detection of laryngeal cancer. *Ann Otol Rhinol Laryngol*. 1948;57:245–256.

56. Roberts SE. A self retaining dual distal lighted laryngoscope with screw driven fulcrum lift. *Laryngoscope*. 1952;62:215–221.

57. King NE. Direct laryngoscopy aided by a new laryngoscope "stabilizer." *Arch Otolaryngol*. 1951;53:89–92.

58. Sommers KE. Direct laryngoscopy and description of a self-retaining attachment for the laryngoscope. *Arch Otolaryngol*. 1952;55:484–488.

59. Priest RE, Wesolowski S. Direct laryngoscopy under general anesthesia. *Trans Am Acad Opthalmol Otolaryngol*. 1960;64:639–648.

60. Jackson C, Jackson CL. Difficulties of direct laryngoscopy. In: *The Larynx and Its Diseases*. Philadelphia, Pa: WB Saunders; 1937:37–43.

61. Jackson C, Jackson CL. Direct laryngoscopy. In: *Cancer of the Larynx*. Philadelphia, Pa: Saunders; 1939:10–29.

62. Thomas GK. Suspension apparatus for laryngeal microsurgery. *Arch Otolaryngol*. 1971;94:258–259.

63. Grundfast KM, Vaughan CW, Strong MS, De Vos P. Suspension microlaryngoscopy in the Boyce position with a new suspension gallows. *Ann Otol Rhinol Laryngol*. 1978;87:560–566.

64. Vaughan CW. Vocal fold exposure in phonosurgery. *J Voice*. 1993;7:189–194.

65. Zeitels SM. Premalignant epithelium and microinvasive cancer of the vocal fold: the evolution of phonomicrosurgical management. *Laryngoscope*. 1995;105(3, pt 2, suppl 67):1–51.

66. Hochman II, Zeitels SM. Exposure and visualization of the glottis for phonomicrosurgery. *Operat Tech Otolaryngol Head Neck Surg* (Phonosurgery Part 1). 1998;9:192–195.

67. Hochman II, Zeitels SM, Heaton JT. An analysis of the forces and position required for direct laryngoscopic exposure of the anterior vocal folds. *Ann Otol Rhinol Laryngol*. 1998;108:715–724.

68. Scalco AN, Shipman WF, Tabb HG. Microscopic suspension laryngoscopy. *Ann Otol Rhinol Laryngol*. 1960;69:1134–1138.

69. Jako GJ. Laryngoscope for microscopic observation, surgery, and photography. *Arch Otolaryngol*. 1970;91:196–199.

70. Kleinsasser O. Mikrochirurgie im Kehlkopf. *Arch Ohren Nasen Kehlkopfheilkunde*. 1964;183:428–433.

71. Jako GJ. Correspondence documents between Geza Jako and the Stumar Instrument Company; 1962.

72. Kleinsasser O. *Microlaryngoscopy and Endolaryngeal Microsurgery*. Philadelphia, Pa: WB Saunders; 1968:48–62.

73. Polanyi T, Bredermeier HC, Davis TW Jr. CO_2 laser for surgical research. *Med Biol Eng Comput*. 1970;8:548–558.

74. Jako GJ. Laser surgery of the vocal cords. *Laryngoscope*. 1972;82:2204–2215.

75. Strong MS, Jako GJ. Laser surgery of the larynx: early clinical experience with continuous CO_2 laser. *Ann Otol Rhinol Laryngol*. 1972;81:791–798.

76. Vaughan CW. Transoral laryngeal surgery using the CO_2 laser: laboratory experiments and clinical experience. *Laryngoscope*. 1978;88:1399–1420.

77. Zeitels SM. Laser versus cold instruments for microlaryngoscopic surgery. *Laryngoscope*. 1996;106:545–552.

78. Isshiki N, von Leden H. Hoarseness: aerodynamic studies. *Arch Otolaryngol*. 1964;80:206–213.

79. von Leden H, Moore P, Timcke R. Laryngeal vibrations: measurements of the glottic wave: Part III. The pathological larynx. *Arch Otolaryngol*. 1960;71:16–35.

80. von Leden H. The electronic synchron-stroboscope: its value for the practicing laryngologist. *Ann Otol Rhinol Laryngol*. 1961;70:881–893.

81. von Leden H, Moore P. The mechanics of the cricoarytenoid joint. *Arch Otolaryngol (Stockh)*. 1961;73:541–550.

82. von Leden H, Moore P. Vibratory pattern of vocal cords in unilateral paralysis. *Acta Otolaryngol (Stockh)*. 1961;53:493–506.

83. von Leden H. Plastic surgery of the larynx. *Revista Panam Otorrinolaringol Broncoesofagol*. 1963;1:7–11.

84. von Leden H, Le Cover M, Ringel RL, Isshiki N. Improvements in laryngeal cinematography. *Arch Otolaryngol*. 1966;83:482–487.

85. von Leden H. Surgery for the improvement of vocal function. *Revista Panam Otorrinolaringol Broncoesofagol*. 1969;3:137–143.

86. Koike Y, Hirano M, von Leden H. Vocal initiation: acoustic and aerodynamic investigations of normal subjects. *Folia Phoniatr*. 1967;19:173–182.

87. Hirano M, Koike Y, von Leden H. Maximum phonation time and air usage during phonation. *Folia Phoniatr*. 1968;20:185–201.

88. Hirano M. Phonosurgery: basic and clinical investigations. *Otologia (Fukuoka)*. 1975;21:239–442.

89. Hirano M. Structure and vibratory behavior of the vocal fold. In: Sawashima M, Cooper F, eds. *Dynamic Aspects of Speech Production*. Tokyo, Japan: University of Tokyo; 1977:13–30.

90. Bishop J. Experimental researches into the physiology of the human voice. *The London & Edinburgh Philosophical Magazine & Journal of Science*. 1836.

91. Fournie E. *Physiologie de la Voix et de la Parole*. Paris, France: Adrien Delahaye; 1866.

92. Zeitels SM, Sataloff RT. Phonosurgery: considerations for the performing artist and voice teacher. *J Singing*. 1998;54:45–48.

93. Hochman I, Sataloff RT, Hillman RE, Zeitels SM. Ectasias and varices of the vocal folds: clearing the striking zone. *Ann Otol Rhinol Laryngol*. 1998;108:10–16.

94. Hillman RD, Montgomery WW, Zeitels SM. Appropriate use of objective measures of vocal function in the multidisciplinary management of voice disorders. *Curr Opin Otolaryngol Head Neck Surg*. 1997;5:172–175.

95. Czermak JN. *On the Laryngoscope and Its Employment in Physiology and Medicine*. London: New Sydenham Society, 1861;11:1–79.

96. Elsberg CA. Clinical experiences with intratracheal insufflation (Meltzer), with remarks upon the value of the method for thoracic surgery. *Ann Surg*. 1910,52:23–29.

97. Elsberg CA. Zur Narkose beim Menschen mittelst der kontinuierlichen intratrachealen Insufflation von Meltzer. *Berlin Klin Wochenschrift*. 1910;23:957–958.

98. Elsberg CA. The value of continuous intratracheal insufflation of air (Meltzer) in thoracic surgery. *Med Rec*. 1910;493–495.

99. Carrel A. Experimentelle intrathorakale Chirurgie mittels der Methode von Meotzer und Auer. *Berlin Klin Wochenschrift*. 1910;13:555–557.

100. Janeway HH. Intratracheal anesthesia from the standpoint of the nose, throat and oral surgeon with a description of a new instrument for catheterizing the trachea. *Laryngoscope*. 1913;23:1082–1090.

101. Bruck A. Diseases of the larynx and trachea: methods of examination. In: Forbes W, trans-ed. *Diseases of the Nose, Mouth, Pharynx, and Larynx: A Textbook for Students and Practitioners of Medicine*. New York, NY: Rebman; 1910:375–376.

102. Johnston RH. Some original endoscopic methods. *Laryngoscope*. 1913;23:607–617.

103. Corbridge RJ, Harries ML. A new method of applying external laryngeal pressure during microlaryngeal surgery: the laryngeal strap. *Laryngoscope*. 1996;101:499–500.

104. Zeitels SM, Vaughan CW. A submucosal vocal fold infusion needle. *Otolaryngol Head Neck Surg*. 1991;105:478–479.

105. Kass ES, Hillman RE, Zeitels SM. The submucosal infusion technique in phonomicrosurgery. *Ann Otol Rhinol Laryngol*. 1996;105:341–347.

106. Colden D, Zeitels SM, Jarboe J, et al. Stroboscopic assessment of vocal fold atypia and early cancer. *Ann Otol Rhinol Laryngol*. In press.

107. Koufman JA. The otolaryngologic manifestations of gastroesophageal reflux disease (GERD). *Laryngoscope*. 1991;(suppl 53): 1–78.

108. Koufman JA, ed. Gastroesophageal reflux and voice disorders. In: Sataloff RT, Rubin JS et al, eds. *Diagnosis and Treatment of Voice Disorders*. New York, NY: Igaku-Shoin; 1995:166.

109. Zeitels SM, Hillman RD, Bunting GW, Vaughn T. Reinke's edema: phonatory mechanisms and management strategies. *Ann Otol Rhinol Laryngol*. 1996;106:533–543.

110. Zeitels SM, Desloge R, Doyle P, Hillman RD. Phonomicrosurgery in singers and performing artists. Presented at: The Annual Meeting of the American Laryngological, Rhinological and Otological Society; 1999.

111. Fagell PL. Tuning up musicians. *Harvard Med Alumni J*. 1999;Summer:28–35.

112. Jackson C. Instruments. In: *Peroral Endoscopy and Laryngeal Surgery*. St. Louis, Mo: The Laryngoscope Co; 1915:11–51.

113. Jako GJ, ed. Laryngeal endoscopy and microlaryngoscopy. In: Paparella M. Shumrick D, eds. *Otolaryngology*. Philadelphia, Pa: WB Saunders; 1980:2410–2430.

114. Pilling GP & Son Company. *Pilling Eye, Ear, Nose, Throat, and Bronchoscopic Instruments and Equipment* [catalog]. Philadelphia, Pa; 1941.

115. Weerda H, Pederson P, Wehmer H. Braume H. A new laryngoscope for endolaryngeal microsurgery. *Arch Otorhinolaryngol*. 1979;225:103–106.

116. Berci G, Ward P. A new universal bivalved speculum direct laryngoscope. *Ann Otol Rhinol Laryngol*. 1981;90:344–345.

117. Jackson C. *Instrument in Tracheo-Bronchoscopy, Esophagoscopy and Gastroscopy*. St. Louis, Mo: The Laryngoscope Co; 1907:15–34.

118. Holinger PH. Presentation of instruments: fiber-optic laryngoscopes, bronchoscopes and esophagoscopes. *Ann Otol Rhinol Laryngol*. 1965;74:1164–1167.

119. Broyles EN. Address of the guest of honor. Presented at: The Annual Meeting of the American Broncho-esophagological Association; 1962:42.

120. Ossoff RH, Sisson GA, Shapshay SM. Adult subglottiscope for laser surgery. *Ann Otol Rhinol Laryngol*. 1988;97:552–553.

121. Zeitels SM, Vaughan CW. The adjustable supraglottiscope. *Otolaryngol Head Neck Surg*. 1990;103:487–492.

122. Desloge RB, Zeitels SM. Microsurgery at the anterior glottal commissure: controversies and observations. *Ann Otol Rhinol Laryngol*. 2000;109:385–392.

123. Holinger PH. An hour-glass anterior commissure laryngoscope. *Laryngoscope*. 1960;70:1570–1571.

124. Fine J. Microlaryngoscopy with a new laryngoscope. *Arch Otolaryngol Head Neck Surg*. 1967;85:112–113.

125. Killian G. Suspension laryngoscopy. JA Hageman, trans. In: Jackson C, ed. *Peroral Endoscopy and Laryngeal Surgery*. St. Louis, Mo: The Laryngoscope Co; 1915:133–154.

126. Lynch RC. Suspension laryngoscopy and its accomplishments. *Ann Otol Rhinol Laryngol*. 1915;24:429–446.

127. Lynch RC. A resume of my years work with suspension laryngoscopy. *Trans Am Laryngol Assoc*. 1916;38:158–175.

128. Andrews AH. Suspension handle for laryngoscopes. *Ann Otol Rhinol Laryngol*. 1977;86:626.

129. Webster M. *Webster's Collegiate Dictionary*. Springfield, Ill: G & C Merriam Co; 1947:55.

130. Jackson C. Direct laryngoscopy by lateral and oblique methods. In: *Peroral Endoscopy and Laryngeal Surgery*. St. Louis, Mo: Laryngoscope Co; 1915:101–103.

131. Brünings W. Technique of autoscopic operations. In: *Direct Laryngoscopy, Bronchoscopy, and Esophagoscopy*. London, UK: Bailliere, Tindall, & Cox; 1912:118–120.

132. Zeitels SM. The origin and development of chest-support torsion laryngoscope holders. In: Premalignant epithelium and microinasive cancer of the vocal fold: the evolution of phonomicrosurgical management. *Laryngoscope*. 1995;(105, pt 2, suppl 65):14–15.

133. New GB, Dorton HE. Suspension laryngoscopy in the treatment of malignant disease of the hypopharynx and larynx. *Mayo Clin Proc*. 1941;16:411–416.

134. LeJune FE. Suspension laryngoscopy. In: Jackson C, Jackson CL, eds. *Diseases of the Nose, Throat and Ear*. Philadelphia, Pa: WB Saunders; 1959:178–180.

135. LeJune FE. Intralaryngeal operation for cancer of the vocal cord. *Ann Otol Rhinol Laryngol*. 1946;55:531–536.

136. Webster M. *Webster's Collegiate Dictionary*. Springfield, IL: G & C Merriam Co; 1947:1004.

137. Brünings W. *Direct Laryngoscopy, Bronchoscopy, and Esophagoscopy*. London, UK: Bailliere, Tindall, & Cox; 1912.

138. Brünings W. Endoscopic technique. In: *Direct Laryngoscopy, Bronchoscopy, and Esophagoscopy*. London, UK: Bailliere, Tindall, & Cox; 1912:36–37.

139. Jako GJ. Microscopic laryngoscopy. Presented at: The Annual Meeting of the New England Otolaryngological Society; 1964.

140. Strong MS. Microscopic laryngoscopy. *Acad Med Bull*. 1968; 14:181–184.

141. Strong MS. Microscopic laryngoscopy: a review and appraisal. *Laryngoscope*. 1970;80:1540–1552.

142. DeSanto LW, Carney FW. Microlaryngoscopic surgery. *Arch Otolaryngol*. 1970;91:324–326.

143. Kleinsasser O. Development of microlaryngoscopy and endolaryngeal microsurgery. Stell PM, trans. In: *Microlaryngoscopy and Endolaryngeal Microsurgery: Techniques and Critical Findings*. Baltimore, Md: University Park Press; 1979:3.

144. Hirano M. Phonosurgical anatomy of the larynx. In: Ford C, Bless D, eds. *Phonosurgery*. New York, NY: Raven Press; 1991:25–41.

145. Bouchayer M, Cornut G. Instrumental microscopy of benign lesions of the vocal folds. In: Ford C, Bless D, eds. *Phonosurgery*. New York, NY: Raven Press; 1991:143–165.

146. Zeitels SM. Microflap excisional biopsy for atypia and microinvasive glottic cancer. *Operat Tech Otolaryngol Head Neck Surg* (Phonosurgery ed). 1993;4:218–222.

147. Sataloff RT, Spiegel JR. Endoscopic microsurgery. In: Gould WJ, Sataloff RT, Spiegel JR, eds. *Voice Surgery*. St. Louis, Mo: CV Mosby; 1991:227–267.

148. Sataloff R, Spiegel JR, Heuer RJ, et al. Laryngeal mini-microflap: a new technique and reassessment of the microflap saga. *J Voice*. 1995;9:198–204.

149. Courey MS, Stone RE, Gardner GM, Ossof RH. Endoscopic vocal fold microflap: a three year experience. *Ann Otol Rhinol Laryngol*. 1995;104:267–273.

150. Bastian RW. Vocal fold microsurgery in singers. *J Voice*. 1996;10:389–404.

151. Zeitels SM. Phonomicrosurgical treatment of early glottic cancer and carcinoma in situ. *Am J Surg*. 1996;172:704–709.

152. Zeitels SM. Phonomicrosurgical techniques. In: Sataloff R. *Professional Voice: The Science and the Art of Clinical Care*. San Diego, Calif: Singular Publishing Group; 1997:647–658.

153. Zeitels SM, ed. Endoscopic management of the larynx for benign and malignant disease. In: Myers E, Bluestone CD, eds. *Advances in Otolaryngology—Head and Neck Surgery*. Chicago, Ill: CV Mosby; 1998:1–40.

154. Shapshay SM, Healy GB. New microlaryngeal instruments for phonatory surgery and pediatric applications. *Ann Otol Rhinol Laryngol*. 1990;98:821–823.

155. Ford CN. A multipurpose laryngeal injector device. *Otolaryngol Head Neck Surg*. 1990;103:135–137.

156. Zeitels SM. Transoral treatment of early glottic cancer. In: Smee R, Bridger P, eds. *Laryngeal Cancer: Proceedings of the 2nd World Congress on Laryngeal Cancer*. Amsterdam, The Netherlands: Elsevier; 1994:373–383.

157. Hochman II, Zeitels SM. Phonomicrosurgical management of vocal fold polyps. *J Voice*. 2000;4:112-118.

158. Zeitels SM, Hillman RD, Radu A. Salient characteristics of patients with posterior laryngeal granulomas and ulcerations. Presented at: The 26th Annual Symposium: Care of the Professional Voice; June 1997; Philadelphia, Pa.

159. Nasri S, Sercarz JA, McAlpin T, Berke GA. Treatment of vocal fold granuloma using botulinum toxin type A. *Laryngoscope*. 1995;105:585–588.

160. Isshiki N, Morita H, Okamura H, Hiramoto M. Thyroplasty as a new phonosurgical technique. *Acta Otolaryngol (Stockh)*. 1974; 78:451–457.

161. Isshiki N, Tanabe M, Sawada M. Arytenoid adduction for unilateral vocal cord paralysis. *Arch Otolaryngol*. 1978;104:555–558.

162. Zeitels SM, Hochman I, Hillman RE. Adduction arytenopexy: a new procedure for paralytic dysphonia and the implications for medialization laryngoplasty. *Ann Otol Rhinol Laryngol*. 1998;107(suppl 173):1–24.

163. Netterville JL, Coleman JR, Chang S, et al. Lateral laryngotomy for the removal of Teflon granuloma. *Ann Otol Rhinol Laryngol*. 1998;107:735–744.

164. Coleman JR, Miller FR, Netterville JL. Teflon granuloma excision via a lateral laryngotomy. *Operat Tech Otolaryngol Head Neck Surg*. 1999;10:29–35.

165. Zeitels SM, Sataloff RT. Phonomicrosurgical resection of glottal papillomatosis. *J Voice*. 1999;13:1323–1327.

166. Gray S, Titze IR, Alipour F, Hammond E. Biomechanical and hisological observations of vocal fold fibrous proteins. *Ann Otol Rhinol Laryngol*. 2000;109:77–85.

167. Gray S, Hammond E, Hanson DF. Benign pathologic responses of the larynx. *Ann Otol Rhinol Laryngol*. 1995;104:13–18.

168. Pierce NL. Leuoplakia laryngis. *Ann Otol Rhinol Laryngol*. 1920;29:33–56.

169. Cragle SP, Brandenburg JH. Laser cordectomy or radiotherapy: cure rates, communication, and cost. *Otolaryngol Head Neck Surg*. 1993;108:648–653.

170. Vaughan CW, Strong MS, Jako GJ. Laryngeal carcinoma: transoral treatment using the CO_2 laser. *Am J Surg*. 1978;136: 490–493.

171. Koufman JA. The endoscopic management of early squamous carcinoma of the vocal cord with the carbon dioxide surgical laser: clinical experience and a proposed subclassification. *Otolaryngol Head Neck Surg*. 1986;95:532–537.

172. Eckel H, Thumfart WF. Laser surgery for the treatment of larynx carcinomas: indications, techniques, and preliminary results. *Ann Otol Rhinol Laryngol*. 1992;101:113–118.

173. Thomas J, Olsen KD, Neel HB, DeSanto LW, Suman VJ. Recurrences after endoscopic management of early (T1) glottic cancer. *Laryngoscope*. 1994;104:1099–1104.

174. Olsen K, Thomas JV, DeSanto LW, Suman VJ. Indications and results of cordectomy for early glottic carcinoma. *Otolaryngol Head Neck Surg*. 1993;108:277–282.

175. Davis RK, Jako GJ, Hyams VJ, Shapshay SM. The anatomic limitations of CO_2 laser cordectomy. *Laryngoscope*. 1982;92: 980–984.

176. Lehman JJ, Bless DM, Brandenburg JH. An objective assessment of voice production after radiation therapy for stage I squamous cell carcinoma of the glottis. *Otolaryngol Head Neck Surg*. 1988;98:121–129.

177. Hellquist H, Lundgren J, Olofsson J. Hyperplasia, keratosis, dysplasia and carcinoma in situ of the vocal cords—a follow-up study. *Clin Otolaryngol*. 1982;7:11–27.

178. DeSanto, LW, ed. Selection of treatment for in situ and early invasive carcinoma of the glottis. In: Alberti PW, Bryce DB, eds. *Workshops from the Centennial Conference on Laryngeal Cancer*. New York, NY: Appleton-Century-Crofts; 1976:146–150.

179. Myers EN, Wagner RL, Johnson JT. Microlaryngoscopic surgery for T1 glottic lesions: a cost effective option. *Ann Otol Rhinol Laryngol*. 1993;103:28–30.

180. Kirchner JA, Carter D. Intralaryngeal barriers to the spread of cancer. *Acta Otolaryngol (Stockh)*. 1987;103:503–513.

181. Kirchner JA. What have whole organ sections contributed to the treatment of laryngeal cancer? *Ann Otol Rhinol Laryngol*. 1989;98:661–667.

182. Wolfensberger M, Dort JC. Endoscopic laser surgery for early glottic carcinoma: a clinical and experimental study. *Laryngoscope*. 1990;100:1100–1105.

183. Wetmore SJ, Key M, Suen JY. Laser therapy for T1 glottic carcinoma of the larynx. *Arch Otolaryngol Head Neck Surg*. 1986; 112:853–855.

184. Krespi Y, Meltzer CJ. Laser surgery for vocal cord carcinoma involving the anterior commissure. *Ann Otol Rhinol Laryngol*. 1989;98:105–109.

185. Casiano R, Cooper JD, Lundy DS, Chandler JR. Laser cordectomy for T1 glottic carcinoma: a 10-year experience and videostroboscopic findings. *Otolaryngol Head Neck Surg*. 1991; 104:831–837.

186. Zeitels SM. Infrapetiole exploration of the supraglottis for exposure of the anterior glottal commissure. *J Voice*. 1998;12: 117–122.

187. Hartig G, Zeitels SM. Optimizing voice in conservation surgery for glottic cancer. *Operat Tech Otolaryngol Head Neck Surg* (Phonosurgery part 1). 1998;9:214–223.

188. Benninger M, Gillen J, Thieme P, Jacobson B, Dragovich J. Factors associated with recurrence and voice quality following radiation therapy for T1 and T2 glottic carcinomas. *Laryngoscope*. 1994;104:294–298.

189. Mendenhall W, Parsons JT, Stringer SP, Cassisi NJ. Management of Tis, T1, T2 squamous cell carcinoma of the glottic larynx. *Am J Otolaryngol*. 1994;15:250–257.

190. Steiner W. Results of curative laser microsurgery of laryngeal carcinomas. *Am J Otolaryngol*. 1993;14:116–121.

191. Rudert HH, ed. Transoral CO_2 laser surgery of early glottic cancer (CIS-T2). In: Smee R, Bridger P, eds. *Laryngeal Cancer: Proceedings of the 2nd World Congress on Laryngeal Cancer.* Amsterdam, The Netherlands; 1994:389–392.

192. Hirano M, Hiarde Y, Kawasaki H. Vocal function following carbon dioxide laser surgery for glottic carcinoma. *Ann Otol Rhinol Laryngol.* 1985;94:232–235.

193. McGuirt WF, Blalock D, Koufman JA, Feehs RS. Voice analysis of patients with endoscopically treated early laryngeal carcinoma. *Ann Otol Rhinol Laryngol.* 1992;101:142–146.

194. Zeitels SM, Jarboe J, Hillman RD. Goretex medialization for aerodynamic glottal incompetence. Presented at: The 28th Annual Symposium: Care of the Professional Voice; June 2000; Philadelphia, Pa.

195. Steiner W. Transoral microsurgical CO_2 laser resection of laryngeal carcinoma. In: Wigand ME, Steiner W, Stell PM, eds. *Functional Partial Laryngectomy: Conservation Surgery for Carcinoma of the Larynx.* New York, NY: Springer-Verlag; 1984:121–125.

196. Zeitels SM, Vaughan CW, Domanowski GF. Endoscopic management of early supraglottic cancer. *Ann Otol Rhinol Laryngol.* 1990;99:951–956.

197. Jackson C. Malignant disease of the epiglottis. In: *Peroral Endoscopy and Laryngeal Surgery.* St. Louis, Mo: The Laryngoscope Co; 1915:438–439.

198. Jackson C, Jackson CL. Endoscopic removal of cancer of the epiglottis. In: *Cancer of the Larynx.* Philadelphia, Pa: WB Saunders; 1939:52.

199. Jackson C. Malignant neoplasms of the larynx. In: *Peroral Endoscopy and Laryngeal Surgery.* St. Louis, Mo: The Laryngoscope Co; 1915:637.

200. Davis RK, Shapshay SM, Strong SM, Hyams V. Transoral partial supraglottic resection using the CO_2 laser excisional biopsy of early supraglottic cancer. *Laryngoscope.* 1983;93:429–432.

201. Davis RK, Kelley SM, Hayes J. Endoscopic CO_2 laser excisional biopsy of early supraglottic cancer. *Laryngoscope.* 1991;100: 680–683.

202. Zeitels SM, Vaughan CW, Domanowski GF, Fuleihan N, Simpson GT. Laser epiglottectomy: endoscopic technique and indications. *Otolaryngol Head Neck Surg.* 1990;103:337–343.

203. Zeitels SM, Koufman JA, Davis RK, Vaughan CW. Endoscopic treatment of supraglottic and hypopharynx cancer. *Laryngoscope.* 1994;104:71–78.

204. Steiner W. Experience in endoscopic laser surgery of malignant tumours of the upper aerodigestive tract. *Adv Otorhinolaryngol.* 1988;39:135–144.

205. Lutz CK, Johnson JT, Wagner RL. Supraglottic cancer: patterns of recurrence. *Ann Otol Rhinol Laryngol.* 1990;99:12–17.

206. Levendag P, Sessions R, Bhadrassin V, et al. The problem of neck relapse in early stage supraglottic larynx cancer. *Cancer.* 1989;63:345–348.

207. DeSanto LW. The "second" side of the neck in supraglottic cancer. *Otolaryngol Head Neck Surg.* 1990;102:351–361.

208. Zeitels SM, Vaughan CW. Preepiglottic space invasion in "early" epiglottic cancer. *Ann Otol Rhinol Laryngol.* 1991;100:789–792.

209. Wolf GT, Dept of Veterans Affairs Laryngeal Cancer Study Group. Induction chemotherapy plus radiation compared with surgery plus radiation in patients with advanced laryngeal cancer. *New Engl J Med.* 1991;324:1685–1690.

210. Shapiro J, Zeitels SM, Fried MF. Laser surgery for laryngeal cancer. *Operat Tech Otolaryngol Head Neck Surg.* 1992;3:84–92.

211. Rudert HH, ed. Transoral CO_2 laser surgery in advanced supraglottic cancer. In: Smee R, Bridger P, eds. *Laryngeal Cancer: Proceedings of the 2nd World Congress on Laryngeal Cancer.* Amsterdam, The Netherlands; 1994:457–461.

212. Kirchner JA. *Pressman and Kellman's Physiology of the Larynx* [monograph series]. Washington, DC: American Academy of Otolaryngology—Head and Neck Surgery Foundation. 1986; 78:689–709.

213. Zeitels SM, Davis RK, ed. Cancer of the supraglottis: endoscopic laser management. In: Smee R, Bridger P, eds. *Laryngeal Cancer: Proceedings of the 2nd World Congress on Laryngeal Cancer.* Amsterdam, The Netherlands: Elsevier; 1994:444–456.

214. Kashima HK, Lee DJ, Zinreich SJ. Vestibulectomy in early vocal fold carcinoma. *Trans Am Broncho-Esophagol Assoc.* 1991;71: 28–32.

215. Davis RK, Zeitels SM. Laser laryngoscopy cordectomy, supraglottic resection, and arytenoidectomy. In: Johnson M, Mondell-Brown M, Newman R, eds. *Instructional Courses: American Academy of Otolaryngology—Head and Neck Surgery.* St. Louis, Mo: Mosby-Yearbook Inc; 1992:178–180.

216. Shapshay SM, David LM, Zeitels SM. Neodymium-yag photocoagulation of hemangiomas of the head and neck. *Laryngoscope.* 1987;97:323–330.

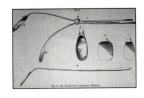

Index

ISBN 0-7695-0131-2

90000

9 780769 301310